Dancing the Body of Light

The Future of Yoga

Dona Holleman

Orit Sen-Gupta

Published by Pegasus Enterprises

Published by Pegasus Enterprises.
Lay out, cover design and photo editing by Walter Goyen, Liqua Amersfoort (NL).
Photographs by Andrea Gennari and Naama Odenheimer.
Printed in The Netherlands by Drukkerij Bariet, Ruinen.

ISBN 90-805113-1-5

For the cover design a photo of Dona Holleman was digitally 'painted' on a water-colour artwork of S. Bob Tomanovic, artist.

Dancing the Body of Light
The Future of Yoga

Dedication

This book is dedicated to those adventurous spirits for whom yoga is a leap beyond the known.

Acknowledgments

Even though in this book the old-fashioned 'he' form has been used instead of the modern 's/he' form, this has been solely for convenience and to facilitate reading. The authors, both women, are aware that the world of yoga is populated for the largest part by women, and that, in spite of this, it is ruled by men. This book is an attempt to bring the work and knowledge of women to the foreground, and to give yoga the dimension of a more fluid vision of the body and the asanas.

The authors wish to express their gratitude to all the people who have helped in the process of creating this book and with enthusiasm and dedicated work have given their support as well. Thanks to Johanna van der Schaft, our book agent, for insisting from the beginning to self-publish, and then to find the channels to enable this. To Buro Klik, Siebren van Hoog for intermediation. To Liqua, Walter Goyen for lay out, cover design and photo editing. To Judith Wolters for having spent days (and nights) sorting through hundreds of photographs and chosing the right ones to go with the text, and to Andrea Gennari for taking the photographs of Dona in her studio in Florence, and to Michel Ardisson for modelling in the Pranayama photographs. Our thanks also to Micha Odenheimer, Shirley June Johannesen, Leslie Young and many others who have been of assistance. Special thanks to Toni Montez for her endless support and financial management of the American version, and to Sylvia Strike for generously offering her services as distributor and contact person.

Orit would like to thank all those who have been an inspiration for her. Teachers who she never met, but whose words have echoed through the tunnel of time to open body and mind to the adventure of consciousness - Patanjali, Dogen and Aurobindo. Also those teachers who have taught her directly, Dr Vijay Pratap who taught her the yoga sutras, and Dona Holleman who showed her that ultimately the knowledge is in the body itself. She also thanks her family - her parents, her partner and friend Michel and their two daughters who are always there for her.

Of all the people who have helped Dona, directly or indirectly, she would like to give special thanks to Jiddu Krishnamurti, who taught her to see the beauty of the world with religious eyes. To B.K.S. Iyengar, who taught her the asanas and kindled her love of yoga. To Vanda Scaravelli, who taught her to play the piano with relaxation, using the body as an instrument of music. To Carlos Castaneda, who showed her that the world is not what we think it is. And finally to D.F., who thought that he could learn to fly, using the energy body, and who, from beyond the veil of death, showed her the beauty and freedom of a body whom gravity has granted a pardon for a moment to fly.

Introduction

The ancient yoga texts tell us that true, transforming benefits are acquired only through uninterrupted practice over a long period of time. How are we to maintain the quality of our practice, full of the fire and light that invigorate our bodies and inspire our lives, if transformation is to take place only at the end of the path?

We will make an attempt to answer this question by presenting a new and radical kind of yoga, which, from the beginning, includes all aspects of the self - body, mind and heart. Although our approach seems new, we believe that it is very old; that we are returning to the way it was practiced at its beginning. The practitioners, who founded this great tradition, saw themselves as pioneers exploring the far reaches of consciousness in order to blaze a path for human evolution.

We too believe that yoga has the potential to play a key role in the further evolution of human consciousness and human civilization, even to help redefine what man is and what he can become. Therefore, each one of us, teachers and students alike, have a crucial role to play. Each one of us must experience and recreate the art of yoga within ourselves, until we can claim it as our own, thus transforming ourselves and the world around us. Every student is a potential teacher, who carries within him a gateway to a new kind of consciousness for mankind.

Though the various components of yoga should form one organic unit, they are too often taught in isolation, both in India and in the West. The basic premise presented in this book is that, whatever the Universe is made of, it is made of one thing, and one thing only. In order to account for the myriad of manifestations, including ourselves, we have to postulate that this 'substance' assumes different gradations, different dimensions. The physical body, in this way, is not conceived of as something new and different from the mind or spirit, but only as a different composition of the same 'substance'.

The first Chapter of **Part One**, called "Healing the Mind-Body Split", traces the history of the split between Hatha Yoga - the physical exercises or *asanas* - and Raja Yoga - *meditation*. For yoga to succeed in our time as a powerful tool for realization and transformation, its practice needs to be taken beyond this split.

Watching the body, one can say that it consists of two different levels: the purely physical part, and the energy which gives it life. We have called this life giving energy the *Energy Body* or *Light Body*. Though the two are merged throughout life, we are usually not aware of this Energy Body, much less do we know how to employ it. In the *Yoga of the Future,* we learn how to become aware of it, and enhance it.

Whereas the physical body is connected to our normal daily consciousness, the Energy Body is connected to a deeper level of consciousness. To reach this Energy Body, mind and body have to meet in a simultaneous attitude of what we have called *Empty Mind* and *Perfect Pose,* which allows the dimension of the Energy Body to become manifest in a way that can be felt and experienced.

In the second Chapter, called "The Seven Vital Principles: Revealing the Body of Light", we give an outline of how this can be achieved. For the sake of clarity we have given a series of steps, called the *Seven Vital Principles*, which form a guide to turn the practice of the asanas, as well as such basic activities as sitting, standing and walking, into profound tools for activating and experiencing the Energy Body and for creating a different flow of energy throughout the body. Simple as they are, they offer the practitioner a new way of directing the mind, body and breath, and are founded on the understanding of the body/mind complex and its interaction with the basic laws of nature.

The first two Vital Principles deal with achieving a certain quality of quietness and emptiness of body and mind in which the hidden intelligence within, the Energy Body, can reveal itself. The third Vital Principle, *intent*, invites the Energy Body into a posture or movement. The Principles of *rooting, connecting, breathing* and *elongating* are the tools of the Energy Body to guide the physical body through those postures or movements.

These Seven Vital Principles, when applied correctly, lead to a qualitative shift in practice and realization. Even though they are described separately, they form one inseparable unit and, welded together in one action, form the key to transforming the mere physical postures into postures of light and beauty.

Part Two contains three Chapters which focus on the technical aspects. There is a tendency in some yoga circles to sacrifice technical precision for so-called higher ideals, while in other circles these higher ideals are neglected in an obsessive search for physical precision. We believe this is a mistake. By merging technical precision with the inner work of the Energy Body through the focus of the mind, we believe that the fullest potential of yoga as a transforming art can be realized.

The third Chapter deals with the *bandhas* and *kriyas* as they are described in the classical texts. In addition to these classical bandhas we have added a few new ones to facilitate the understanding and the practice of the Seven Vital Principles, and we have offered a new view on their function. The integration of the bandhas into the practice of the asanas is also explained in detail.

The fourth Chapter deals with technical instructions regarding the *seven groups of asanas:* Standing Poses, Sitting Poses, Forward Bendings, Twists, Back Bendings, Hand Balancings and Inverted Postures. These instructions are given together with a detailed explanation of the anatomy of the body and include a manual for daily practice. This Chapter ends with an explanation of how the various asanas are interconnected and together express a deep vocabulary formed by the body and filled with the light of consciousness.

The fifth Chapter deals with *pranayama, savasana* and *sitting meditation*. This Chapter includes technical instructions, as well as the original texts, translated from Sanskrit, in which these exercises are described. The addition of these classical texts opens a window for us into the origins and development of these exercises, thus helping us to understand better how to carry this tradition into the future, within the world in which we live.

Part Three deals with the concept that if yoga is truly to touch and transform us, it must be a path of the heart as well as of the body and the mind. In the sixth Chapter, called "Becoming a Yogi", we introduce some of the basic practices dealing with our emotional life. This includes the relationship between student and teacher, interpersonal relationships, and ethical practices. This Chapter ends with "The Yogi Artist", in which the relationship between yoga and creativity is explored.

The book ends with an Epilogue called "Mounting Pegasus". If we dedicate ourselves, body, heart, and mind, to seeking the inner meaning of yoga, we will indeed be able to fly up towards the heavens and become one with the luminous dance of the Universe.

Chapter 1.
Healing the Mind/Body Split

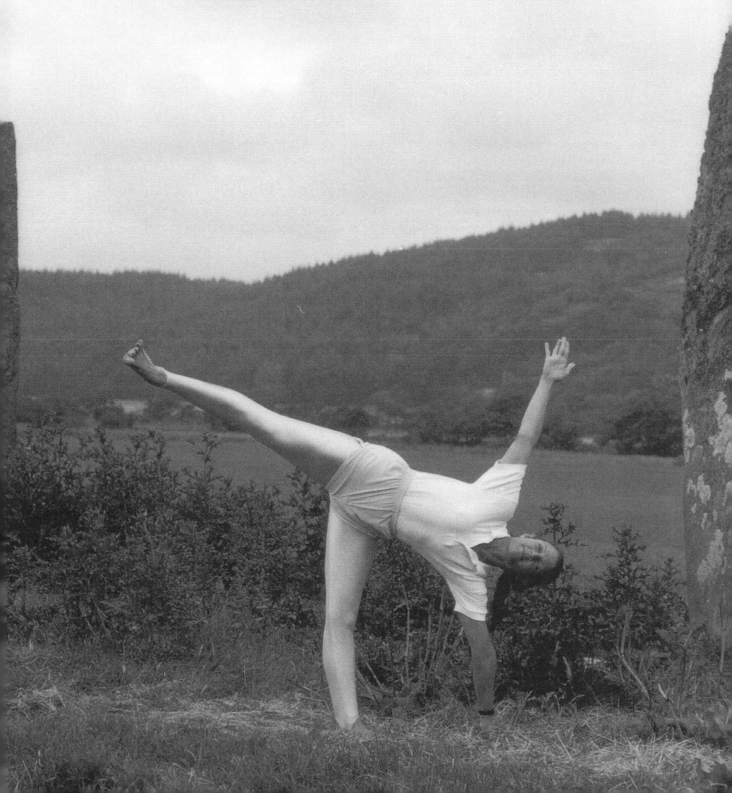

1.1   The History of the Mind/Body Split in Yoga

Many of us understand yoga as a set of physical exercises in which we learn to control, form and manipulate our bodies, gaining flexibility, beauty, vigor and health. Others see it as essentially a path to meditation, to the inner worlds of the mind, where gateways open into the Absolute. According to these it is a path leading beyond the world, a means not of strengthening or beautifying the body, but of transcending it.

Neither of these views expresses adequately what yoga is about. Emphasizing the mind alone, or the body alone, cannot be true to the intentions of the great and adventurous spirits who founded this discipline, and cannot provide what the world desperately needs now, and in the future.

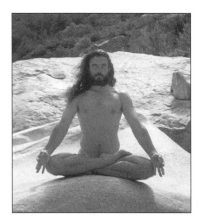

Yoga is not about the body or about the mind. It is about the synthesis of body and mind, and the transformed self that is the result. It is an adventure in human potential, in going beyond the split identity that either body alone or mind alone provides, in discovering a new kind of energy and life. By uniting body and mind, a new kind of vocabulary is created, a new language of consciousness. Ultimately, this new consciousness can only be experienced, not described adequately in words. Yet words can help us create the conditions necessary for experience, can warn us against pitfalls and false starts, and can urge us gently forward on the path.

Like any great art, yoga is a discipline in need of constant renewal. In essence - and this is a subject we will touch upon later in the book - every generation of students must be involved in renewing it, in making it come alive within themselves, in their own time, in their own bodies and minds. In a broader sense, yoga has a complex history, in which historical conditions, intellectual and spiritual influences, and the stamp of great and charismatic personalities, have shaped the way it is practiced and perceived till this day.

A close reading of the earliest texts shows the extent to which body and mind were seen as one inseparable unit. In the Upanishads, that followed the Vedas, the ancient seers stressed the point that everything was *Brahman*, that there was non other than Brahman, that Brahman existed in every blade of grass: "In Him are woven the Sky and the Earth and all the regions of the air, and in Him rest the mind and all the powers of life," says the Mundaka Upanishad, adding: "Where all the subtle channels (nadis) of the body meet, like spokes in the center of a wheel, there He, Brahman, moves."

Yet, later on, probably under the influence of Buddhism, which was founded in India and at one point nearly replaced Hinduism as the dominant religion, a profound disillusionment about the physical world became the primary motif in Indian philosophy. Even though Hinduism eventually re-asserted itself as the religion of most Indians, Buddhist ideas had already penetrated deeply into Indian consciousness. The mainstay of Vedanta philosophy, as expounded by Shankaracharya and others until this day, states that only the Absolute (Brahman) exists, and that all the rest, including everything we see as real, is but a mirage.

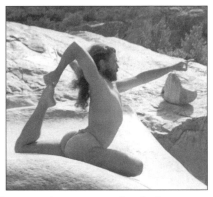

This idea was taken very seriously in India, and had a profound effect on the attitude of Indian philosophers and yogis towards the physical world. It led to the devaluation and denial of the body and to the neglect of social needs and responsibilities to the world as a whole. Yogis renounced worldly life and retreated to the forests and caves, where they practiced mostly meditative techniques in order to leave their bodies and merge with the Infinite. Even the Hatha yogis, who did practice the physical *asanas* or postures, did so with the ultimate intention of separating the soul from the body and uniting with the Absolute. Though they used their body as an instrument in their quest, it was unimportant to them, as was the world itself. Their main endeavor was to sweep the mind clean and wipe out all memories of the past, so that their consciousness would become transparent and reflect only the Absolute, the Unmanifested, That which never changes.

This obsessive denial of the body and of life finally proved destructive. Concentrating exclusively on the mind in order to obtain Oneness damaged man's delicate relationship to the world. The quest for a consciousness, centered only on the Absolute, was rooted in a deep religious drive for truth. But eventually, the one-sided, obsessive nature of this drive, and a failure to fully think through its implications, caused profound damage to Indian society. The overall affect was exactly the opposite of what the Vedanta philosophers would have wished. Instead of encompassing all of life within the Absolute, a split was created. While some yogis and spiritual seekers lived out their dream of transcending this world, the material world itself did not recede into nothingness, but was neglected by those who should have provided moral direction. The value of the body and of the individual was denied, and the great spiritual traditions of India and its people were thrust into an even greater duality.

1.2   The Return of the Body: Iyengar and Yoga

In a fascinating turn of history, interest for the physical aspect of yoga was renewed through its introduction into the West. In general, when a science, art, or discipline is introduced into a new culture, it will inevitably go through changes in form and content. In the twentieth century we witnessed the flow of Eastern traditions to the West, and it would be a mistake to take these passages for granted.

There are three conditions necessary for a spiritual tradition to stay alive in an alien culture. First of all, it must nurture the essential principles and techniques that it brings over. Second, it must shed unnecessary paraphernalia that are incomprehensible to its newly adopted society. Third, it must strive to integrate its essential principles into the cultural context of its new home, while insuring that these principles are not diluted or lost.

More than any other teacher, B.K.S. Iyengar renewed Hatha Yoga in the process of bringing it to a Western audience. In the West, Iyengar encountered a very different mentality than in India. People were enthusiastic about Hatha Yoga, thirsty for knowledge, and willing to work hard to attain it. Iyengar's personality was amply suited to the task of adapting this tradition to new surroundings. Rather than repeat mechanically what he had learned from his teacher, Krishnamacharya, he inquired deeply into each of the postures in order to perfect them. This inquiry was his great innovation: he continuously attempted to arrive at a more perfect performance of the yoga postures.

Iyengar, while remaining always a demanding teacher, learned to adjust his transmission of yoga to the needs of his students. In the beginning, the Westerners who learned and practiced with him, were expected to imitate his movements as he went through the sequences. When they had difficulties, he would place them manually into the poses. Explanations were scarce, and external tools nonexistent. Iyengar expected his students to reach his level on their own; eventually, some of them succeeded, to a greater or lesser extent.

When his greatness as a teacher and practitioner became more widely known, the size of his classes grew, and his teaching had to adjust to this new reality. First of all, as his classes grew larger, it was impossible for Iyengar to reach each individual and physically place him in the proper alignment. Second, he began to encounter different kinds of physical problems among the students, for which he developed special kinds of props and asanas. Thus he opened yoga up to everyone, regardless of age or physical condition. Most significantly, though, Iyengar began to respond to the need of Western students to understand the poses, rather than perform them blindly, and to adapt the postures to their bodies in a conscious way. Hence he developed a more verbal form of teaching to complement his finely tuned sensitivity to the body and its movements. The total effect of his work was to transmit to the Western world a method for developing what Iyengar himself called 'the intelligence of the body'.

Yet yoga, as we have already emphasized, is about the fusion of the mental and the physical, and work on the physical body has to be accompanied by equal intelligent work on inner states of consciousness. One of the earliest texts states that 'controlling the whirls of the mind' is essential (Patanjali "Yoga Sutras", 1,2). According to these texts, yoga is much more than an intelligent physical exercise, and its success is not measured merely by the beauty of the asanas, but also by the lucidity of the mind that is achieved through these movements. We would like to believe that this calm and lucid state of mind is the fruit of practice, and will ripen over the years as its spontaneous outcome. But this should not be taken for granted. We know from experience that what is not nurtured in daily practice may never be fully realized or internalized.

Should the precision and intelligence, that have gone into perfecting the asanas, be accompanied by equally serious effort to develop the mental and spiritual aspects of yoga? This is not a philosophical question, but an existential one. The future is at stake, for whatever we learn and pass on will be the *Yoga of the Future*. For yoga to survive and grow in the West, we must work consciously on the fusion of mind and body, on the integration and transformation of all aspects of our being.

1.3 Getting It All Together: Aurobindo and Integral Yoga

Iyengar has been the ideal model for many people regarding Hatha Yoga techniques. In our search for foundations on which to base the *Yoga of the Future*, we can use another important model, Aurobindo Ghose, an Indian philosopher and saint, who lived in Pondicherry, India, and died in 1950.

Aurobindo was born in India in 1872. England and Europe were at the peak of their glory, or so it seemed to Aurobindo's father, a doctor who had been educated in England. If the future lay in the West, it was important to give the younger generation a European education, and with this in mind he sent his three sons to England. Aurobindo was then seven, and by the time he finished public school it was evident that he was a student with outstanding abilities. As a result he was sent on a scholarship to Cambridge, where he won most of the prizes for Greek and Latin verse. Here, Aurobindo and some of his Indian friends discovered Indian Nationalism. As a result he returned to India in 1892, to spend twenty years fighting for Indian independence. Refusing to join the prestigious Civil Service, without a profession, penniless, Aurobindo nurtured many antagonistic feelings towards the British; but, although he resented them, his way of thinking and acting had been greatly molded by Western culture. As such, he was a living synthesis between East and West, which was the reason why his understanding of yoga in later years would be so unique and powerful.

Aurobindo was gifted with an intense belief in the power of dedicated action to change the world. Initially, when a friend invited him to practice yoga, he replied that a discipline, which required giving up the world, was not for him. But it often happens that chance occurrences effect the way we see things. Once, when Aurobindo's brother Bharin had a high fever which would not go down, a sadhu came to the house. Seeing the sick man, he asked for a glass of water, cut through it with a knife while chanting a mantra, and gave it to Bharin to drink. A few minutes later the sick man was cured. Although Aurobindo had a skeptical nature and till then did not believe in God, he realized in that moment the power of yoga.

He began to practice, not to achieve liberation, but rather to gain strength in his resistance work against the British. When he was thirty-five years old and had been in India for fourteen years, he met a yogi for the second time in his life. The two men spent three days in a quiet place, where the yogi taught him how to meditate, telling him: "Don't think, look at your mind. You will see thoughts coming into it. Before they can enter, throw them away from your mind, till it is capable of silence." Aurobindo had never heard of thoughts entering the mind from outside, but did not question it. He simply sat down and did what the yogi told him. According to his later accounts, this experience brought him an inexpressible peace, a silence, a feeling of release and freedom.

Four months after this meeting, Aurobindo was arrested by the British government and charged with masterminding a plot to kill a certain high judge. He was imprisoned for one year, and it was in these adverse conditions that he deepened his understanding of yoga. According to him, the first realization he had was that of God's overwhelming presence. Wherever he looked - at the walls of the prison, at the tree outside his window, at the guards, at the thieves and murderers - he saw God, Krishna. Even while he was in court, sitting in his iron cage in the middle of a hostile crowd, he had the same vision. He saw the judge, the prosecutor - they too were Krishna. This skeptical man, who had until then combined a great capacity for knowledge with a passion for action, now found himself overcome by a powerful emotion of universal love (Bhakti).

When he was found not-guilty and released, Aurobindo, no longer inclined to political activism, left for Pondicherry, a French enclave in what was then British India. It was the year 1910, and he was thirty-eight years old. From then on, until the end of his life, he devoted himself to creating a new kind of yoga to form the basis for the future. Aurobindo called his new synthesis of yoga philosophy *Integral Yoga*.

The word 'radical' means 'to return to the root', and like many profound innovators, Aurobindo saw his work as a return to the original intentions of the Vedas and the early philosophers. Earlier, we wrote about the denial of the body and of this world which, under the influence of Buddhism and Vedanta, had become the norm. Aurobindo was deeply sensitive to this negative aspect of the direction yoga had taken, and set out to recover what he felt had been lost.

Yogis in India had, for generations, become specialized in *Jnana Yoga* (the Yoga of Knowledge), *Bhakti Yoga* (the Yoga of Devotion), and *Karma Yoga* (the Yoga of Action), each of which were pursued as separate paths. Aurobindo, relying on the ancient texts of the Vedas and Upanishads, believed that originally there was only one path, not three, and that this path raised the whole of the individual towards spiritual maturity, not just part of him. Again integrating these three disciplines into one path, Aurobindo took also Vedanta philosophy and, in true yoga fashion, stood it on its head. If the only thing that is 'real' is the Absolute, then the Absolute is everything, and everything that exists is part of the Absolute. Thus the body and the world too are divine and part of the plan of existence.

In this way, both the human body and human society were re-consecrated, made holy again, and metaphysical building blocks were laid down to serve as a foundation for a more balanced practice, in tune to the rhythms of life. Yoga was no longer seen as liberation from life (mukti), but also as celebration of life (bukti). Life and liberation were no longer opposites that excluded each other, but were rather seen as two aspects of a larger whole.

Yet Aurobindo did not stop there. Like several other great twentieth-century philosophers and mystics, he believed in evolution. Not in Darwin's theory of evolution, in which life achieves new forms through chance mutations and the survival of the fittest, but in an evolution in which life gradually unfolds towards God, towards a higher consciousness and energy. His belief in this kind of evolution gave him the audacity to imagine a man who had succeeded so completely in transforming himself that he would go beyond being an ordinary mortal and would initiate the next stage in human evolution. Aurobindo's belief was that this quantum leap in evolution could be achieved by a collective of yogis simultaneously. He did not give any actual techniques to achieve this bold step, however. Realizing that he was speaking for the future, he limited himself to only broadly outlining the direction.

Chapter 1: Healing the Mind/Body Split
1.4 Hatha and Raja Yoga: Tools for the Next Evolutionary Leap?

15

1.4 Hatha and Raja Yoga: Tools for the Next Evolutionary Leap?

One important key to the *Yoga of the Future* is indicated, paradoxically, by what Aurobindo left out of his synthesis. As mentioned before, *Integral Yoga* fused three different disciplines - Bhakti Yoga, Jnana Yoga and Karma Yoga - into one spiritual path. Yet *Hatha Yoga* (the Yoga of the Body), and *Raja Yoga* (the Yoga of the Mind) were left out. These two disciplines were considered highly effective and powerful by Indian philosophers and yogis. Why did Aurobindo leave them out of his vision of Integral Yoga?

In his book "Synthesis of Yoga" he devotes quite a few pages to Hatha and Raja Yoga, outlining their aims and practices, and explains why he left them out of his new integration of yoga: as he knew them, the practices of Hatha and Raja Yoga were long, laborious, and world negating. In Hatha Yoga, the practitioner aimed at the purification of his body to such an extent that mastery was often accompanied by the development of *siddhis* or supernatural powers. But the cost was often too high. True achievement usually came at the expense of other parts of the practitioner's being. If done exclusively, Hatha Yoga left neither time nor inclination for participation in worldly life. Aurobindo had the same objection to Raja Yoga. Its practitioners were often consumed in meditative trances, and were equally unwilling or unable to function in the world, neglecting their bodies, their families, and the world in general.

In Aurobindo's days, Hatha or Raja Yoga usually did involve withdrawal from the world. In the last few decades, here in the West, these disciplines have developed along different lines. Both Hatha and Raja Yoga are now practiced mainly by people who function in society and are fully integrated in it. Often they have families and are high level professionals in science, medicine, and the arts. To make Hatha and Raja Yoga accessible to these people, modifications had to be made, most significantly in the number of hours per day in which meditation and asanas were practiced.

But is this new way of practicing valid? Perhaps these two disciplines do indeed require a withdrawal from the world. Is this 'abridged version' of real value in an authentic spiritual quest? Or perhaps they, cut down to Western size, serve mainly as sedatives, soothing and tranquilizing us so that we can go about our modern, frenzied lives with a sense of distance and calm, but without creating the conditions for real transformation. This does not have to be the case. The practice of these disciplines need not be one's exclusive occupation in order to be a powerful and effective spiritual path. In fact, the danger of spiritual mediocrity and inauthenticity lies in *not* being able to connect our practice to our daily lives, to living in this world.

Our challenge today is to find the means to accomplish what Aurobindo set out to do: to create an *Integral Yoga* that uplifts and transforms daily life - ours and that of the world around us. Hatha and Raja Yoga can be practiced within the context of our modern world, but only within the broader framework of a total commitment to the *Yoga of the Future*, which is also the yoga of the ancient past. A dualistic philosophy, which leads us back to where we have to choose between yoga and worldly life, must be rejected. Instead, we must embrace a yoga which unites transcendental Reality with life in this body, in this world, in this time. Far from being an 'abridged version', this is a yoga that demands all of us, asks of us a commitment, not to elevate only ourselves, but to transform all of life. For not only do we need the world; the world needs us too.

The profound power of Hatha and Raja Yoga can be the ideal tool for the acceleration of human evolution. Not practiced in isolation from life, but together with the commitment to action, emotion, and knowledge, which are at the root of the other three forms of yoga: Karma, Bakhti and Jnana Yoga. It is up to us modern-day practitioners to find a way to integrate all five of them together into our lives as a means towards personal and global transformation.

1.5   Uniting Body and Mind

How are we to practice Hatha and Raja Yoga in a new way that will spur our spiritual evolution forward, rather than separate us from life? Most of the time, we tend to think of modern culture as an environment unfriendly to spiritual understanding. With its rampant consumerism, its secular bias, and its frenzied pace, it is certainly an easy place to lose one's path in life and one's peace of mind. But in one area at least, at the cutting edge of modern sciences, the understanding of the basic structure and functioning of the physical universe is coming closer to that of the ancient spiritual traditions, including yoga. These sciences, in turn, can actually help us verbalize that Reality which advanced yoga practitioners experienced directly.

In the twentieth century, science began to paint a picture of a Reality that is far more unified than was once known. Certain disciplines such as particle physics and quantum mechanics have yielded a wealth of evidence that what we think of as physical Reality is not as 'hard' and 'solid' as was once believed. The divisions between states of being, once thought of as absolute, are now understood to exist along a continuum or spectrum. For example, light, under certain conditions, can oscillate between existence as a particle - a hard, solid, point - and a wave, something much harder to define, nearly spiritual in its essence. Quantum mechanics has revealed that Reality, at the subatomic level, seems to be based as much on principles of mind, as on solid physical reality. Even materials, such as rocks, that seem to us dense and hard, are in reality almost entirely empty and porous, their 'realness' based on the utterly unpredictable paths of infinitesimal particles, which pulsate in and out of existence a million times per second, as well as on our perception of them.

For centuries, yogis have maintained that the division between the physical and the mental is not absolute. Still, most people practice yoga in a way which divides Hatha Yoga from Raja Yoga, contrasting the 'physical' body with the 'spiritual' mind. In reality, body and mind are merely different expression of one 'substance', expressed in 'particle' form as body, and 'wave' form as mind, in the same way as light oscillates back and forth between these two forms. The key to the Yoga of the Future is to experience our body and mind as merely two sides of one coin, so that these two seemingly distinct parts of our being can begin to operate as one totality, indivisible from the other. In this way, Hatha Yoga can be considered as focusing on the 'particle' side of us - the body, and Raja Yoga on the 'wave' side - the mind. The true art is to unite these two focuses into one, where body and mind begin to act in unison, as a 'unified field', opening up into something that is more than body and more than mind. Only by fusing the precision of Hatha Yoga asanas with the flow of *Raja Yoga meditative practices*, of 'particle' yoga with 'wave' yoga, can we transcend the body/mind split and again integrate yoga and ourselves into one unified whole.

1.6   **The Body of Light Emerges**

According to the ancient texts, the physical body, which is nourished by the food we eat, is akin to an outer shell, or casing. This outer body is animated by an inner body, called the *Energy Body,* which gives 'life' to the physical body. Both the physical body and the Energy Body are made of energy, but the physical body, like molten lava that has hardened into rock, has lost the fluidity, warmth, and light which characterizes the Energy Body. All of us have the capacity to see this Energy Body. Some people may be more sensitive than others, but something in us, something in the body itself, is aware of this 'life' energy. Thus one may look at a certain person and observe that this person looks 'gray' and 'miserable', while somebody else looks 'radiant' and 'full of life.' This 'grayness' or 'radiance' does not simply describe a physical phenomenon, having to do with skin color, but something else. It is the capacity of our own 'life' force to measure the 'life' force in another human being, its strength or weakness. In this context it is interesting to note that this awareness expresses its opinion in terms of light, its weakness ('grayness'), or its strength ('radiance'). Therefore we have called this Energy Body the *Body of Light*.

The Body of Light is usually 'locked' within the physical body. Although it gives life to us at every moment, we are not consciously aware of it. By becoming aware of it, we can learn to lure the Body of Light out of its captivity, and to let it take the lead. This is done through the integration of physical and mental yoga. The asanas are practiced assiduously, with careful attention paid to the proper alignment and positioning of the muscles and bones, and at the same time, the busy mind of daily activity is allowed to settle down into a deeper and quieter state. In this state we can become aware of the Body of Light; as it radiates outward and softens the boundaries between 'inside' and 'outside' our skin becomes permeable, transparent, and the body becomes open to the great waves of energy emanating from the Earth below and from the Sky above. When the Body of Light moves the physical body in this way, not only is there no muscular effort or fatigue involved, but the movements themselves are expanded into a fuller expression of the self. This is the *Yoga of the Future,* when body and mind ride on the energy of the Body of Light.

1.7   **Perfect Pose, Empty Mind**

We have coined the phrase above to help point us in the direction we have described: the integration of body and mind. The first two words indicate performing the asanas in the spirit of perfection; the second two words indicate the state of consciousness which is at the base of this perfection. *Perfect Pose* and *Empty Mind* are like reflections in a mirror, twin expressions of the same mode of being: the one cannot exist without the other.

Let us first see what we mean by *Perfect Pose*. During the past three decades there has been a renaissance in the art of the asanas: the pendulum has swung for many practitioners towards a concern for and appreciation of the minutia of Hatha Yoga postures. This attention to the precision of the asanas is a blessing, a much-needed corrective to the tendency to neglect the body, which had become one of the outstanding features of yoga in India. But there is also a danger: that we end up doing the same thing with the body as the Indian yogis did with the mind: magnifying it at the expense of everything else, at the exclusion of everything else.

There is obviously a right way of doing the pose as opposed to a wrong way, which may harm the body. Working on the precision in the poses, refining each pose ever further, however, brings one sooner or later to the 'point of no return': refining beyond this point leads to obsession, not to Perfect Pose. At the same time, concentrating exclusively on correct alignment and structure, there is the danger of forgetting the other components of the practice: breathing, harmony, connectedness within the body and, more than anything else, the quality of a calm and still mind.

The second danger is that, by obsessively searching for perfection in the basic poses, without being sure that we are ever going to find it, we postpone proceeding to the more advanced ones.

Thus we are caught in a vicious circle of working on beginner poses, unable to break through to new ones. We do not realize that sometimes the only way to perfect a basic pose is by doing a more advanced one imperfectly. This is because the body does not always learn best under the glare of the spotlight of conscious effort. The attempt to perform a more advanced pose often carries the body beyond itself, and stimulates the intelligence inherent in the body, which is part of our subconscious awareness. Returning afterwards to the basic pose, we find ourselves performing it differently. This process, in turn, enhances our faith in the subconscious intelligence of the body, and further breakthroughs become possible. Abandoning our obsessive search for perfection, paradoxically, will help us find Perfect Pose.

There is something else at stake here. It is important, for us as well as for future generations, to save the greatest variety of poses possible so that they do not die of neglect. Each pose sheds a different light on the beauty of the body and its infinite possibilities, and is therefore vital to the whole. Each asana is an expression of a certain insight or understanding; a certain part of the intelligence of the body reveals itself in each movement, in each pose, therefore they are precious.

Moreover, the physical postures are not only physical; they are also vehicles for subtle changes, like shades or colors, in states of consciousness. For example, the Forward Bendings sensitize us to the feeling of surrendering and giving. The Bird Poses create a feeling of compactness and intensity, like a bird before it is about to take flight. The Back Bendings reveal a potential in consciousness for expansion and openness, for going beyond. This process, like everything else in the mind/body continuum, is a two-way street. As the poses reveal new dimensions of consciousness, this consciousness, in turn, begins to color the texture of the muscles, joints and skin, thereby transforming them.

However, as we said before, to progress in the direction of Perfect Pose, we have to lose our tendency for 'obsessive' perfection, and rather learn to practice the asanas from a deeper place within ourselves, the place from which perfection simply emerges when the conditions are right. We have called this place *Empty Mind*.

1.8 Finding Empty Mind

Some modern philosophers teach that the structure of human consciousness includes at least three levels. The first level is that of the ego. This is our social and psychological identity as a father, a mother, a lawyer, a businessman, an American, or any other identity. Next is the existential level, which includes both body and mind.; it is what we feel ourselves to be underneath our social identity, underneath our self image. Finally, there is the level of mind, which involves a feeling of being one with the Cosmos.

Western society, for the most part, treats only ego consciousness as real, and Western psychology is directed in general towards the level of ego and its memories, while Eastern spiritual teachings often tend to deride the ego, and offer ways to break or escape ego identity altogether. The ego cannot be denied, however; it forms an important and integral part of the totality of the human being. Integrated into a fuller understanding of the potential of human consciousness, and of our connection to all that exists, the ego, which consists of our individuality, our social persona, our thoughts and emotions, can and should be an important tool for deepening our spiritual life. Who can deny the profound experience of being a mother, brother, child, doctor, artist, teacher, Italian, Jew, African, of loving and caring for this world?

Yet, we will suffocate spiritually if we do not find ways to temper the ego; not to let it run rampant, but to put it in perspective, so that we can open up to the full spectrum of our consciousness. Finding Empty Mind means discovering the inner gate through which we can leave the level of ego and enter into an awareness of other dimensions of existence. The Yoga of the Future, the yoga which the world needs, can help us integrate these different levels of consciousness, the superficial ones and the deeper ones. Our goal is not to abandon this world for higher realms, but to raise this world up in its totality - right from the physical level upwards.

Empty Mind means, first of all, emptying the mind of all the everyday concerns of what is called the level of ego. If we think of the mind's conscious awareness as the surface of a lake, the everyday concerns which so often occupy us are like waves blowing across it. The sense of anxiety we have about events and outcomes where we try to control the future, and sometimes, as if we could, the past, is a syndrome called *disturbed mind*. Our mind flits from thought to thought, without being able to focus with clarity. Another kind of unfocused awareness, characterized by passivity and depression, is also given a name: *dull mind*.

To reach Empty Mind, we have to withdraw our attention from the anxieties (disturbed mind) or the passivity (dull mind) of normal ego consciousness. We tend to believe that if we are not 'thinking' all the time - filling ourselves with the urgencies and emotions connected to the level of ego - we will cease to exist. This thinking is the *doing* of the mind. When we stop this doing, we reach a place of mental depth and clarity which has always been there, as the deep and quiet waters of the lake are always there underneath the surface waves. It is this deep and empty quietness that swallows up the rolling waves on the surface of the mind. The consciousness is no longer disturbed, dispersed or dull, but is quiet and one-pointed; this is called *Empty Mind*.

Practicing the asanas from this state of *Empty Mind* is essential to attaining *Perfect Pose.* Out of this quiet and one-pointed consciousness, the mind projects its *intent*, which guides the breathing and the movement of the asana with unwavering intensity. There is no loss of balance when intent is released and the movement is performed; rather, the mind remains calm, wide, rooted. Mind is the fastest and smallest element that exists in our world. It can go through walls and be at various places simultaneously. This ability of the mind is superior to mere physical strength or speed, and needs to be acknowledged and mastered as one of the most important tools in the practice of yoga.

How deep should we dive into the lake of our consciousness? There is a potential danger in not going deep enough, but thinking that one has. Likewise, there is a danger in going too deep within and thus losing the ability to function outwardly. The right depth means that the mind, rather than taking flight from the body, is able to work with the body, but from *within*. In this, the mind keeps a finely tuned balance between the distractions of the exterior world and the attraction of too much inwardness. Mind and body become one indistinguishable unit, in which the intelligence of the body becomes fully activated as conscious awareness travels freely through all parts of the body.

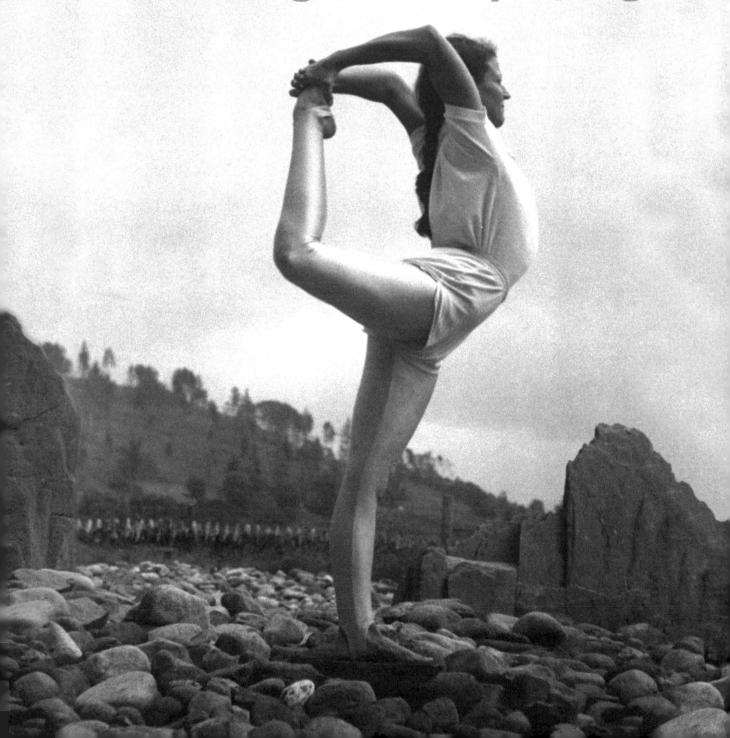

Chapter 2.
The Seven Vital Principles:
Revealing the Body of Light

2 Introduction

The future of yoga, so we have stated, lies in integrating Hatha and Raja Yoga into a new form of practice that fuses the mind and the body into one unit, greater than both of its parts. Until now, we have offered a mainly theoretical basis. In this Chapter - the most important one in the book - we will provide a set of *Principles* that can help each student practice the asanas in a new way, combining physical precision, mental intensity, and a direct connection to the surrounding space of which we are a part.

The technique of the asanas with its precision is one aspect of practicing yoga, but if this becomes the only aspect, then yoga loses half of its meaning. The other half is the poetic side, where the body loses its sharp division line between it and the surrounding space, and the asana becomes part of the *unified field*, the continuum of space/time in which we all have our being. Thus, finding the balance between precision and flow, is to go beyond the body - mind split and again integrate yoga and ourselves into an un-fragmented whole.

Practicing yoga, hence, means that the poses and the breathing exercises are done with a certain mental attitude in which mind and body are one, not two, and in which the body and the poses are not something imposed on the surrounding space, but in which both the body and the asanas are flowing *events*, dynamic happenings in space/time, expressions of a fluid mind which does not have a fixed position that has to be defended at all cost. A mind that does not have a fence around it, but has a boundless curiosity to explore the Universe at large as well the personal universe that each one of us carries along.

In Taoist literature, the term *wei-wu-wei* means *doing-without-doing*. *Doing* belongs to our external, superficial layer, or, in modern terms, to the ego, which is for ever searching for its own enhancement and expression. Underlying the ego, however, is the intelligence of the body which, bypassing the ego and the brain, has different sources and resources. At the crucial moment, when the mind and the ego are made quiescent through *wu-wei* or *not-doing*, this body intelligence will take over.

We are all acquainted with this body intelligence. For instance, when we want to throw something in the wastepaper basket, chances are that it will miss the basket, unless you are a basketball player. On the other hand, if you throw it without aiming and, more important, without 'caring' whether it gets in or not, chances are that you will make a perfect 'goal'.

In wu-wei or not-doing (actually wei-wu-wei or doing-without-doing) there is a threefold sequence. The first is a conscious wish to achieve something. The second is the internal lull, where we stop worrying about the outcome of this wish; in other words, when the ego has given up 'hope' and expectations. The third is that, in this vacuum, the deeper intelligence of the body takes over, 'fulfilling' the wish.

This not-doing is the negative side of the coin, the positive side being that the wish itself remains strong and clear. Many traditions deal with this dual aspect of doing versus not-doing, connecting doing with the physical body, and not-doing with the *Energy Body* (the *Body of Light*). In this context yoga has two dimensions. On the one hand it deals with physical bones and muscles, and positions done with these. On the other hand, we are more than bones and muscles. We are creatures of energy, of Light.

The technical instructions given in **Part Two** concerning the asanas, bandhas, kriyas and breathing exercises, belong in the realm of the physical body. They form the frame and should be done under the guidance of a competent teacher to avoid hurting the physical body by anatomically wrong movements. Together with learning these techniques, however, we have to learn to invite the Energy Body or Body of Light, which is usually latent, to emerge and to even take the lead. This is the art of yoga, when body and mind ride on the energy of the Body of Light.

There are certain principles that one can use to accomplish this. They are called: *The Seven Vital Principles of Practice.* As stated above, these Principles do not substitute the precision of the physical postures, but are rather added to them to bring the postures into a different dimension.

2.1 The First Vital Principle: Relaxation or Undoing the Body

In the *First Vital Principle, relaxation*, the body is swept clean of the past, which is expressed in tensions and blockages in joints and muscles. Throughout the day and over the years, as the body accumulates the 'fall-out' of emotional experiences and physical stress, it stores this 'fall-out' in various parts of the body, such as the shoulders, the neck, the lumbar region, and the hip joints. Many authors have written about the connections between negative emotional experiences and specific parts of the body. Although we will not go into details, it is important to realize that there is a deep connection between our physical body and our emotional and mental life.

Suffice to say here that, once the body has stored these negative energies, they become stuck to the point that most people are not even aware that they have a 'problem'. Before we can imprint a new type of awareness in the body, we have to relax the physical body, in whichever position it happens to be. This does not necessarily have to be a yoga position, but can be while walking, sitting or in any other activity.

Relaxation is not the same as letting the body go limp in its totality. It means, in the first place, relaxing the muscles while maintaining the integrity of the body, in whichever position one is. The accumulated tensions, for the most part unconscious, should be brought to the surface and released consciously. In this way the body is upheld by its skeletal structure and the muscles closest to it, not by the big, peripheral muscles, where most of the tensions are stored. For instance, while standing or sitting, the back should be held absolutely straight, using the deepest muscles close to the spinal column, while the muscles of the shoulders and arms are allowed to hang relaxed from the shoulder joints.

Hence, the first thing in relaxation is to become aware that there are tensions or blockages of energy in certain muscles and joints. One has to become aware of them, as it were, from 'inside'. Many people say: "Oh yes, I have stiff shoulders, but there is nothing I can do about it."

This means that they look at the problem from 'outside', as an external observer. This, in general, has the opposite effect from relaxation, as it fixes the blockage even more in the mind and body, till it becomes "my stiff shoulders, my stiff hips". Each repetition of the affirmation further aggravates the situation. This, in the language of the Energy Body, is called *doing*.

There is another way, however, which, in the language of the Energy Body, is called u*ndoing*. In this undoing, the tension is not confirmed by external observation and affirmation. On the contrary, the mind 'crawls', as it were, inside the muscle or joint, without naming the problem, without even calling this tension 'a problem'. The mind, from 'inside' the muscle or joint, merely observes the tension, the blockage, quietly and with a great deal of clarity and affection. In this quiet observation the body will, by itself, unfold and unwind, gradually allowing air and space to come back into the tense parts. This is called u*ndoing*, when the muscles and joints unfurl like a tightly closed leaf, to let in the sunlight and the air.

The skin is also included in this process. In the course of the years, the skin tends to become a defensive barrier, protecting the body from the onslaughts of the world, like cold or heat, or from the energies of other people. It becomes like a sharp dividing line between the inner and outer energies, keeping the outer energies out, and the inner energy in.

In deep relaxation the skin becomes again transparent, translucent, like in early childhood, so that the body becomes vulnerable again to the outside energies, and no longer constricts the inner energy or Body of Light. This is one of the most important aspects of relaxation: reconnecting to the surrounding space by, as it were, 'taking the skin away', making it so transparent that it does not obstruct the free flow of energy from the inside towards the outside, and vice versa. In this state of transparency, we can deliberately expand the Body of Light beyond the skin.

2.2   The Second Vital Principle: Empty Mind or Undoing the Mind

In the *Second Vital Principle, empty mind,* the mind too is swept clean of the past, which is expressed in all the preconceptions that we have, all the prejudices, the ideas, the likes and dislikes, even our thoughts and beliefs. Throughout the day and over the years, the mind accumulates these thoughts, concepts, likes and dislikes, and stores them as memories. Anytime we are confronted with an experience, we pull out these memories and see in which 'category' the experience falls: pleasurable, unpleasant, easy, difficult, etc. The mind is constantly occupied with this activity: confronting the present experience with the memory of past ones and seeing into which 'category' the experience falls, so that it can then react to it according to the stored memory. We almost never confront new experiences directly, but always view them through the looking glass of the past. This is the 'doing of the mind', its day-long activity: looking back and confronting, looking back and confronting.

In yoga, the mind too, like the body, needs to 'undo' itself. Thoughts, emotions and memories are necessary tools for living in the body and functioning in the daily world; they originate from the surface of our being and serve the ego in order to survive in the world.

Below these surface concerns - thoughts, emotions and memories - however, there exists a deeper level of consciousness that can be brought to the surface. Useful as the thoughts and emotions are in daily life, when we want to reach that deeper level of consciousness they become obstacles, preventing us from moving towards the other side of ourselves, the internal body intelligence or the Body of Light.

After relaxing the physical body, the mind too needs to take a step back and sink into the quiet and alert state which underlies thought and emotion. Here too, as in physical relaxation, it is not enough to look at the mind from 'outside'; we need to observe it from 'inside', with a great deal of patience and affection. In this way the mind becomes aware of its activity, and how this activity isolates it from the body and from the surrounding space. Letting go easily and gently of its activity, it sinks into a deeper state and becomes empty. It is only in this Empty Mind that something new can come, something new can surface. From here it is a small step to *intent*.

2.3 The Third Vital Principle: Intent

At the root of the *Third Vital Principle*, *intent*, lies the idea that movement, acrobatics, dance, and *asanas*, are inherent in the human body and psyche. When the forefathers of the human race left the ape phase behind to become 'Homo erectus' (upright people), they not only liberated the hands, which resulted in the development of the frontal brain, but the spinal column as well, allowing it thus to bend in ways that no animal could. We can see in prehistoric cave paintings and in the arts of the Egyptian, Cretan, Mayan and Siberian cultures, that human beings have always done acrobatics. Behind these acrobatic movements was probably a kind of ecstatic state of mind; even today, ecstatic dances can be observed as a communal ritual of native peoples all over the world.

On the basis of this observation, we have to review the idea that one is 'learning' postures and breathing techniques in yoga. In reality, there is nothing that the body can 'learn' which is not already there, pristine and innocent, in its complete form. Inviting this form to emerge is *intent*.

Intent is the projection of a clear picture of the movement that we want to perform, while keeping the body in a state of relaxation and the mind in a state of quiet alertness: empty mind. This picture that we visualize, invites the Body of Light to pull the physical body into the movement or pose with the help of a specific kind of breathing, called *Mula Bandha Breathing*: before we begin any movement or pose, we visualize it, quietly and precisely. This does not have to take a long time; in an experienced practitioner, visualization takes place in just a split second. The more clearly we are able to visualize the movement leading to the pose and the pose itself, the more the result will be *Perfect Pose*. It is interesting to notice that the poses, which are difficult for us to perform, are also difficult for us to visualize.

The next four Principles help and guide the Body of Light in the actual performance of the postures, resulting in Perfect Pose. If we compare this whole sequence to gardening, relaxation and Empty Mind would be like preparing the soil, and intent like putting the seed in the ground. *Rooting* would be when the plant puts down its roots, *connecting* when it unfurls its leaves and flowers, and *breathing* when it takes in the air to grow upwards towards the sun *(elongating)*.

2.4   The Fourth Vital Principle: Rooting

The *Fourth Vital Principle* is *rooting*, of reconnecting ourselves to the Earth. Even though human beings believe themselves to be special, different from all the other creatures that walk, swim, crawl and fly, this is illusionary. We are an integral part of nature; like all the other creatures we are children of this Earth, our feet are walking on the Earth, our roots are connected to the Earth. Wearing shoes and living in apartment buildings and concrete cities, we are cut off from this connection, and therefore our energy level will always be limited, as both the physical body and the Body of Light are caught in a closed-circuit energy system. Opening this closed-circuit system by learning to reconnect to the Earth and drawing its energy up into our bodies, is the principle of rooting.

We have to first realize that the Earth and the body are not two different entities, hard and closed within themselves; rather, we need to experience the Earth as a kind of soft sponge or dense cloud, into which the energy of the body can 'sink', like the roots of a plant into the soil. Depending on the position, this is done through the soles of the feet (Tadasana, Standing Poses), through the palms of the hands (Full Arm Balance), through the top of the head (Head Balance), or through any other part of the body which is in direct contact with the Earth.

This 'sinking' is the first aspect of rooting. It is the act of connecting the energy of the Body of Light, (after having 'dissolved' the muscles and skin of the physical body), to the energy of the Earth. Underlying this principle is the idea that the Earth, like the human body, is an energy field, even though an energy field of gigantic proportions. When lying on one's back in a field of grass or on the beach, or putting one's hands in the soil while gardening, one can feel the Earth's mothering energy, soothing, healing, cleansing and rejuvenating.

We are, of course, all day long in touch with this energy as we are, literally, Earth-bound creatures. This contact is on an unconscious level, though, and whatever is on an unconscious level has little power compared to what is brought to the surface. Therefore, this contact should not only be made conscious, but it should even be *intentional*. From a purely physical point of view this is felt as a heaviness, a pressing downwards on the surface of the Earth of those parts of the body which are in direct contact with it. From an energy point of view it is felt as an elongation of the internal energy into the Earth through those physical contact points.

Allowing the energy of the Earth to rebound back into the body is the second aspect of rooting. This rebounce effect is inherent in the 'sinking' process, and is called Newton's law of the 'Normal Force'. According to this law, an object which is pulled down by gravity, is also pushed up against it with the same amount of energy. As a result of this law, the human body stands lightly on the Earth; it is not flattened against the Earth, which would be the effect of gravity only, and it is not levitating either, which would be the case if the rebounce force exceeded the gravitational pull.

By *intentionally* riding on the downwards pulling force of gravity with a small part of the body, we can deliberately build up its opposite force to create lightness in the rest of the body. A small portion of the body has to be 'sacrificed' and become heavier; this is the part which roots. Next, we use the first suitable joint above this rooting part to 'split' the force: the rooting part going down, the rebounce force rebouncing the rest of the body back up, making it light. For example, in Standing Poses this 'splitting' of the gravity-rebounce force occurs in the lower and upper spring joints (with the soles of the feet and the bottom of the toes constituting the rooting parts). In Sitting Poses the 'splitting' occurs in the femur joints (with the buttock bones, pubic bone and coccyx as the rooting parts). In Hand Balancings the 'splitting' is in the wrist joints (hardly noticeable) and the shoulder joints. In Head Balance the 'splitting' is in the joint between the skull and the atlas, etc.

As the rebounce force is directed upwards from those joints, it expands them from inside, creating a feeling of elasticity and space in those joints. Lightness and youthful elasticity are important objectives of yoga to enhance the quality of daily life.

2.5   The Fifth Vital Principle: Connecting

In rooting, the part of the body which rests on the Earth becomes a conduit through which our energy flows down into the Earth's energy field, and the Earth's energy in turn flows back up into us. In this reciprocal process, the quality and intensity of the energy flowing from us into the Earth is matched by similar energy flowing up from the Earth: the *rebounce effect*. The joint closest to the point of contact between body and Earth is where the energy flows in both directions, where it 'splits'.

The rebounce energy, flowing upwards from the Earth, does not stop at this first joint. Through the practice of the *asanas,* this energy is distributed throughout the entire body. To facilitate this, the physical body, which is the vehicle of the *Energy Body*, must be aligned in a way that will enable the energy to flow easily through a connecting chain of muscles and joints. This is the *Fifth Vital Principle, connecting.*

Before describing these energy pathways through the muscles and joints, we can go a little deeper into the connecting principle. First of all, the body should always move in opposite directions simultaneously to gain maximum space and ease in the joints. We need to consciously create these simultaneously opposing directions as we move. For example, when we lift our hands above our heads while rooting our feet into the Earth, the movement has more power and grace than when we lift our hands merely from the shoulder area, without any connection to the legs or feet. As we lift our hands, we should therefore be aware that this movement comes from all the way down, from the feet; to the extent that we are aware of this connection between the hands and the feet will we be able to draw the energy from the rooting feet through the legs, the trunk and the arms, up into the hands.

Each of the poses creates a specific chain of muscles and joints through which energy flows. In general terms, the energy travels through all the major joints: the ankles, knees, hips, spinal column, shoulder joints, elbows and wrists. These joints should not only be in contact with each other through our awareness, but they should also be physically aligned with one another. This enables them to receive the energy and, in turn, send it on to the next joint. For this to function best, these joints should be open and aligned on smooth straight or round lines, never on angular lines. This will allow the energy to travel on in an even flow, without being held up or even cut off by sharp angles; therefore, all movements in yoga are done on round, generous lines.

The muscles form another, no less important energy pathway, as they connect certain places in the body where energy is gathered. These gathering places are called *bandhas*. Energy is collected in these bandhas and sent on to the next bandha or gathering point through specific muscle chains. Even though all muscles serve as a conduit for energy in the asanas, to simplify things one can isolate the large, obvious muscles, through which the connections between the bandhas occur. These muscle chains will be discussed later in the book. Even though we are dealing with energy, and thus with the Energy Body or Body of Light, the physical conduits - the joints, the muscles and the bandhas - are of paramount importance.

This whole process, which we have called *connecting,* should be done consciously while performing the poses. There are two ways to be aware of the chain of connections through which the energy flows. One is to be aware of the entire connecting chain in the body, joint to joint, muscle group to muscle group, bandha to bandha. The other way is to be fully aware of the relationship between the two extremities through which the energy is flowing - the rooting place and the point farthest away from this rooting place. For example, in standing upright, the movements we make in the rest of the body need to be connected to the feet so as not to interrupt the current of energy. We should never forget that our whole body is one unit, and that each part is connected to all the other parts, both on a physical as well as on an energy level. Only by being constantly aware of these natural connections do we overcome the tendency to move the body in a fragmented way.

2.6   **The Sixth Vital Principle: Breathing**

Breathing forms the true bridge between the physical body and the Body of Light. At the moment of birth, human beings draw their first breath, and at the moment of death, when the Body of Light withdraws from the physical body, it does so with the last breath. It is an art which, when understood fully, can unite the physical body and the Body of Light and turn them into one functioning unit. When practiced and perfected, it is like a wave which fuels the Body of Light and pulls it through the movements and into the postures. In the wake of this wave, the Body of Light pulls the physical body through those same movements.

Breathing is a fundamental tool throughout our practice of the Principles. During the undoing of body and mind, we release tensions and excess energy and go deep within on the waves of the exhalations. On the waves of the inhalations we take in energy to counteract dullness and fatigue, thus giving power to our intent.

To enhance this in the actual asanas, we use a specific kind of breathing called the *Mula Bandha Breathing.* This type of breathing runs along the entire length of the spinal column, elongating and energizing the entire body. It begins with the inhalation, in which we let the air descend into the lower abdomen. Then, we move the air or lower abdomen backwards towards the sacrum in a wave-like action. When it comes into contact with the sacrum, as it cannot go further backwards, the breath turns back upwards again along the inner line of the spine in a wavelike motion, 'ironing out', as it were, the spinal column, and elongating it. Hence, it lifts and widens the kidney region, and, on reaching the upper part of the spine, it lifts and widens the upper part of the rib cage, the shoulders and the shoulder blades. Finally it moves into the back of the neck, through the base of the head, and forward over the top of the head. This is the line of the *inhalation*.

The line of the *exhalation* is from the forehead down again through the base of the throat into the lower abdomen, after which the new cycle of breathing starts. Thus the total curve of the inhalation and the exhalation is elliptical.

Through this breathing the Body of Light is elongated and expanded from the lower abdomen through the spinal column towards the periphery of the body, and then beyond the skin, to mingle with the surrounding space, connecting Earth and Sky in one wave of breath.

2.7   The Seventh Vital Principle: Elongating

In *elongating* the body moves in an open, non-constricted way, as a natural outcome of practicing the first six *Vital Principles*. As energy, enhanced by the breathing, flows downwards through rooting, and upwards along the connecting pathways, it elongates the body. As always, the conscious awareness of the movement of elongating enhances its power.

In this context it is important to be aware that there is a profound difference between stretching and elongating. Stretching is a mechanical lengthening of a certain muscle, produced by shortening another muscle, and takes place on a purely physical level. Therefore, there is a limit to stretching, beyond which the muscle will rip. This ripping happens when the power of the shortening muscle exceeds the capacity of the other muscle for being stretched.

Elongating is something entirely different. Deep within the fibers of the muscles there is a hidden door. This hidden door is opened by breathing and, once opened, allows the muscle to undo itself, that is, to elongate without the aid of another muscle shortening itself. For example, whereas in order to stretch the biceps muscle of the arm we contract the triceps, and vice versa, in elongating we experience both muscles undoing themselves simultaneously and elongating. The result is extraordinary.

Whereas in stretching there is the danger of ripping, in elongating there seems to be no limit at all. Rather, both muscles seem to simultaneously abandon all striving and ride on the flow of energy. Thus, not only is there no danger involved, but there is also no fatigue or residue, as in the case of stretching, where the shortening muscle is left with the residue of lactic acid.

The process of elongating comes about by rooting, connecting and breathing, in which breathing is both the connecting glue as well as the fuel which pulls the body through the movements and asanas.

2.8 Summary

We begin to dance the *Body of Light* when the physical vehicle, with all its joints and muscles, rides on the energy flow of the Body of Light. Performing all the asanas in that way, there is no fatigue and effort, but rather an increased amount of energy. The body elongates and reconnects, not only all its own internal parts, but reconnects itself to the surrounding space as well, in which we live and breathe. In that there is beauty, and power, and grace, and above all, joy.

The Seven Vital Principles, even though they have been described separately, form one inseparable unit and are welded together in each action, in each movement. Although they are presented here as a sequence in time, this is partially misleading. It is true that the process of undoing the body and mind, and intent, precede the other Principles, but in a seasoned practitioner the whole process takes only a split second. Rooting, connecting, breathing and elongating happen simultaneously in the same way that our bodies perform multiple functions, like breathing, digesting and moving, all at the same time.

The Principles are the tools, which help us activate the Energy Body; they form the key to transforming the mere physical posture into a posture of light, of beauty. Only by transforming the posture, the body itself in this way, can we express fully our potential as creatures of Light, of life. This is the *Yoga of the Future*, in which the physical body is not discarded, but is pulled up to the level of the Body of Light, as a vehicle of joy.

2.9 From Transparent Body to the Body of Light

When learning how to work with these Seven Vital Principles you can start with a simple exercise: *Sitting*.

Sit in Siddhasana or Padmasana with the back straight and the hands on the knees, the palms facing upwards. In this position one has to first work on *rooting*. At all times the body forms a living link between the Earth and the Sky. The body has to feel, in the first place, the contact with the Earth, whether it is in a sitting, a standing or a lying down position, and from there the awareness has to move upwards.

In Padmasana, the back of the thighs and the buttock bones form that part of the body which is in contact with the Earth, and thus these parts have to utilize the force of gravity. Establish that link, feel the contact of the back of the thighs and the buttock bones with the Earth, and then yield them to the force of gravity, following the line of gravity down into the Earth. The buttock bones and the thighs should gradually, as it were, sink into the Earth.

The bowl of the pelvis should be held completely vertical, neither tilted backwards nor forwards. This means that the two frontal hip bones are in a vertical alignment with the groins, at an angle of ninety degrees with the femurs. As you keep the pelvis firmly vertical, without collapsing, you have to 'grow' the buttock bones downwards. The body is like a tree. If one considers the hip joints, the groins and the sacro-iliac joints as 'ground level', then the part which is below this 'ground level' has to 'grow' downwards, just like the roots of a tree, while the part which is above it has to 'grow' upwards, like the trunk of the tree.

This 'growing upwards' is done when the body picks up the rebounce force from the downward 'growing' roots (buttock bones). The exchange of the downward and upward forces takes place in the sacro-iliac joints, the hip joints and the groins.

One can divide the body roughly into three compartments: the pelvis, the chest and the head. Most people hold the body up from the chest or from the head, shoulders and neck. This means that the support for the weight of the body comes from the diaphragm or even from the shoulders.

In the first place, the body has to counteract that tendency by dropping the point of support into the third, the basic, compartment, the lower abdomen. Draw a line from hip joint to hip joint, and another one, a front-back line, from the mid point between the navel and pubis to the sacrum: where those two lines cross is the center of gravity. It is from here that the body should be upheld. Thus the energy in the neck and the shoulders, which is often used to hold the body up, has to be brought down into the lower abdomen. This is a question of internal weight, it is not a question of dropping the spinal column. It is the force with which the body is upheld which is lowered.

In the second place, the body has to shift the internal weight backwards as well, into the backside of the body. The frontal side of the body is in contact with the frontal brain and the eyes; it is that part of the body that we can see and think about. The backside of the body, on the other hand, is that part which we cannot see, with which we don't have a relationship, and which is in contact with the back brain. Our actions are always focused on the front of the body, on the front of the face. If one says: "Let me think", one points to the forehead. If one says: "I feel", one points to the chest. If one says: "I am afraid", one points to the diaphragm. This shows that we feel or experience our emotions on the front of the body. On the backside of the body we do not feel anything. Thus, after having lowered the internal weight of the awareness into the lower abdomen, you have to bring it also from the frontal side of the body into the backside, towards the sacrum, the 'sacred' bone.

It is easy to feel how the awareness is lodged on the frontal side of the diaphragm. The diaphragm, which is a negative emotional center, is hot. It is here that we find the solar plexus, the 'sun knot', where we experience fear and anxiety, which, when excessive, the body expresses as 'ulcers. On the backside of the body, we find the kidneys which, in most Oriental disciplines, are associated with water, with the moon, with coolness.

One of the most important acts in yoga is to bring the hot, solar energy of the frontal diaphragm, and the cool, lunar energy of the kidneys, into balance. This the meaning of the word 'Hatha Yoga', *ha* and *tha* meaning 'the sun' and 'the moon'. The internal weight of awareness, the internal Energy Body, which is lodged against the frontal wall of the abdomen, has to be brought backwards towards the kidneys, without disturbing the physical body, and without bending the spine.

In the chest, too, the awareness has to be moved backwards. The sternum is the center of positive emotions (love, affection) as the diaphragm is the center of negative emotions (fear, anger). From the sternum, the internal weight, the awareness of the Body of Light, has to be brought backwards into the shoulder blades, without bending the chest or the thoracic spine.

In this way the whole back of the chest, the shoulder blades, and even the kidneys, widen. The shoulder blades are the wings of the body. Use them!

The most difficult area for shifting the awareness is the head. Our emotions and thoughts are engraved on the front of the face, in the grooves and wrinkles, in the worry lines or in the laughing 'crow's feet' wrinkles next to the eyes. Here too, we have to draw the weight of the internal energy backwards into the back of the head. This is particularly important for the energy of the eyes and ears.

Normally the 'I' which looks out through the eyes is standing, so to speak, right behind the eyeballs, peeking out through the holes of the eyes. The physical result of this is that the eyes have a certain hardness to them, are dry, round, and their focusing attention is driven through the inner corners of the eyes, giving the eyes an impression of narrowness. Drawing the awareness into the back of the head has the immediate effect of widening the eyes, of making them soft and 'liquid', and of diffusing their focusing attention through the outer corners, giving them an almost Egyptian slant.

The same applies to the ears. Here too the 'I', which habitually stands, as it were, right behind the ear holes, has to move backwards into the back of the head, leaving the ears soft and open and more vulnerable, not only to sounds, but also to the empty spaces in between the sounds.

These are the first two acts the body has to perform: after rooting the buttock bones, the upholding force of the body is lowered into the lower abdomen, and then shifted backward into the backside of the body, the part of the body that is unknown, mysterious.

The third act of the body is to become aware of the surrounding space, especially the space above the head. The body is a conduit for electrical energy, which passes between the Earth and the Sky, like lightning which goes from the Earth to the clouds and back down again. Starting with the vertical space above the head, you can actually feel the weight of the Sky on your head, pressing down on you. Part of this weight is gravity pulling the body down, and part is the actual weight of the air molecules pressing down on the head. Instead of struggling to elongate the body upwards against this weight, there is a much simpler way. This is by visualization.

In your imagination, 'take the Sky away', the air above the head, as if you create a vacuum above the head. In this vacuum the spinal column will unfurl itself upwards, without any muscular effort. It is just the image of having 'taken the weight of the Sky away' that makes the spine go up like a cork surfacing above water level after having been pressed underneath it and then released. Thus, you have to bring the inner awareness not only into the back of the body, but also deep within, into the skeletal structure, from where it can then expand outwards again.

With the buttock bones growing downwards like the roots of a tree, the spinal column growing upwards like the trunk of a tree, and the branches growing sideways - that is, the rib cage, the shoulder blades, the shoulders, and the kidney region widening - the picture of the human tree is complete. All the energies are in balance, the inner awareness, the awareness of the Body of Light, moves freely in all directions, and the body is light, held up by its own inner expansion.

The last act of the body is to 'take the skin away' all over the body, this barrier between the inner energy and the outer space or energy. The skin is the 'bag' in which we live, like a leather bag, and basically what is inside the skin is the same 'substance' as what is outside, but it is contained. Due to our lifelong thoughts and emotions, the skin becomes tough to the point of brittleness, a barrier to hold the outer energies at bay, and to 'protect' the inner being from these outer energies. Thus the Body of Light, the inner energy, is trapped within this hard skin, and cannot mix with the energy which is outside, the sun and air which nourish it. Therefore, through visualization, the skin has to be 'taken away'.

To practice this, start with the hands. With the palms facing upwards, relax the hands and carefully 'take away' the skin. In doing this, you feel as if the hands swell and become big. One can compare this sensation to a sponge. When the sponge is squeezed, it is small and tight, but when it is released, it immediately swells up, filling itself with air. As the hands become big, they also become warm and begin to tingle, as the energy within the hand spills out and mixes with the energy outside, till there comes a moment in which you no longer clearly feel where the hands end and the space around the hands begins. No longer feeling the boundaries of the hands, you do not feel whether they are resting on your knees, on the Earth, or on nothing at all.

After the hands, you can do the same thing with the arms, 'taking the skin away', feeling the swelling, the warmth, the tingling, and the melting of boundaries. Then move up to the shoulders, the shoulder blades, the neck and the chest. You can clearly feel how the skin holds the inner energy, the inner body, tight, so that when you 'take the skin away' from the shoulders, the shoulder blades, the sternum, and the rib cage, they become big, wide, open, vulnerable. Watch carefully that the skin dissolves everywhere evenly, that there are no hidden parts where it refuses to melt. Those are the places where the body has collected tensions, so you have to spend a little extra time 'undoing' the skin in those parts.

Then move to the pelvis, the legs, the feet. Keeping the skeletal frame straight, upright, 'take the skin away' everywhere. It is like making an X-ray picture of your body, where the skeleton is outlined clearly, but the muscles and the skin are only vague shadows, transparent. The most difficult area to make transparent is the head, the face. Carefully dissolve the skin on the face till it is transparent, like a clear piece of quartz crystal, through which the inner Light can shine out.

Once the body is rooted in the Earth, has made the connection with the Sky and the surrounding space and has become, as it were, transparent, by dissolving the tensions in the muscles and the skin, we can turn our attention to the breathing. As we mentioned before, there is a special type of breathing, which forms the true link between the physical body and the Body of Light, and which is used to move the Body of Light in the asanas, and even in daily life itself. This breathing is called the *Mula Bandha Breathing*.

Let us trace the trajectory of this breathing.

As we said, there are three main compartments in the body: the pelvis, the chest and the head, with three 'gates' or diaphragms. When you inhale, the air enters the body through the first 'gate', the throat. The throat is a tube like structure with an upper part and a lower part.

The upper part should be soft, not constricted, to let the air pass and go straight into the lower part of the throat, right above the sternum. This part should be widened, opened from inside, to draw the air in and send it down into the lower abdomen. Letting the air enter through the bottom part of the tube of the throat, and not through the top part, makes the breathing soundless.

Sound in breathing is produced when the air is forced through the upper part of the throat, which is held constricted for this purpose. This 'noisy' type or breathing is used for various Pranayamas, such as Ujjayi, as well as in fast movements when we need to use the air as a kind of 'jet' to propel us through those movements. For the purpose at hand, though, which is to connect and elongate the Body of Light and expand it beyond the skin, we have to use the lower throat breathing. The upper throat breathing is 'extrovert', the air is thrown out of the body with the sound and is thus lost. In the lower throat breathing the air is 'introvert', revolved backwards into the body and the Body of Light, giving strength and fuel to that body for expansion and movement.

When the inhalation reaches the lower abdomen, this should not push forward, but, on the contrary, should pull backwards. As it moves backwards, the wave of the breathing encounters the sacrum and, not being able to go further backwards, returns upwards along the inner line of the spine.

One can compare this to a tidal wave or 'tsunami', where the water is first sucked backwards, to then become a wave which climbs higher and higher, till in the end it topples over forwards in a graceful curve. The movement of the breathing is exactly like that. As the wave starts in the lower abdomen, and involves first of all the pelvic diaphragm, this particular type of breathing is called the *Mula Bandha Breathing*. *Mula* means 'root' in Sanskrit, and *bandha* 'to bind', 'to gather'.

As the wave of the inhalation moves upwards along the inner line of the spine, it elongates it, till it meets the second diaphragm, the one which divides the abdomen from the chest: the thoracic diaphragm. This too is widened and lifted by the wave of the inhalation, in a modified version of *Uddiyana Bandha*.

Still moving upwards, the wave finally reaches the third diaphragm, at the top of the sternum. This results in a lifting and widening of the whole upper part of the rib cage, the shoulders and the shoulder blades. From here the wave continues through the cervical spine and the base of the head over the top of the head, to finally fall forward, like the tidal wave, in a graceful curve: *Jalandhara Bandha*. This is the line of the *inhalation*.

The line of the *exhalation* is from the forehead down again through the base of the throat into the lower abdomen, after which the new cycle of breathing starts.

Thus the total curve of the inhalation and the exhalation is elliptical. This movement is not just a movement within the physical body. As you have expanded the Body of Light like a cloud by 'taking the skin away', the Mula Bandha Breathing is done within this cloud, within this expanded body. Breathe through the cloud, watch that the whole cloud is breathing.

As you inhale, as you exhale, do not re-create the skin. All movements, all asanas, should be done with this breathing.

Now practice the Seven Vital Principles in *Standing and Walking:*

Stand with the back straight and the arms hanging loosely down, keeping the feet at hip width. Now it is the feet which are the roots. Feel the soles of the feet on the Earth, as if you are spreading the skin of the feet on the Earth. The heels, the balls of the feet, the toes, everything is rooting into the Earth. Feel how the energy of the feet actually sinks down, as if the Earth is not there at all, or is like a spongy material, in which the soles of the feet sink.

As the soles of the feet 'grow' downwards into the spongy Earth, the legs have to pick up that same force and turn it up to elongate upwards. Here the 'ground level', the division line between rooting and elongating upwards, is in the center bones of the feet, the ones between the ankles and the metatarsals, the lower spring joints, or the talocalcaneonavicular joints. This is where the rebounce force is picked up and utilized to elongate the legs, so that there is only minimum muscular effort involved, as it is the energy of the legs which elongates. The Body of Light, fueled by the Mula Bandha Breathing, draws the physical legs along, up towards the femur heads and the pelvis.

Even though the pelvis is supported by the femur heads, it should not sit heavily on them. By elongating the legs, and especially the upper thighs, the pelvis can pick up that rebounce force in the hip joints and lift up from the femur heads with the help of the Mula Bandha Breathing, to bring the Earth energy into the lower abdomen.

From there the energy moves upwards with the breathing, as described above in the Sitting Position, with a wave-like action that moves along the inner line of the spine, drawing the spine with it upwards. As the wave climbs higher and higher it lifts the whole body up, not only the spinal column, till it reaches the back of the head. From there it spills over, like the crest of the tidal wave, forward over the top of the head, down the forehead and down again with the exhalation into the lower abdomen.

Thus, while standing, the roots are the feet, and the back and the front of the body are on parallel lines, which means that the awareness is equal on the back and the front of the body. Again, to make the body light, you have to use the combination of the Mula Bandha Breathing and 'taking' the Sky or the air above your head 'away', so that the body elongates upwards.

Then 'take the skin away' on your whole body, without collapsing the skeletal frame, till you cannot tell any more where your body is in space. There is no sensation, no feeling. The feeling disappears, because there is no more dividing line between the body and the space around it. Having taken the hard, brittle skin away, there are no more boundaries, and the inner energy expands and merges with the energy outside the body. Not only does the body become light, but again you can feel the warmth and the tingling at the top of the head. That means that the channel is open between the Earth and the Sky and the electrical current moves freely up and down.

Then start to *walk*.

When you move one foot forward, feel the contact with the Earth, let the foot sink into the Earth. The foot and the Earth should not hit each other. Instead you have to visualize the Earth as a kind of spongy material into which the foot sinks the moment it comes into contact with it. The body too should not hit the space around it as it moves forward, it has to move like air moving through air, or as a cloud moving through air. You can initially practice the expansion of the Body of Light in slow motion, but eventually you should be able to do it in one fast movement, like a burst, an explosion of energy. The moment you 'take the skin away' there is a burst of energy. You have to learn to do this instantly, to expand the Body of Light in the twinkling of an eye. All the asanas should be done in that way.

Chapter 3.
Bandhas and Kriyas

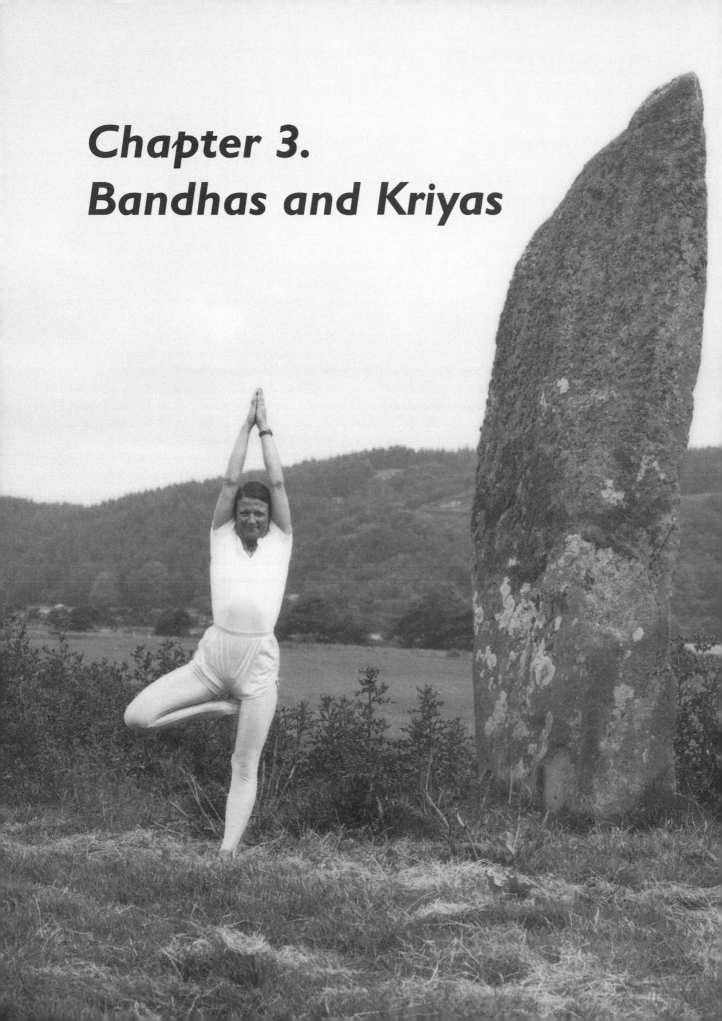

3   Introduction

The word *bandha* in Sanskrit means 'to bind'. The word has been mentioned many times in this book, specially in reference to the Mula Bandha breathing and to the gravity-rebounce action in the poses. We can also find the same root in the English words 'bond', 'bound' and others. Whereas the word 'to bind' has a constrictive meaning, the word 'bound' as found in 'bound for' also carries the meaning 'to go somewhere'.

In general, the easiest way maybe to understand a bandha is to compare it to a cyclone or a whirlwind. In the cyclone or whirlwind, all the action takes place on the rim, on the periphery. In the case of the whirlwind, the rim twirls around a center, called the 'eye' of the cyclone. This one can see very clearly on meteorological charts. Thus the energy is trapped and compressed towards the center. This would be the 'binding' part of the bandha.

However, just 'binding' the energy to a particular spot in the body would not make much sense. As in the cyclone, when the energy is compressed towards the center, the center is consequently pushed upwards. Thus one can see leaves (in a small whirlwind) or clouds (in a cyclone) being pushed up towards the sky. Thus the center or 'eye' of the cyclone is the highest point. People who live in the country know that when there is a thunderstorm, if the raindrops turn from water to hail it means that the 'eye' of the storm is passing straight overhead. The rain from the lower periphery is sucked up into the higher center and turns into ice. This would be the 'bound for' part of the word bandha. After trapping the energy it is then shot through to the next knot or bandha.

In the body a bandha functions in the same way. It is a particular spot in the body where energy is trapped and then sent through to the next bandha. One of the main characteristics of energy is, however, that it can only be trapped in a round container, or an arch. Thus, all the bandhas are found in those parts of the body where there is an arch-construction of bones, with usually a ligamental floor. The sole of the foot, with its arch structure and the ligamental 'stirrup', the arch of the pelvis with the pelvic diaphragm, the arch of the lower ribs with the lower thoracic diaphragm, even the arch of the jaw bones with the floor of the tongue, the palm of the hand with the ligamental plate of the palm, these are the places where we find the bandhas most used in yoga.

To trap the energy within the arch, the peripheral rim of muscles and joints is slightly constricted inwards towards the center. If the arch is in contact with the earth, this rim is also rooted into the earth, creating thus the rebounce force or the Normal Force of Newton. The combination of rooting and constricting the energy towards the center creates the 'eye' of the storm, in other words, the center is lifted and the energy is shot upwards.

One can see this action in Tadasana in the Pada Bandha (the lifting of the lower spring joints of the feet) by the combined action of rooting the rim of the feet (the metatarsals, the toes and the heels) and lifting the stirrups of the medial arches, formed by the four major muscles in the feet, namely the Abductor muscles of the big and small toes, the Peroneus longus and the Tibialis posterior. One can see this action in the Mula Bandha, or the lifting of the pelvic floor through the combined action of the rooting of the buttock bones and the constriction of the outer hips inwards. In Sarvangasana one sees it in the action of the arms and shoulder heads, combined with Jalandhara Bandha.

In Adhomukha Vrksasana the body weight is centered above the center of the palms, which are sucked upwards into Hasta Bandha.

The art of distributing the energy throughout the body is to send it from bandha to bandha, thus connecting all the parts of the body. The simplest pose to do this is to stand in Tadasana and then raise the arms up over the head, so that the connection runs in a straight line from the Pada Bandha through the Mula Bandha, the Uddiyana Bandha, the Jalandhara Bandha to the Hasta Bandha.

Bandhas and Kriyas

Bandhas

1. *Pada Bandha*
2. *Mula Bandha*
3. *Uddiyana Bandha*

6. *Jalandhara Bandha*
7. *Hasta Bandha*
8. *Padma Bandha*

Kriyas

4. *Agnisara*
5. *Nauli*

3.1   Pada Bandha

This bandha is described in detail in the Chapter on Tadasana (see page 49).

3.2   Mula Bandha

This bandha is described in detail in the Mula Bandha breathing in Padmasana (see page 77).

3.3   Uddiyana Bandha

In the "Hatha Yoga Pradipika", Uddiyana Bandha is described in Chapter 3, sutras 55-60:
*   "Uddiyana Bandha is so called by the yogis, for when it is practiced the Prana is arrested and flies through the Sushumna. It is called *Uddiyana Bandha* (uddiyana means 'to fly up'), because the great bird Prana flies up incessantly. The drawing back of the abdomen above the navel is Uddiyana Bandha. It is the lion that kills the elephant of death..."

Of all the bandhas, Uddiyana is the most excellent. When this has been mastered, liberation follows naturally'.

The old Hatha Yoga texts tend to generally exaggerate the benefits of specific practices, but Uddiyana is beneficial for a number of reasons.

1.   When it is performed successfully, the other two bandhas (Mula Bandha and Jalandhara Bandha) follow naturally. One can actually feel the area of the Mula Bandha and its upward movement. One can also feel how the chin and chest unite to perform Jalandhara Bandha without any effort.
2.   This bandha and the kriyas that follow it (Agnisara and Nauli) strengthen the abdominal muscles and the diaphragm.
3.   By pulling the inner organs of the abdomen up and squeezing them inward, they become less prone to sagging and are cleansed due to a major circulation of blood.
4.   This internal massage of the intestines makes them more supple and improves elimination.
5.   According to Indian tradition, the area of the abdomen just below the navel functions as the stove of the body. In Chinese tradition this point is called 'Dantien', in Japanese 'Hara' and in yogic tradition 'Manipura chakra'. The practice of Uddiyana Bandha strengthens this extremely important area where the body stores heat and energy.

This bandha is best performed in the early morning, either before elimination of the bowels, or immediately afterwards. For beginners it is better afterwards, as it is easier to control the involuntary muscles of the abdomen when the intestines are empty.

Technique
*   Stand with the feet slightly wider than the hips. Place the hands on the thighs, just above the knees, with the fingers pointing outwards. Keep the knees slightly bent and the torso inclined forward at an angle of about thirty degrees.
*   Inhale, and then exhale forcefully through the nose, emptying the lungs of air.

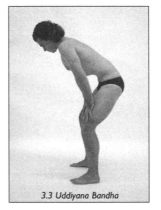

3.3 Uddiyana Bandha

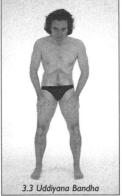

3.3 Uddiyana Bandha

By exhaling forcefully (without inhaling afterwards) you create a vacuum in the chest cavity. This vacuum is necessary in order to be able to draw the diaphragm and the inner organs of the abdomen upwards.

- Then draw the abdomen in and up in one swift movement. When Uddiyana Bandha is complete, the area of the diaphragm and abdomen will be completely hollow. When the practice of this bandha becomes more fluent, you will feel that it includes Mula Bandha and Jalandhara Bandha.
- Hold it for as long as you can, keeping the inward and upward drawing of the abdominal muscles. Then release by lightly lifting the chin, widening the throat muscles and simultaneously relaxing the abdominal muscles in a gradual way. After which air will automatically enter the lungs. Make the inhalation as slow and smooth as possible.
- Inhale and exhale until the breathing is even again.

Repeat Uddiyana Bandha three times.

3.4 Agnisara

Agnisara is a natural continuation of Uddiyana Bandha, but you should only begin to practice it after you feel fairly confident with Uddiyana Bandha. *Agni* means 'fire'. By practicing this kriya one is fanning the fire in the Hara.

Technique
- Do Uddiyana Bandha (as described above from 1-4)
- Do not release the Jalandhara Bandha but, keeping the lungs empty, push the abdominal muscles forcefully out.
- Draw the abdominal muscles again back into full Uddiyana Bandha (still without breathing) and repeat this process a few times until you feel the need to breathe again.
- Then release by lightly lifting the chin,

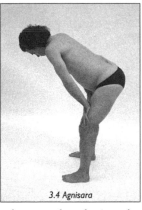 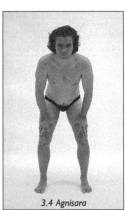

3.4 Agnisara   *3.4 Agnisara*

widening the throat muscles and simultaneously relaxing the abdominal muscles in a gradual way. After which air will automatically enter the lungs. Make the inhalation as slow and smooth as possible.
- Inhale and exhale until your breathing is even again.

Repeat Agnisara three times.

3.5 Nauli

Nauli is a natural continuation of Uddiyana Bandha and Agnisara, but you should only begin to practice it after you feel fairly confident in those. Nauli is a refining of Agnisara in the sense that we do not push simply all the abdominal muscles out, but, isolating the Rectitudinal muscles of the abdomen, push only those forward and out, while keeping the Oblique abdominal muscles.

Technique

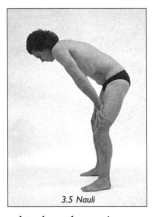
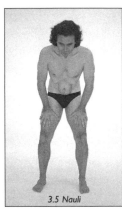

3.5 Nauli   3.5 Nauli

- Do Uddiyana Bandha (as described above from 1-4).
- Do not release the Jalandhara Bandha but, keeping the lungs empty, push the Rectitudinal muscles of the abdomen forward and out. When you do this action correctly, the muscles bulge out in a long line.
- Draw the abdominal muscles again back into full Uddiyana Bandha (still without breathing) and repeat this process a few times until you feel the need to breathe again.
- Then release by lightly lifting the chin, widening the throat muscles and simultaneously relaxing the abdominal muscles in a gradual way. After which air will automatically enter the lungs. Make the inhalation as slow and smooth as possible.
- Inhale and exhale until your breathing is even again.

Repeat Nauli three times.

When this initial Nauli becomes easy, you can elaborate it further by moving the protruding (Rectitudinal) muscles of the abdomen to the right and to the left, rotating them round and round fairly fast. Eventually, in both Agnisara and Nauli, one can build the amount of rounds up to twenty-five to thirty rounds at a time (all without breathing). These twenty-five or so rounds (after an exhalation) constitute one cycle.

The most important thing here is not to be in a hurry, but to build up the amount of rounds performed in one cycle gradually over a period of a few months. In this way the practice is revitalizing and the muscles gain strength and tone in a gradual way, without too much effort.

> ### Counter indications for the bandhas and kriyas
> For any major disease it is recommendable to consult a doctor before starting to practice these bandhas or kriyas. In general they should not be practiced under the following conditions:
> - During periods of menstruation or pregnancy
> - With high blood pressure
> - With heart problems in general
> - With ailments of the abdominal organs.

3.6 Jalandhara Bandha

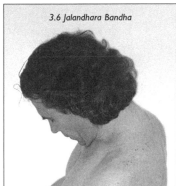

3.6 Jalandhara Bandha

Jalandhara Bandha is slightly more complex than Mula Bandha and Uddiyana Bandha, as we can discern two levels or planes of action:

- The *lower level*, which is circumscribed by the two collar bones at the front of the chest and the promontory (the first thoracic vertebra) at the back of the neck. This level, in Jalandhara Bandha, is raised vertically.
- The *upper level*, which is circumscribed by the jaw bones at the front of the face and the atlas vertebra at the back of the neck. This level slides horizontally forward in Jalandhara Bandha.

How do we perform Jalandhara Bandha? The classical texts only tell us to bring the chin down to perform the chin lock. To quote the "Hatha Yoga Pradipika": "Contract the throat and hold the chin firmly against the chest". The question is how to do this without creating pressure and discomfort in the neck and upper back muscles. Often the chin cannot reach the chest unless we push it down forcefully at the expense of straining the neck and upper back muscles.

In order to perform this bandha correctly we have to do two things.

- The first thing is to do the Mula Bandha breathing. In this breathing the inhalation starts at the bottom of the spinal column, in the region of the sacrum, and then moves upwards through the kidney area. Thus, as the interior part of the spine is elongated, the upper chest lifts and the shoulder blades widen.
- The second thing is to take the head down. In order not to create a strain in the neck and upper back muscles this should be done in a special way.

Instead of taking the head straight down, one has to first slide it horizontally forward on the first cervical vertebra, and then bend it down. In this case, not only is there no strain in the Trapezius muscle, but there is actually a release as the shoulder blades widen and descend.

Let us look more closely at this technique of taking the head down. The muscle where the tension is mainly felt is the Trapezius muscle, which covers the spine from the fifth cervical vertebra to the second thoracic vertebra. When the thoracic spine is elongated due to the Mula Bandha breathing, the frontal upper ribs are lifted and spread together with the sternum and the collar bones. In order to lift those thoracic vertebrae, the Trapezius muscle has to be kept fairly relaxed, which is not possible if the chin is brought down at a sharp angle. The joint surfaces between the atlas or first cervical vertebra and the skull permit a horizontal sliding movement forwards and backwards. These joints are different from most joints in the body and resemble most the joints between the sacrum and the ileum, the sacro-iliac joints. Both these pair of joints have roughly the shape of a bean, and permit a slight sliding action. It is interesting to note that these two sliding joints are at the extreme ends of the spinal column, and are actually the first and last joints that connect the spine to the rest of the body.

If the chin is brought sharply down to the sternum, this movement starts from a backward position of the joint. As a result the upper cervical vertebrae are pushed out backwards (you can feel this very clearly with your fingers) and there is a strong tension in the Trapezius muscle. If, on the other hand, one slides the head *first* forward horizontally in the joint in between the atlas and the skull (the so-called 'swan neck movement') and *then* bends the head down, the bending starts from a more forward position of the skull in respect to the atlas vertebra. The result of this is that there is much less strain on the muscles and ligaments of the neck and in the Trapezius muscle, and the upper cervical vertebrae are *not* pushed out backwards, but remain in, concave, the way they should be according to their natural curve (again you can feel this easily with your fingers). Thus the word 'chin lock' is, in a way, misleading. It is not so much that one brings the chin down to lock it, but one has to rather elongate the corners of the jaws (right underneath the ears) forwards. Then, keeping that length of the jaws and the freedom and openness in the fleshy part underneath them, one has to bring the chin to meet the upcoming sternum. Thus chin and sternum meet halfway and there is no strain anywhere.

3.7 Hasta Bandha

hasta=hand

This bandha is used in all the poses where the palms of the hands are in contact with the earth (as in the Hand Balances) and the body needs to get its rebounce energy from this contact. This energy then travels through the arms and shoulder joints to lift the body up from those shoulder joints.

In Hasta Bandha we have to apply the same principle as for Pada Bandha. That is, as the weight of the body in Pada Bandha has to be shifted from the heels (the upper spring joints) to the central bones of the feet (the lower spring joints), so also in Hasta Bandha the weight of the body has to be shifted from the wrists (which correspond to the upper spring joints) to the central bones of the palms (which correspond to the lower spring joints). Then the center of the palms is sucked upward in the same way as for the Pada Bandha, thus trapping the energy in the typical arch construction and sending it upward through the arms and shoulder joints. The fingers are kept long and flat on the earth and they root together with the wrists, forming the rim of the cyclone or bandha. This corresponds to the action in the Pada Bandha, where the toes are elongated on the earth and root together with the heel bones.

3.8 Padma Bandha

padma=lotus

This is not really a bandha in the usual form and sense. At the top of the head, at the place of the fontanel, is what the Buddhists and Hindus call the *thousand-petalled lotus*. It is the last and uppermost opening in the body, the telescope with which human beings, being upright creatures, look at the Universe and acknowledge their participation in the *Great Dance*. The fontanel, anatomically speaking, is the exact place where the two side plates and the front plate of the skull meet, and which in newborn babies is still completely open and vulnerable. As the child grows, this opening closes as the plates come closer together.

In all ancient cultures the fontanel has a mystical sense. It is supposed to be the place where the soul enters the body at birth and leaves it at death. It is the place where Pallas Athene, the great goddess of wisdom, was born of the head of Zeus, and where the Ka leaves the body of the dying Pharaoh. In Sanskrit the fontanel is called the *Brahmarandhra,* the Gate of Brahma, while in the Kahuna religion of Hawaii it is the place where the Aumakua dwell, the divine double being, half male, half female, which guards over the person. The Hopi Indians have an interesting story. According to their legends the earth has been destroyed several times in the past (by flood and fire), and is due again to be destroyed. The reason for these destructions is always the same: human beings have become wicked, and their 'wickedness' is due to the fact that the hole at the top of the head closes up. As said before, in Buddhist and Yogic literature the fontanel or the thousand-petalled lotus is the last gate to be opened in order to reach 'enlightenment' (the total 'explosion' of the *Luminous Body*). Therefore we have named this last bandha the Padma Bandha.

In the normal upright position this lotus points straight up towards the sky, channeling the energies which come from above and connecting them to the feet which, rooting in the earth, channel the earth energy, creating thus a kind of magnetic or electrical current through the body.

It is interesting to note that the ancient yogis probably thought that it was important to reverse this electrical current every now and then, rendering the north pole the south pole, and vice versa. Thus they invented the *Head Balance*, in which the fontanel dips into the earth energy, while the soles of the feet receive the current from above. Thus, in Head Balance, the fontanel becomes the place where the body roots, but as the opening is so small and there is not really a rim around it as in the case of the other bandhas, it is here only the case of the energy moving up and down, without the muscular and skeletal structure around it.

Thus we have listed six bandhas which are used on a regular basis in yoga. Three on the extreme ends of the body (the feet, the hands and the top of the head), and three in the middle (Mula Bandha, Uddiyana Bandha and Jalandhara Bandha). Try to cultivate, not only in the yoga practice, but also in daily life, a feeling of warmth and tingling in the palms of the hands, on the soles of the feet and on the top of the head, so that these gateways between the inner and outer energies are always open, permitting a smooth exchange of energy.

Chapter 4.
Technique of the Asanas

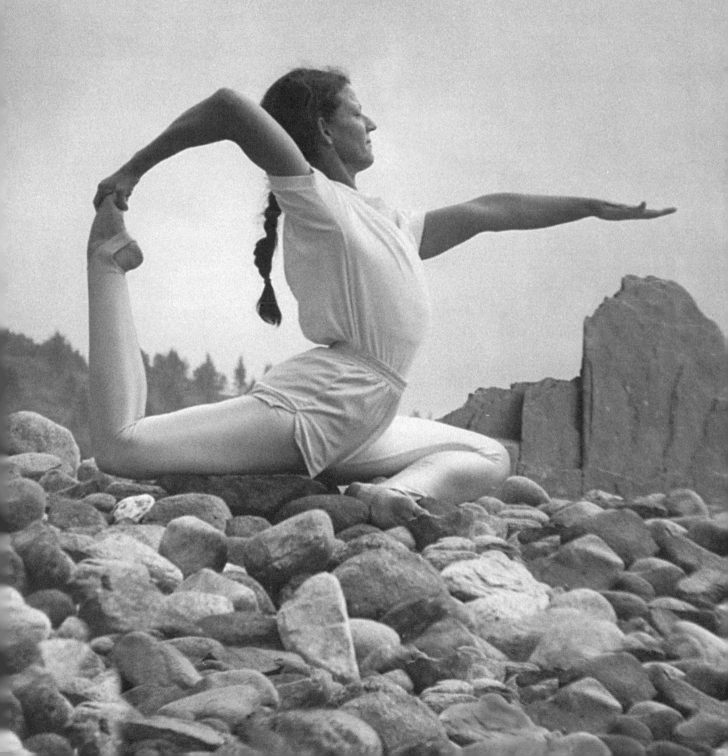

4   Introduction

This chapter gives the technique of the *asanas*. If you cannot study with a competent teacher, it will give you a fairly good understanding of how to practice the poses on your own.

All the asanas are done on a yoga mat. For some positions, though, like Head Balance and Shoulder Balance, it is advisable to use a padding for the head, like a folded blanket. Otherwise, no aids and props are mentioned in this book. External tools, aids and props tend to distract the attention from the real pose, and give a false sense of accomplishment. It is better to do the poses slowly and to your capacity, even if that capacity is limited, rather than force the body with the aid of props to do what its own innate intelligence is not yet capable of handling.

The second issue not tackled in this book is that of physical problems and diseases. If treated well, the body is a self-healing organism. As such, yoga in itself is the greatest aid there is. Without going into specific details, just practicing the whole of yoga, including the breathing, creates the ideal condition for the body to take care of most normal physical problems. For major diseases, one should refer to a qualified doctor and eventually practice yoga under his or her guidance.

The third issue is that of dealing with physical and mental fatigue due to stressful living. The body is not only a self-healing organism, but it thrives on a finely tuned balance between exercise and rest. This balance is provided by the method of practicing yoga as described in this book. The feeling of resting is provided by the relaxation, the breathing and the elongation described in the *Seven Vital Principles*. Practicing all the following asanas, guided by the Seven Vital Principles, gives the body the balance which it needs to feel in optimum health and vitality.

The last issue is that of aging. In the "Hatha Yoga Pradipika", it is written that anybody can practice yoga, old, young, healthy and ill. There is no need to fear the effect of aging; the body can be as young as you want it to be. Disease and age are held at bay by cultivating the habit of happiness and joy, and above all, by a real love for this marvelous instrument, the body, and for this greatest gift of all, yoga.

Before going into the various groups of asanas, it is interesting to have a closer look at the basic posture, Tadasana or Straight Standing Pose, which contains all the postures in the same way as white light contains all the colors of the rainbow.

4.1   Tadasana / Standing straight
tada=mountain

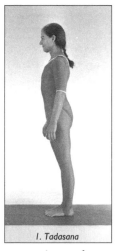

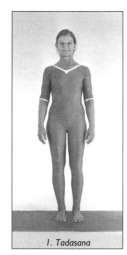

1. Tadasana

1. Tadasana

Technique

The feet

Stand with the feet at hip width, parallel to each other. Keep the feet even, and the toes straight forward; do not turn them in or out. On the back of the body, the fibers of the latissimus dorsi and those of the gluteus maximus cross over the lumbar vertebrae with a strong ligamental plate, the fascia thoraco-lumbaris. If the feet are turned outward, these fibers slacken and the lumbar spine sags inward, exaggerating the natural curve. To protect the lumbar spine from sagging, the feet must be parallel to each other, or even slightly turned inward for those who have a weak or excessively curved lumbar spine. This tightens the fibers of the gluteus maximus and consequently tightens the fascia thoraco-lumbaris. The weight of the body is evenly distributed between the two feet; the soles of the feet should be conscious of their contact with the earth, as if the feet had roots going deep into the earth with the force of gravity (rooting, the fourth of the Seven Vital Principles).

The foot has three arches: the inner (long) arch, the outer (short) arch and the frontal or transverse arch. The inner arch is supported by the abductor hallucis, which runs from the heel to the big toe and abducts it. The outer arch is supported by the abductor digitis minimus, which runs from the heel to the little toe and abducts it. The transverse arch is supported mainly by two muscles, the peroneus longus and the tibialis posterior. The longus runs underneath the sole of the foot and up on the outer side of the lower leg to the head of the fibula. The tibialis posterior runs from the navicular bone in the foot over the heel up to the back of the lower leg. These two muscles together form a kind of stirrup which supports the transverse arch. These three arches must be raised to rebounce the weight of the body back upwards against the downward pull of gravity. The arches of the feet form the ultimate point where the weight of the body is received. As the upper body weight falls onto the pelvis, it divides into two, flowing through the hip joints into the thigh bones. The weight divides again in the knee joints and flows downwards through the fibula and tibia into the ankles and arches, where it is divided over the many bones of the feet. As the feet are small compared to the rest of the body, they need a special structure in order not to collapse under the weight of the body. This structure is the arch.

Arches are also used in architecture to hold great weights. For instance, the dome of a cathedral is copied from the arch of the feet; only thus can the weight of the roof of the cathedral be supported. In the body we find many domes. Two of them are key points in bearing the weight of the body: the feet and the pelvis. It is interesting to note that the central point of gravity is in the dome of the pelvis, while the dome of the feet is the place where the body roots into the earth. Thus the first rebounce action takes place in the arches and ankles, the second in the pelvis and the third in the spinal vertebrae.

To lift the three arches, the distance between the big and little toes has to increase by abduction of these toes: the big toe continues the curve of the inner arch and the little toe the curve of the outer arch, so that the triangle of the foot (heel-big toe-small toe) occupies the maximum floor space and the toes are fully spread. In the beginning, the hands can be used to spread the toes. Bend forward; with the fingers spread the toes and elongate them away from the metatarsals, so that the toes are straight, not curled (the result of wearing shoes). Animals have four points to stand on, but we have only two, which makes for a difficult balance while standing and walking. Therefore the toes serve to maintain the equilibrium of the body. We have to learn to use our feet like hands in all the postures, so the toes are like fingers on the earth, especially the big toes and the little ones. To check how the toes serve for balance, sway to right and left, and feel how each time the toes correct the balance of the body. Then try the same thing while walking. Walking is a form of controlled 'falling'; when you walk, you 'fall' from the ball of one foot onto the heel of the other one. Here too, you can feel how the toes serve to keep the balance in this unstable movement. The bottom of the toes, the distal heads of the metatarsals (especially those of the big and little toes) and the heels should be rooted in the earth. Without disturbing the toes, pull the cushions underneath the heels backwards with your fingers, so that the heels are extended on the earth Then lift the central metatarsals up to form the transverse arch.

Learn to use both the outer and inner arches evenly. With weak inner arches, the outer ankles are caved in, so that the inner ankles are pushed out, towards each other. To lift the inner arches, you have to root the base of the big toes into the earth and elongate the other toes. Then bring the body weight diagonally towards the outer heels, so that the inner ankles move in and the outer ankles move out. Keeping that action, bring the body weight onto the center bones of the feet, in particular the talus bone (between the metatarsals and the ankles), and raise the outer arches up. To check the arches, you can experiment with a pen. Most people are aware of the long inner arch, but few people are aware of the short outer arch. Lifting the arches, see if you can pass the pen underneath them from the outer edge of the foot towards the inner edge, through the outer and the inner arches. Lift the inner and outer ankles of both feet evenly. As the weight of the body is transmitted through the legs to the ankles, the ankles have to rebounce that weight back upwards together with the arches; they should not be passive. The inner and outer ankles should have the same height.

The legs
Elongate the back of the knees. The knee caps are embedded within the knees, but do not overstretch the back of the knees; the legs should not be bowed backwards. The knees face straight forward, with the inner knees in line with the inner ankles and the outer knees in line with the outer ankles. Create space in the knee joints, they continue rebouncing the weight of the body back upwards.

The pelvis
Anatomically the shoulder joints, hip joints and ankle joints should be aligned vertically, so that the lower legs are at right angles to the soles of the feet. Thus the weight of the body is transmitted to the feet in a straight line. As described later in this Chapter, for the purpose of making the body light we will change this angle. For the moment, however, we will base the rest of the description on this classical anatomical alignment.

Keeping these three joints in line and keeping the knees straight, the next step is to assess the position of the pelvis. The pelvis is a bowl-like construction at the lower end of the spinal column. It is attached to the spinal column in the sacro-iliac joints, which connect the ileum part of the pelvis to the sacral part of the spine, and to the legs in the hip joints, which connect the ilea with the femurs.

These are the two pair of joints where the pelvis moves in relation to the spine and legs. However, these joints are also heavily protected, the sacro-iliac joints by the irregularity of their joint surfaces, and the hip joints by their strong ligaments and muscles. As a result, the pelvis usually moves in relation to the rest of the trunk in the lumbo-sacral joint, where there is very little protection. This joint connects the sacrum with the lumbar spine and is already a stress point for most people. Eventually this joint and the rest of the lumbar spine weaken, which can lead to damage of its vertebrae and discs.

The pelvis can assume three positions. The correct one is the neutral position, in which the pelvis is vertical and the buttock bones point straight down. When the hip joints, knees and ankles are in line, the hip joints are thus fully extended (a hundred and eighty degrees). This position is quite rare. Sometimes the pelvis is rotated too far backward, causing the lumbar spine to come too far back, and sometimes it is rotated too far forward, causing the lumbar spine to curve too far inward as the sacrum and coccyx are tilted up, in which case the abdominal muscles become slack as the angle between pelvis and femur is less than a hundred and eighty degrees.

In both cases the pelvis has to be brought to a vertical position. The most common incorrect posture is the one in which the pelvis is rotated forward around the femur heads. This can easily be checked in the following way: choose an outer corner where two walls meet and stand with the back against it. Keep the heels two inches away from the corner, but rest the sacrum and the back of the head against it. Then put the hands in the small of the back. If there is a wide gap between the lumbar area and the corner, the pelvis is rotated forward, thus pulling the lumbar spine into the body. To correct this, practice as follows: move the feet forward until they are about a foot away from the corner, but keep the sacrum and the back of the head on the corner. Bend the knees a little and rotate the pelvis back around the femur heads, until the lumbar spine is in touch with the corner. Then straighten the knees again. Repeat this movement for a couple of weeks, gradually moving the heels closer to the corner as the mobility in the hip joints increases, until the heels are two inches away from the corner. It is not the intention to eliminate the natural curve of the lumbar spine, but only to reduce it. Thus a gap can remain of about two inches between the lumbar spine and the corner.

This is a see-saw action. Rotating the pelvis backward around the femur heads means that the two frontal hip bones move *up* towards the ribs, while the coccyx moves *down* and forwards towards the pubic bone. Many people cannot do this without bending the knees. This shows that the hip joints are unable to extend fully and therefore the knees have to give in to allow the pelvis to rotate backward. This is the see-saw action of pelvis and knees at the periphery around the central axis of the hip joints. Thus, when the knees are fully extended and the hip joints are in line with the ankle joints, the pelvis is stuck in that forward rotated position.

There are two points in the pelvis where the body often resorts to see-saw action:

I.   See-saw action around the hip joints
This is the action described above. To open the hip joints, the following movements are
necessary:
a. Rotate the pelvis backwards until it is vertical and the buttock bones point straight down
    to the earth.
b. At the same time, straighten the knees fully.
c. Constrict the following muscles around the pelvis slightly inwards towards each other:
    the tensor fascia lata muscles, which run from the frontal hip bones through the ileo-tibial
    tract of the fascia latas to the outer sides of the knees, the adductors on the inside of the
    thighs, the iliopsoas muscles and the rectus abdominus. When these muscles are toned,
    they stabilize the pelvis and lift it up from the femur heads. Do not tighten the gluteus
    maximus.

Steps a. and b. are simultaneous peripheral dynamic movements in opposite directions around
the static axis of the hip joints. As a result, these joints open fully and the groins and sides of the
hips are extended. Thus, in the correct movement the two frontal hip bones move up and
the knees resist backwards simultaneously. Just resisting the knees backwards tends to cause the
pelvis to rotate forwards, while just lifting the two frontal hip bones up towards the ribs
without resisting the knees tends to cause the pelvis to rotate backwards (see-saw action I).

II. See-saw action around the sacro-iliac joints
To open the sacro-iliac joints the following movements are necessary:
a. Keeping the pelvis (the compound bone of ileum, ischias and pubis) vertical, move the
    two frontal hip bones forward and up towards the ribs, and the knees back (see-saw
    action I).
b. At the same time, the compound bone of sacrum and coccyx has to make a movement
    which is called counter-nutation, that is, it has to rotate backwards in relation to the pelvis.
    This means that the coccyx moves forward towards the pubic bone and the sacrum
    becomes vertical.
c. Constrict the tensor fascia lata muscles and the adductors of the inner thighs slightly
    inwards towards each other and tighten the iliopsoas and rectus abdominus.

Steps a. and b. are simultaneous peripheral dynamic movements in opposite directions around
the static axis of the sacro-iliac joints. As a result, these joints open and the - now vertical -
sacrum moves forwards into the space between the two ilea, wedging them slightly apart.
The entire pelvis widens laterally and lifts vertically up from the femur heads.

Moving the two frontal hip bones forwards without anchoring the coccyx would cause the
entire pelvic bowl to rotate forwards and the coccyx to be tipped back and up. On the other hand,
moving the coccyx forward towards the pubic bone without also moving the two frontal hip
bones forward would cause the entire pelvic bowl to rotate backwards. Thus, in the correct
movement the pelvis (ilium+ischias+pubis) and the sacrum (+coccyx) move separately,
rotating in opposite directions: the pelvis rotates forward and the sacrum rotates backward
around the axis of the sacro-iliac joints. Thus these joints are opened.

The result of movements I and II together is that the pelvis becomes vertical, is widened laterally, moved vertically forward against the femur heads and lifted up from those femur heads.

The spine and chest

The upper rim of the sacrum is connected to the lumbar spine in the lumbo-sacral joint. When the pelvis and sacrum become vertical through the dual action in the hip and sacro-iliac joints, the lumbo-sacral joint is pulled slightly backward and down. This causes the rest of the lumbar vertebrae to come back too and thus the whole lumbar spine is elongated.

Thus, the first action of rebouncing the weight of the body back up takes place in the arches of the feet and the ankles. Lifting the pelvis up from the femur heads is the second rebounce action. The elongation of the spinal column, which starts in the lumbar vertebrae and continues through the thoracic and cervical vertebrae, is the third.

When the lumbar spine moves back, the shoulders move neither forward nor backward, but the shoulder joints remain in line with the hip and ankle joints. Do not bend the spine in the lumbar or thoracic area and do not collapse the chest or abdominal area between the navel and the lower ribs.

The weight of the body is brought onto the back and the pelvis and back are widened laterally. At the same time the distance between the two frontal hip bones widens, so that the lower abdomen moves in and up towards the navel. This tones the muscles of the lower abdomen and strengthens the internal organs.

As the pelvis and back widen laterally, the spine 'grows' out of the pelvis by itself. If the spine is pulled up by the rib cage, the shoulders and the shoulder blades, the body is not centered in the pelvis and the pelvis has not widened. It is important to learn this movement first, as all the other asanas depend on it.

As the lumbar spine 'grows' out of the pelvis, the thoracic spine continues that movement. Move only the spine, elongating it upward; do not push the lower ribs forward in the mistaken idea that you are lifting the spine. The spine elongates up through its own internal liberating force and the rib cage is merely suspended from it, without any strain or tension on the solar plexus: as the spine elongates, the rib cage is also lifted, but vertically and passively. The result is the same as in the pelvis: the rib cage widens laterally.

Summarizing

Keep the ears, shoulder joints and hip joints in a line with the ankle joints, and the knees straight. Then move the top of the sternum (corresponding to the first two thoracic vertebrae) and the pubic bone (corresponding to the coccyx) forward. At the same time move the lower ribs (corresponding to the lower thoracic vertebrae) and the navel (corresponding to the lumbar vertebrae) backward. Do not bend any part of the spine. As a result, the whole back is widened laterally and the spine is elongated vertically. When you practice this on the corner between two walls, the sacrum and the back of the head are in touch with the corner, but not the thoracic vertebrae or the heels.

<u>*To open the upper part of the chest do as follows*</u>
a. Keep the ears in line with the shoulder joints, the hip joints and the ankles.
b. Keep the lower ribs down and in as described above.
c. Elongate the neck upward as if you were balancing a book on the head. Keep the face vertical, do not tilt the chin up.

Steps a. and c. are the two simultaneous peripheral actions around the axis of the upper chest. As a result, the upper chest opens.

A healthy and harmoniously developed spine shows an even groove from the sacrum to the first thoracic vertebra. Many people have a deep groove in the lumbar area and none on the sacrum or between the shoulder blades. This shows an unhealthy and uneven development of the spine. To get an even groove, center the body in the pelvis and draw the groove down to the sacrum, at the same time drawing it up through the area between the shoulder blades to the first thoracic vertebra with the movements described above.

The shoulders, shoulder blades and arms hang passively; do not pull the shoulders back forcefully, and do not pull the shoulders and arms up. The arms and hands are suspended passively from the shoulder joints, held to the body by their ligaments, not by the muscles above the shoulders (the trapezius muscles). As the back and rib cage widen, the shoulders and shoulder blades widen too and go down automatically if the arms are dropped, in other words, if one gives the full weight of the arms to the force of gravity.

<u>*The neck and head*</u>
Elongate the neck up, keeping the face vertical. Do not tilt the chin up and do not push the head forward. The ears remain in line with the shoulder joints. The neck can only elongate if you are aware of the tensions which shorten the muscles at the back of the neck. Gently 'undo' these tensions from inside and ease the neck upwards. The correct position of head, neck and shoulders is that adopted by women in more primitive cultures when carrying water basins on their heads.

Tadasana is the basic position for all the other ones, and, if understood fully, will greatly facilitate the understanding of the other positions. The above description is the purely anatomical explanation. This has to be understood first, before one can, as it were, explode the physical frame, so that the Body of Light can take over. This goes for all the other techniques given in this book. Note that the words 'earth' and 'sky' have been used, instead of the usual 'floor' and 'ceiling'. This is to maintain a certain awareness of the human body as a link between the energy of the earth and the energy of the sky. After all, the physical body is made of the substance of the earth, but the Body of Light, the Energy Body, is made of the light of the sun, the light of the stars, lighting up the earth body from within.

The anatomical posture is, taken literally, a limiting posture. How can we make the transition from this purely physical description of the pose into the liberation of the Energy Body, loosening the grip of gravity on the body. What is the key, if there is a key?

A key there is, and a very interesting one too. At this point we need to take a closer look at the bones of the feet, and especially the joints. The bones of the lower legs, the tibia and the fibula, end in what is commonly known as the ankles, the inner and the outer ankles. The inner and outer ankles form a kind of vice into which is wedged a particular bone, called the talus. You can compare the talus to a wooden horse in a gym, with somebody (the lower leg bones) sitting astride on it. This joint is called the talocruralis joint, and is more commonly known as the *upper spring joint*. It is vital in the movements of walking, running and jumping, as it permits the lower legs to bend forward in relation to the foot. The entire weight of the body is transmitted from the tibia and the fibula through the talocruralis joint to the talus. Underneath and on the front of the talus are two other joints. The one underneath is called the subtalar or talocalcanean joint. It connects the talus to the heel bone (the calcaneus). The one on the front of the talus is connected both to the frontal part of the heel bone as well as to the first bone in the arch of the foot, the navicular bone. Therefore it is called the talocalcaneonavicular joint. It is also called the *lower spring joint* and is situated slightly forward from the ankles, on top of the arch. It permits the sideways rocking movement of the bones of the foot necessary in walking, running and jumping, to maintain the balance (the word 'navicular' comes from *nava*, which means 'boat').

The job of the talus is to divide the weight of the body over the heel and the bones of the arch, respectively through the subtalar joint and through the talocalcaneonavicular joint. Not only are these joints used for dividing the weight of the body, but they are also used for walking, running and jumping, hence their name *spring joints*.

Of the two, the talocalcaneonavicular joint is the more complex. As described previously, it is supported by the peroneus longus and the tibialis posterior. The tibialis posterior has the function of shortening the distance between the navicular bone and the heel bone, in which process the navicular bone slips partially under the talus, thus raising the arch. The fibers of the two muscles are intertwined, and the force of the action of the tibialis posterior is thus transmitted to the peroneus longus.

These two muscles form a kind of stirrup underneath the medial arch of the foot, supporting and lifting the lower spring joints. This action of lifting is called *Pada Bandha (pada* is 'foot' in Sanskrit and *bandha* means 'bound'). Pada Bandha is the first of the major Bandhas in the body and at once supports and motivates the other Bandhas. Seen from this point of view, the rest is easy to deduce.

The key to lightness is to not keep the pelvis aligned with the upper spring joints or talocruralis joints, but to keep it aligned with the lower spring joints or talocalcaneonavicular joints. One can compare this to the stance of Olympic ski jumpers. The angle of the ski jumper to his skis is never ninety degrees, but less. In the case of Tadasana, the entire body is kept at an angle of about eighty degrees forward. This brings the lower abdomen vertically above the lower spring joints.

As described earlier, most people follow the anatomical description and stand completely vertical, with the shoulder and hip joints aligned with the ankles or upper spring joints. Thus the weight of the body falls on the talocruralis joints and through the subtalar joints onto the heels. In this way it is very difficult to rebounce the weight of the body back upwards. Leaning the physical body slightly forward, so that more of the body weight is transmitted by gravity to the talocalcaneonavicular joints permits those joints to take responsibility for the rebounce action by using the tibialis posterior and the peroneus longus, pulling the arches up and continuing that action up to the knees. In this action these two muscles are supported by the abductors of the big toes and the little toes, and the result is not only that the body is extremely 'bouncy', but also stable at the same time.

Thus the real rebounce action is not in the ankles or lower legs, but in the lower spring joints, the talocalcaneonavicular joints.

As mentioned before, this is the result of leaning the *physical body* slightly forward over the arches of the feet. However, the *inner energy*, the weight of the inner awareness, has to move backward, towards the back of the body (see also the description of Padmasana, Sitting and Savasana). This double action of moving physically forwards and energy-wise backwards, coupled with the action of the spring joints, liberates the energy from the rooting feet towards the lower abdomen and from there up along the spine towards the top of the head. This is what is called, in the Seven Vital Principles, *connecting*.

4.2 Surya Namaskar / Sun Salutation

Surya Namaskar or the *Sun Salutation* is a classical way to connect the various asanas into one continuous, flowing event. Combined with the breathing, it helps the body to perform all the asanas without interruption and therefore without a break in the flow of energy. We have suggested in this book that most groups of asanas can be done in this way, as an alternative to the start-stop-start method, in which each pose is performed separately from the other, with a break in between. This last method is fruitful in order to learn the precision of the asanas but, as indicated above, it also involves an inevitable break in the rhythm of the body and the breathing, as well as in the flow of energy.

Even though the practice of yoga in general is not conditioned by physical states such as disease or aging, or by mental states, such as depression, Surya Namaskar in particular has a beneficial effect on the minds and bodies of people who tend to have minor physical diseases, or who struggle with the physical and mental effects of aging, due to its influence on the blood circulation and the flow of the breath and the energy. Specially in the case of aging, the start-stop-start method not only tends to cool the body off in between the asanas, but also makes it hard to start up the energy, the motor, each time again. Combining the various asanas with a mild form of Surya Namaskar, without straining, can help the body - and the mind - to retain its heat, the flow of the breath and of the energy, as well as the physical and mental concentration necessary to perform the asanas. This is the purificatory effect of the flow, after which the body and mind feel refreshed and optimistic, having, as Patanjali states, burned the impurities of the body and the nervous system in the fire (tapas) of the practice.

In the sequence of Surya Namaskar it is important to concentrate on the synchronization of the breathing and the movement, so that the two form one, uninterrupted unit. We have coined Surya Namaskar in combination with the asanas Mala.

A *mala*, in Sanskrit, is a necklace, a rosary, a circle of beads or pearls (the asanas) strung together on a string (Surya Namaskar).

The sequence

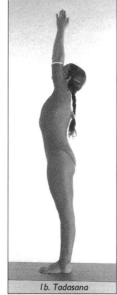
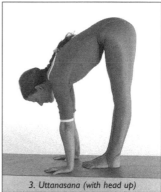

1. Stand in **Tadasana** (*tada=mountain*) on a mat with the feet together. Keep the body slightly slanted forward so that the weight of the body falls directly onto the lower spring joints. On a Mula Bandha inhalation, raise the arms over the head, using the rebounce action in the lower spring joints (Pada Bandha) to trigger off the Mula Bandha (photo 1b).

1a. Tadasana — *1b. Tadasana*

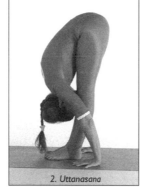
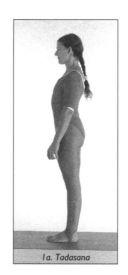

2. On the exhalation bend forward, keeping the legs perpendicular, and place the hands on the mat next to the feet. Bring the trunk and head to the thighs and shins. This position is called **Uttanasana** (*uttana=intense stretch*).

3. On the inhalation, raise the head and curve the whole spine up, from the sacro-iliac joints to the first cervical vertebra.

2. Uttanasana — *3. Uttanasana (with head up)*

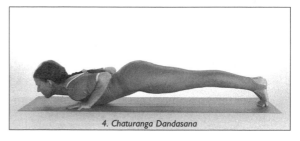

4. On the exhalation, lean the body weight on the hands and jump with the feet backwards. At the same time bend the arms and lower the chest, till the shoulder joints are above the hands with the elbows pointing backwards and the upper arms parallel to the earth. The head, trunk

4. Chaturanga Dandasana

and legs are parallel to the earth and the weight of the body is supported only on the hands and the balls and toes of the feet. This position is called **Chaturanga Dandasana** or *Crocodile Pose* (*chatur=four; anga=limb; danda=staff*).

5. On the inhalation, raise the head and chest till the arms are straight and perpendicular, rooting the hands and performing Hasta Bandha. Keep the legs parallel to the earth. Pull the pubic bone slightly forward, so that the trunk can curve upwards and backwards. Elongate the neck as in Jalandhara Bandha, so that the sternum is raised high, and then curve the head backwards. This position is called **Urdhvamukha Svanasana** or *Upward Facing Dog Pose* (urdhva=upwards; mukha= face; svana=dog).

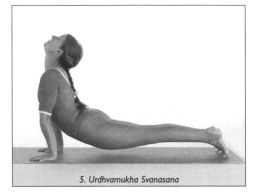

5. Urdhvamukha Svanasana

6. On the exhalation, raise the pelvis and thighs and bring them backwards, keeping the arms straight and the hands and feet *rooted,* till the chest, the head and the spinal column form one line with the arms. Thus the whole body forms a triangle, with the coccyx as the highest point. This position is called **Adhomukha Svanasana** or *Downward Facing Dog Pose* (adho= downwards; mukha=face; svana=dog).

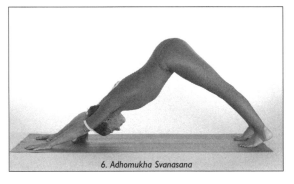

6. Adhomukha Svanasana

7. On the exhalation, bend the knees and jump forward into Uttanasana, rooting the hands as in Adhomukha Vrksasana (see page 184) and shifting the weight of the body to the hands as you jump. Lift the head and keep the bending of the knees minimal, so that when the feet land in between the hands the hips are high and the knees can straighten immediately. Bring the trunk and head to the thighs and shins in Uttanasana.

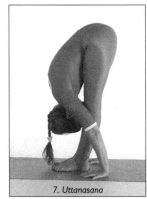

7. Uttanasana

8. On the inhalation, stand up again straight in Tadasana (see 1a).

4.3   Standing Poses

These positions can be done in <u>three different modes</u>:

a.   Performing each position separately and holding it for one minute.

b.   Vinyasa
Connecting two or more positions by flowing from one into the other, using the breathing. For example:
*   Utthita Trikonasana » Parsvottanasana » Parivrtta Trikonasana
*   Utthita Trikonasana » Ardha Chandrasana » Virabhadrasana III
*   Virabhadrasana II » Virabhadrasana I » Virabhadrasana III
*   Utthita Hasta Padangusthasana » Urdhva Prasarita Ekapadasana » Virabhadrasana III
Use your imagination to make your own combinations and keep each position for three breaths.

c.   Mala
Connecting all the positions, through Surya Namaskar, in the following way, using the breathing, and holding each of the Standing Poses for the duration of three breaths:
*   Tadasana » inhale extend the arms upwards » exhale Uttanasana, inhale raise the head » exhale Chaturanga Dandasana » inhale Urdhvamukha Svanasana » exhale Adhomukha Svanasana, inhale » exhale Utthita Trikonasana on the right side, stay for three breaths, inhale » exhale Adhomukha Svanasana, inhale » exhale Utthita Trikonasana on the left side, stay for three breaths, inhale » exhale Adhomukha Svanasana, inhale » exhale Uttanasana » inhale Tadasana, exhale » inhale extend the arms upwards etc.

Standing poses

1. Tadasana	18. Utthita Hasta Padangusthasana
2. Garudasana	a. Holding the foot with the same side hand
3. Vrksasana I	b. Holding the foot with the same side hand
4. Vrksasana II	and bringing it to the side
5. Ardha Baddha Padmottanasana	c. Holding the foot with the opposite hand
6. Vatayanasana	d. Holding the foot with the opposite hand
7. Utkatasana I	and turning the trunk and head to the
8. Utthita Trikonasana	side of the raised leg
9. Ardha Chandrasana	e. Holding the foot with both hands and
10. Parsvottanasana	bringing the head to the shin
11. Parivrtta Trikonasana	19. Urdhva Prasarita Ekapadasana
12. Parivrtta Ardha Chandrasana	20. Prasarita Padottanasana
13. Virabhadrasana II	a. Hands on earth, head up
14. Utthita Parsvakonasana	b. Hands and head on earth in between feet
15. Virabhadrasana I	c. Holding ankles, head on earth in between feet
16. Virabhadrasana III	d. Namasté II, head on earth in between feet
17. Parivrtta Parsvakonasana	21. Padangusthasana
	22. Padahastasana
	23. Uttanasana

1. Tadasana

tada=mountain

- See page 49.

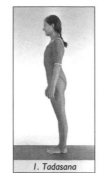
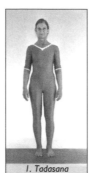

1. Tadasana   *1. Tadasana*

2. Garudasana

garuda=eagle

- Stand in Tadasana.
- Bend the left knee slightly and wrap the right leg around it.
- Cross the right elbow over the left and join the palms of the hands. The fingers point upwards to the sky, and the right palm will be slightly higher than the left.
- Hold for one minute and then repeat on the other side, changing the crossing of the legs and arms.

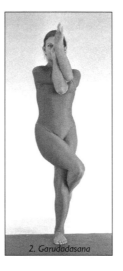
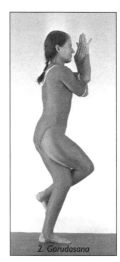

2. Garudadasana   *2. Garudasana*

3. Vrksasana I

vrksa=tree

- Stand in Tadasana.
- Lift the right foot and place it as high as possible against the inner left thigh. Extend the right (bent) knee out of the hip joint, down and back, by pressing the heel firmly against the inner left thigh.
- Do not turn the right side of the pelvis backwards. The pelvis should remain straight, facing forward.
- On a Mula Bandha inhalation lift the arms up over the head. This movement starts with rooting the left foot and performing Pada Bandha. This movement, traveling upwards through the left leg and the hip joints will elongate them and will activate the Mula Bandha. Thus the pelvis and trunk are lifted up from the femur heads. The coccyx should remain pointed down to

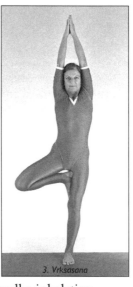

3. Vrksasana

the earth as the lower abdomen moves in and up on the Mula Bandha inhalation.
- Join the palms of the hands. On each inhalation elongate the left leg further and extend the right thigh further sideways and down out of the right hip joint. Lift the pelvis and lower abdomen so that the hands and arms also go further up. On each exhalation maintain that length of the body.
- Hold for one minute and then repeat on the other side.

4. Vrksasana II

vrksa=tree

- Stand in Tadasana.
- Lift the right foot and place it in the groin of the left leg as for Padmasana (see page 77). Extend the right (bent) knee out of the hip joint, down and back, without turning the right side of the pelvis backwards. The pelvis stays straight, facing forward.
- Rotate the right arm around the back and hold the right foot. Do not tilt the pelvis forward, but keep it in a vertical position, and keep the left leg straight.
- On a Mula Bandha inhalation, lift the left arm up over the head. This movement starts with rooting the left foot and performing Pada Bandha in the lower spring joint. This movement, traveling upwards through the left leg and the hip joints will elongate them and will activate the Mula Bandha. Thus the pelvis and trunk are lifted up from the femur heads. The coccyx and the right knee should remain pointed down to the earth as the lower abdomen moves in and up on the Mula Bandha inhalation.
- On each inhalation elongate the left leg further and extend the right thigh further down out of the right hip joint. Lift the pelvis and lower abdomen so that the left hand also goes further up. On each exhalation maintain that length of the body.
- Hold for one minute and then proceed to 5.

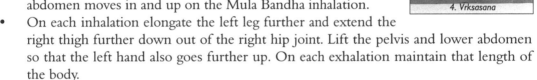

4. Vrksasana

5. Ardha Baddha Padmottanasana

ardha=half; baddha=bound; padma=lotus; uttana=intense stretch

- On an exhalation bend forward, hold the left ankle with the left hand and bring the head to the shin. If the balance is a problem you can keep the left hand on the earth.
- On each Mula Bandha inhalation lift the pelvis up from the left femur head so that the spine elongates further towards the head.

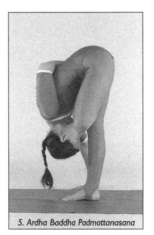

5. Ardha Baddha Padmottanasana

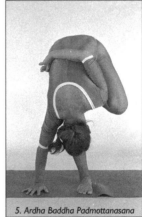

5. Ardha Baddha Padmottanasana

- On each exhalation slide the head further down on the left shin.
- Hold for one minute, raise the head and trunk on an inhalation and then repeat 4 and 5 on the other side.

6. Vatayanasana
vatayana=horse

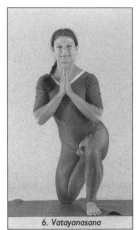
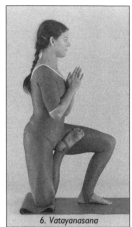

6. *Vatayanasana*   6. *Vatayanasana*

- Stand in Tadasana.
- Lift the right foot and place it in the groin of the left leg as for Padmasana (see page 77). Extend the right (bent) knee out of the hip joint, down and back, without turning the right side of the pelvis backwards. The pelvis stays straight, facing forward.
- On an exhalation bend the trunk forward and place the hands on the earth.
- Bend the left knee and place the right knee on the earth behind you in such a way that there is an angle of ninety degrees in the left knee.
- Lift the hands and stand up, balancing on the left foot and the frontal inner edge of the right knee.
- Bring the pelvis and back to a vertical position and rotate the right hip joint forward to come in line with the left one.
- Join the palms of the hands in front of the sternum in Namasté I and look straight forward.
- Hold for one minute and then change legs.

7. Utkatasana I
utkata=powerful, fierce

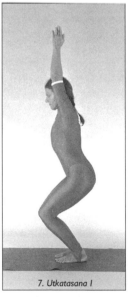

7. *Utkatasana I*

- Stand in Tadasana.
- Spread the feet at hip width and, using a Mula Bandha inhalation, lift the arms up over the head. This movement should start with rooting the feet and performing the Pada Bandha in the lower spring joints. This movement, traveling upwards through the legs and the hip joints will elongate them and will activate the Mula Bandha. Thus the pelvis and trunk are lifted up from the femur heads. The coccyx should remain pointed down to the earth as the lower abdomen moves in and up on the Mula Bandha inhalation.
- Join the palms of the hands. On an inhalation elongate the legs further and lift the pelvis and lower abdomen so that the hands and arms also go further up.
- On the exhalation rotate the pelvis and trunk forward to an inclination of about thirty degrees from the vertical line and bend the knees slowly to an angle of ninety degrees, without changing the inclination of the trunk. The arms stay in line with the trunk.
- Hold for ten seconds and then stand up again.

8. Utthita Trikonasana

utthita=extended; tri=three; kona=angle; trikona=triangle

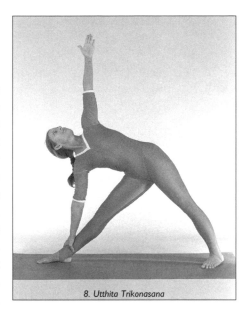

8. Utthita Trikonasana

- Stand in Tadasana and spread the legs.
- The distance between the feet is the same as the length of one leg. Turn the left foot forty-five degrees in and the right foot ninety degrees out to the right. The heel of the right foot should be in line with the center of the inner arch of the left foot. Turn the right shin, knee and thigh to face the same direction as the right foot. The pelvis also turns slightly to the right.
- Turn the left shin, knee and thigh out. This lifts the inner knee and ankle of the left leg and brings the weight on the outer edge of the left foot. For the action in the arches, ankles and knees follow the instructions given in Tadasana. Root the feet and perform Pada Bandha on both the feet to activate the Mula Bandha.
- On a Mula Bandha inhalation elongate both legs and lift the pelvis and trunk up from the femur heads. Lift the arms sideways, in line with the shoulders and parallel to the earth. The palms of the hands face the earth.
- On the exhalation, roll the right side of the pelvis over the right femur head, at the same time extending the right buttock bone towards the left heel. To do this the Biceps muscle of the right thigh has to elongate from the knee to the buttock bone. Thus the coccyx points towards the left heel and the right side of the lumbar spine is elongated. Do not turn the left hip bone forward, but keep rolling it out and back.
- As the right buttock bone moves towards the left heel, you have to elongate the whole right side of the body from the groin to the tips of the fingers. Then place the right hand on the right ankle. The right hip bone, waist and lower side ribs should go down faster than the right hand. Do not put any weight on the hand but keep the weight of the body on the pelvis and upper thighs. Keep the outer edge of the heel and the little toe of the left foot firmly on the earth and the left hip bone, thigh, knee and shin rotating outwards.
- The spine should be in line with the line between the feet, and should divide the back in two equal parts. The left and right side of the waist and rib cage should be equally long and parallel to each other.
- Point the left hand straight up towards the sky with the palm facing forward. Keep the head and neck in line with the spine and look up at the left hand.
- On each Mula Bandha inhalation elongate the body in two opposite directions, splitting in the hip joints. The lower abdomen and spine elongate towards the back of the head, while the right buttock bone, coccyx and left leg extend towards the left heel.
- On each exhalation rotate the left side of the trunk backwards and the left hip bone, thigh, knee and shin outwards. Do not swing the left hand backwards, but keep it pointing straight up towards the sky, and keep the outward rotation of the right thigh and knee.
- Hold for one minute and then proceed to 9.

9. Ardha Chandrasana

ardha=half; chandra=moon

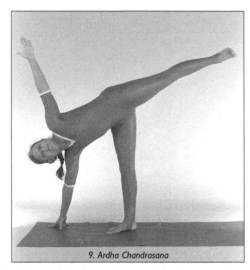

9. Ardha Chandrasana

- On an exhalation bend the right leg and place the right hand on the earth, in line with the feet and about half a meter from the right foot.
- Place the left hand on the left hip, bring the weight of the body forward over the right foot and then straighten the right leg, lifting the left leg up till it is in line with the trunk. The toes point forwards.
- Extend the left arm up and point it straight up to the sky with the palm facing forward. The right arm is parallel to the right leg, so that both the arms are in one line. Keep the head in line with the spine and look up at the left hand. Root the right foot and perform Pada Bandha to activate the Mula Bandha.
- On each Mula Bandha inhalation lift the pelvis up from the right femur head and elongate the body in two opposite directions, splitting in the hip joints. The lower abdomen and spine elongate towards the back of the head, while the coccyx and left leg extend towards the left heel.
- On each exhalation rotate the left side of the trunk backwards and the left hip bone, thigh, knee and shin upwards.
- Do not swing the left hand backwards, but keep it pointing straight up towards the sky, and keep the outward rotation of the right thigh and knee.
- Hold for one minute and then bend the right leg on an exhalation to return to Utthita Trikonasana (8). Repeat 8 and 9 on the other side.

10. Parsvottanasana

parsva=side, flank; uttana=intense stretch

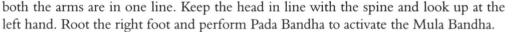
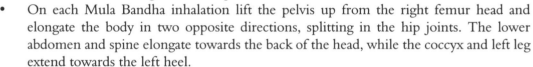

10. Parsvottanasa

- Stand in Tadasana and spread the legs.
- The distance between the feet is the same as the length of one leg. Turn the left foot forty-five degrees in and the right foot ninety degrees out to the right. The heel of the right foot should be in line with the heel of the left foot. Turn the right shin, knee and thigh to face the same direction as the right foot. The pelvis also turns slightly to the right.
- Turn the left shin, knee and thigh out. This lifts the inner knee and ankle of the left leg and brings the weight on the outer edge of the left foot. For the action in the arches, ankles and knees follow the instructions given in Tadasana. Root the feet and perform Pada Bandha on both the feet to activate the Mula Bandha.

- Join the palms on the back in Namasté II and press the knuckles of the index fingers together by taking the elbows back.
- On a Mula Bandha inhalation elongate both legs and lift the pelvis and trunk up from the femur heads. On the exhalation rotate the pelvis and trunk towards the right, rolling over the right femur head, till they face the right foot. The line from hip bone to hip bone across the lower abdomen should be almost perpendicular to the right thigh so that the trunk from the navel upwards faces the same direction as the right foot.
- On a new inhalation lift the pelvis still further up from the femur heads and elongate the Biceps muscle of the right thigh from the knee to the buttock bone, extending that bone towards the left heel. On the exhalation bend the trunk forward till the head rests on the right shin.
- On each Mula Bandha inhalation lift the pelvis up from the right femur head and elongate the body in two opposite directions, splitting in the hip joints. The lower abdomen and spine elongate towards the back of the head, while the right buttock bone, coccyx and left leg extend towards the left heel. On each exhalation slide the head further down on the right shin.
- Keep the elbows raised high and the palms of the hands pressed firmly together.
- Hold for one minute, raise the head and trunk on an inhalation and then repeat on the other side.

11. Parivrtta Trikonasana
parivrtta=turned around; trikona=triangle

- Stand in Tadasana and spread the legs.
- The distance between the feet is the same as the length of one leg. Turn the left foot forty-five degrees in and the right foot ninety degrees out to the right. The heel of the right foot should be in line with the heel of the left foot. Turn the right shin, knee and thigh to face the same direction as the right foot. The pelvis also turns slightly to the right.
- Turn the left shin, knee and thigh out. This lifts the inner knee and ankle of the left leg and brings the weight on the outer edge of the left foot. For the action in the arches,

11. Parivrtta Trikonasana

ankles and knees follow the instructions given in Tadasana. Root the feet and perform Pada Bandha on both the feet to activate the Mula Bandha.
- On a Mula Bandha inhalation elongate both legs and lift the pelvis and trunk up from the femur heads. Lift the arms sideways, in line with the shoulders and parallel to the earth. The palms of the hands face the earth.
- On the exhalation rotate the pelvis and trunk towards the right, rolling over the right femur head, till they face the right foot. The line from hip bone to hip bone across the lower abdomen should be almost perpendicular to the right thigh, so that the trunk from the navel upwards faces the same direction as the right foot.

- On a new inhalation lift the pelvis and trunk still further up from the femur heads and elongate the Biceps muscle of the right thigh from the knee to the buttock bone, extending that bone towards the left heel. Thus the coccyx points towards the left heel and the right side of the lumbar spine is elongated.
- On the exhalation elongate the whole left side of the body from the groin to the tips of the fingers and, rotating the stomach and chest still further towards the right, place the left hand on the right ankle. The left hip bone, waist and lower side ribs should go down faster than the left hand. Do not put any weight on the hand but keep the weight of the body on the pelvis and upper thighs. Keep the outer edge of the heel and the little toe of the left foot firmly on the earth.
- Extend the right arm straight up towards the sky with the palm of the hand facing forward. Keep the head and neck in line with the spine and look up at the right hand.
- The spine should be in line with the line between the feet, and should divide the back in two equal parts. The left and right side of the waist and rib cage should be equally long and parallel to each other.
- On each Mula Bandha inhalation elongate the body in two opposite directions, splitting in the hip joints. The lower abdomen and spine elongate towards the back of the head, while the right buttock bone, coccyx and left leg extend towards the left heel.
- On each exhalation rotate the right side of the trunk backwards and the right thigh, knee and shin outwards, keeping the inner edge of the right foot on the earth. Do not swing the right hand backwards, but keep it pointing straight up towards the sky, and keep the outward rotation of the left thigh and knee.
- Hold for one minute and then proceed to 12.

12. Parivrtta Ardha Chandrasana

parvrtta=turned around; ardha=half; chandra=moon

- On an exhalation bend the right leg and place the left hand on the earth, in line with the feet and about half a meter from the right foot.
- Place the right hand on the right hip, bring the weight of the body forward over the right foot and then straighten the right leg, lifting the left leg up till it is in line with the trunk. The toes point down to the earth.
- Extend the right arm upwards, pointing it straight up to the sky with the palm of the hand facing forward. The left arm is parallel

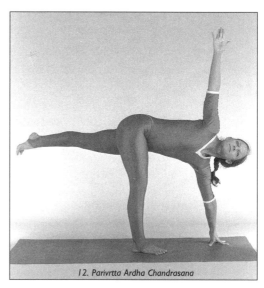

12. Parivrtta Ardha Chandrasana

to the right leg, so that both the arms are in one line. Keep the head in line with the spine and look up at the right hand. Root the right foot and perform Pada Bandha to activate the Mula Bandha.

- On each Mula Bandha inhalation lift the pelvis up from the right femur head and elongate the body in two opposite directions, splitting in the hip joints. The lower abdomen and spine elongate towards the back of the head, while the right buttock bone, coccyx and left leg extend towards the left heel.
- On each exhalation rotate the right side of the trunk backwards and the right thigh, knee and shin outwards, keeping the inner edge of the right foot on the earth. Do not swing the right hand backwards, but keep it pointing straight up towards the sky.
- Hold for one minute and then bend the right leg on an exhalation to return to Parivrtta Trikonasana (11). Repeat 11 and 12 on the other side.

13. Virabhadrasana II
Virabhadra is the name of a hero

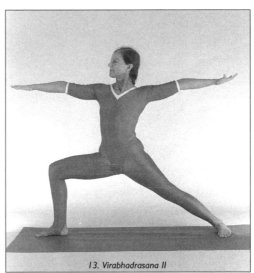

13. Virabhadrasana II

- Stand in Tadasana and spread the legs.
- The distance between the feet is one and a half times the length of one leg. Turn the left foot forty-five degrees in and the right foot ninety degrees out to the right. The heel of the right foot should be in line with the center of the inner arch of the left foot. Turn the right shin, knee and thigh to face the same direction as the right foot. The pelvis also turns slightly to the right.
- Turn the left shin, knee and thigh out. This lifts the inner knee and ankle of the left leg and brings the weight on the outer edge of the left foot. For the action in the arches, ankles and knees follow the instructions given in Tadasana. Root the feet and perform Pada Bandha to activate the Mula Bandha.
- On a Mula Bandha inhalation elongate both legs and lift the pelvis and trunk up from the femur heads. Lift the arms sideways, in line with the shoulders and parallel to the earth. The palms of the hands face the earth.
- On the exhalation bend the right knee at an angle of ninety degrees, so that the thigh is parallel to the earth. The knee is in line with the right groin and foot and the weight of the body is even on both feet.
- Keep the trunk vertical, at an angle of ninety degrees with the right thigh. On each inhalation elongate the body in opposite directions, splitting in the hip joints. The lower abdomen and spine elongate upwards towards the back of the head, the coccyx and right buttock bone drop further down and the left leg elongates towards the left heel.
- On each exhalation maintain the length of the trunk. Keep the head and neck in line with the spine and look at the right hand.
- Hold for one minute and then proceed to 14.

14. Utthita Parsvakonasana
utthita=extended; parsva=sideways; kona=angle

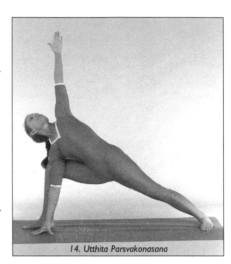
14. Utthita Parsvakonasana

- On an inhalation elongate the Biceps muscle of the right thigh from the knee to the buttock bone and extend that bone towards the left heel, so that the coccyx points towards that heel. At the same time elongate the right side of the body from the right groin to the tips of the fingers and roll the right side of the pelvis over the right femur head.
- On the exhalation place the right hand on the earth on the inside of the right foot. The back of the right arm pit rests against the inside of the right knee. Extend the left arm up towards the sky with the palm of the hand facing forward.
- The right hip bone, waist and lower side ribs should go down faster than the right hand and should close with the thigh in the right groin. Do not put any weight on the right hand but keep the weight of the body on the pelvis and upper thighs. Keep the outer edge of the heel and the little toe of the left foot firmly on the earth.
- The spine should be in line with the line between the feet, and should divide the back from the waist upwards in two equal parts. The left and right side of the waist and rib cage should be equally long and parallel to each other. Keep the head and neck in line with the spine and look up at the sky.
- On each Mula Bandha inhalation elongate the body in two opposite directions, splitting in the hip joints. The lower abdomen and spine elongate towards the back of the head while the right buttock bone, coccyx and left leg extend towards the left heel. On each exhalation rotate the left side of the trunk backwards and the left hip and knee outwards, at the same time keeping the outward rotation of the right thigh and knee.
- Hold for one minute and then repeat 13 and 14 on the other side.

15. Virabhadrasana I
Virabhadra is the name of a hero

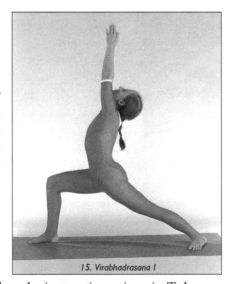
15. Virabhadrasana I

- Stand in Tadasana and spread the legs.
- The distance between the feet is one and a half times the length of one leg. Turn the left foot forty-five degrees in and the right foot ninety degrees out to the right. The heel of the right foot should be in line with the heel of the left foot. Turn the right shin, knee and thigh to face the same direction as the right foot. The pelvis also turns slightly to the right.
- Turn the left shin, knee and thigh out. This lifts the inner knee and ankle of the left leg and brings the weight on the outer edge of the left foot. For the action in the arches, ankles and knees follow the instructions given in Tadasana.

- On a Mula Bandha inhalation lift the arms up over the head. This movement should start with rooting the feet and performing Pada Bandha in the lower spring joints. This movement, traveling upwards through the legs and the hip joints will elongate them and will activate the Mula Bandha. Thus the pelvis and trunk are lifted up from the femur heads. The coccyx should remain pointed down to the earth as the lower abdomen moves in and up with the Mula Bandha inhalation.
- Join the palms of the hands. On an inhalation elongate the legs further, lifting the pelvis and lower abdomen so that the hands and arms also go further up.
- On the exhalation rotate the pelvis and trunk towards the right, rolling over the right femur head. The line from hip bone to hip bone across the lower abdomen should be almost perpendicular to the right thigh so that the trunk from the navel upwards faces the same direction as the right foot.
- On a new inhalation lift the pelvis and trunk still further up from the femur heads. On the exhalation bend the right leg to an angle of ninety degrees, so that the thigh is parallel to the earth.
- Keep the heel and little toe of the left foot firmly on the earth and extend the right femur head slightly back towards the left heel, without bending the left knee. In this way the pelvis stays facing in the direction of the right foot.
- Keep the trunk vertical, at an angle of ninety degrees with the right thigh. On each inhalation elongate the body in opposite directions, splitting in the hip joints. The spine and arms elongate upwards, the coccyx and right buttock bone drop further down and the left leg elongates towards the left heel.
- On each exhalation maintain the length of the trunk and rotate the right side of the trunk and the right femur head further backwards.
- Hold for one minute and then proceed to 16.

16. Virabhadrasana III
Virabhadra is the name of a hero

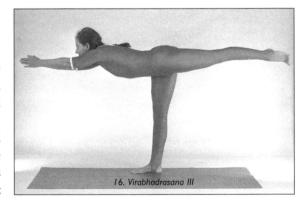
16. Virabhadrasana III

- On a Mula Bandha inhalation lift the pelvis up from the femur heads. On the exhalation bend forwards and place the trunk on the right thigh.
- Bring the weight of the body forward over the right foot and straighten the right leg, lifting the left leg up till it is in line with the trunk. The toes point down to the earth.
- On each inhalation lighten the weight of the trunk on the right femur head by rooting the right foot and performing Pada Bandha, and elongate the body in two opposite directions, splitting in the hip joints. The trunk and arms elongate forwards, while the coccyx, the right buttock bone and the left leg extend backward towards the left heel.
- Keep the hands, head, shoulders, spine, hips and left leg on one line, parallel to the earth and look at the hands.
- Hold for ten seconds. On an exhalation bend the right leg and return to Virabhadrasana I (15). Repeat 15 and 16 on the other side.

17. Parivrtta Parsvakonasana

parivrtta=turned around; parsva=sideways; kona=angle

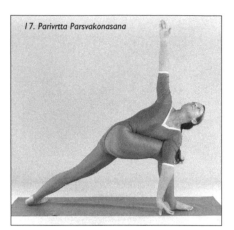

17. Parivrtta Parsvakonasana

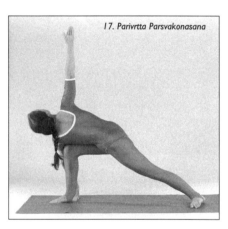

17. Parivrtta Parsvakonasana

- Stand in Tadasana and spread the legs.
- The distance between the feet is one and a half times the length of one leg. Turn the left foot forty-five degrees in and the right foot ninety degrees out to the right. The heel of the right foot should be in line with the heel of the left foot. Turn the right shin, knee and thigh to face the same direction as the right foot. The pelvis also turns slightly to the right.
- Turn the left shin, knee and thigh out. This lifts the inner knee and ankle of the left leg and brings the weight on the outer edge of the left foot. For the action in the arches, ankles and knees follow the instructions given in Tadasana. Root the feet and perform Pada Bandha to activate the Mula Bandha.
- On a Mula Bandha inhalation elongate the legs and lift the pelvis and trunk up from the femur heads. Lift the arms sideways, in line with the shoulders and parallel to the earth. The palms of the hands face the earth.
- On the exhalation rotate towards the right, rolling over the right femur head. The line from hip bone to hip bone across the lower abdomen should be almost perpendicular to the right thigh, so that the trunk from the navel upwards faces the same direction as the right foot.
- On a new inhalation lift again up from the femur heads and on the exhalation bend the right knee to an angle of ninety degrees, so that the thigh is parallel to the earth. Elongate the Biceps muscle of the right thigh from the knee to the buttock bone and extend that bone towards the left heel, so that the coccyx points towards that heel.
- At the same time elongate the whole left side of the body from the left groin to the tips of the fingers and, rotating the stomach and chest still further towards the right, place the left hand on the earth on the outside of the right foot. Turn the arm in the same way as in Savasana, so that the back of the left shoulder near the shoulder blade presses against the outside of the right knee. Do not put any weight on the hand but keep the weight of the body on the pelvis and upper thighs. Keep the left heel on the earth. If you cannot do that, lift it just enough to facilitate the rotation of the body, and then put it back on the earth again after reaching the final position.
- The spine should be in line with the line between the feet, and should divide the back from the waist upwards in two equal parts. The left and right side of the waist and rib cage should be equally long and parallel to each other. Extend the right arm up to the sky with the palm of the hand facing forward. Keep the head and neck in line with the spine and look up at the sky.

- On each Mula Bandha inhalation elongate the body in two opposite directions, splitting in the hip joints. The lower abdomen and spine elongate towards the back of the head, while the right buttock bone, coccyx and left leg extend towards the left heel.
- On each exhalation rotate the right side of the trunk backwards and the right thigh, knee and shin outwards, keeping the inner edge of the right foot on the earth. At the same time keep the outward rotation of the left thigh and knee and the left heel on the earth.
- Hold for one minute and then repeat on the other side.

18. Utthita Hasta Padangusthasana

utthita=extended; hasta=hand; padangustha=big toe

18a. Holding the foot with the same side hand

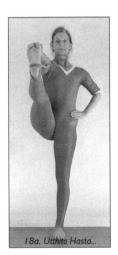
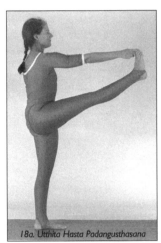

- Stand in Tadasana.
- Place the left hand on the hip, bend the right leg and hold the big toe with the index and middle fingers of the right hand. Extend the leg forward and raise it as high as possible, keeping the left leg and the trunk straight. Root the left foot and perform Pada Bandha to activate the Mula Bandha.
- On each Mula Bandha inhalation elongate the left leg and lift the pelvis and trunk up from the left femur head. On each exhalation raise and elongate the right leg further.
- Hold for one minute and then proceed to 18b.

18a. Utthita Hasta...   *18a. Utthita Hasta Padangusthasana*

18b. Holding the foot with the same side hand and bringing it to the side

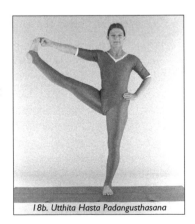

- Take the right foot to the right side.
- On each Mula Bandha inhalation elongate the left leg and lift the pelvis and trunk up from the left femur head. On each exhalation take the right leg further to the side, without turning the pelvis.
- Hold for ten seconds and then repeat 18a and b on the other side.

18b. Utthita Hasta Padangusthasana

18c. *Holding the foot with the opposite hand*

- Stand in Tadasana.
- Place the right hand on the hip, bend the right leg and hold the ball of the foot with the left hand. Extend the leg forward and raise it as high as possible, keeping the left leg and the trunk straight. Root the left foot and perform Pada Bandha to activate the Mula Bandha.
- On each Mula Bandha inhalation elongate the left leg and lift the pelvis and trunk up from the left femur head. On each exhalation raise the right leg further.
- Hold for one minute and then proceed to 18d.

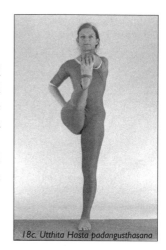
18c. Utthita Hasta padangusthasana

18d. *Holding the foot with the opposite hand and turning the trunk and head to the side of the raised leg*

- On an exhalation turn the trunk and head towards the right till the shoulders are in line with the right leg.
- On each Mula Bandha inhalation elongate the left leg and lift the pelvis and trunk up from the left femur head. On each exhalation raise and elongate

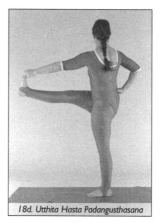
18d. Utthita Hasta Padangusthasana

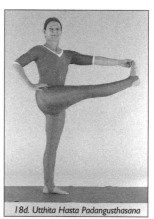
18d. Utthita Hasta Padangusthasana

the right leg further and turn the trunk and head further towards the right.
- Hold for ten seconds and then repeat 18c and d on the other side.

18e. *Holding the foot with both hands and bringing the head to shin*

- Stand in Tadasana.
- Bend the right leg and hold the foot with both hands. Extend the leg forward and raise it as high as possible, keeping the left leg and the trunk straight.
- On an exhalation bring the head to the shin, keeping the back as straight as possible. Root the left foot and perform Pada Bandha to activate the Mula Bandha.
- On each Mula Bandha inhalation elongate the left leg and lift the pelvis and trunk up from the left femur head. On each exhalation raise the right leg further.
- Hold for ten seconds and then repeat on the other side.

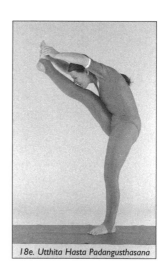
18e. Utthita Hasta Padangusthasana

19. Urdhva Prasarita Ekapadasana

urdhva=above, upwards; prasarita=extended; eka=one;
pada=leg, foot

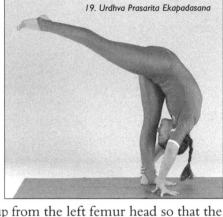

19. Urdhva Prasarita Ekapadasana

- Stand in Tadasana.
- On an exhalation bend forward, place the right hand on the earth and lift the right leg up backwards, without turning the right hip back. Keep both legs straight and both hips at the same height.
- Hold the left ankle with the left hand and on an exhalation bring the head to the shin.
- On each Mula Bandha inhalation lift the pelvis up from the left femur head so that the spine elongates still further towards the head.
- On each exhalation slide the head further down on the left shin.
- Hold for ten seconds and then repeat on the other side.

20. Prasarita Padottanasana

prasarita=spread, extended; pada=leg, foot; uttana=intense stretch

20a. The hands on the earth, the head up

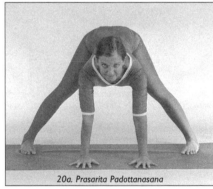

20a. Prasarita Padottanasana

- Stand in Tadasana and spread the legs.
- The distance between the feet is one and a half times the length of one leg. Turn both feet slightly in, rooting them and performing Pada Bandha to activate the Mula Bandha.
- On a Mula Bandha inhalation elongate both legs and lift the pelvis and trunk up from the femur heads.
- On the exhalation rotate the pelvis forward and place the hands on the earth in front of you. Keep the arms straight and the fingers pointing forward. Do not put any weight on the hands.
- Keep the hips in line with the feet and lift the head, elongating the back of the thigh upwards towards the sky.
- On each Mula Bandha inhalation elongate the body in two opposite directions, splitting in the hip joints. The lower abdomen and spine elongate towards the back of the head, while the buttock bones extend backwards.
- Hold for one minute and then proceed to 20b.

20b. *The hands and head on the earth in between the feet*

- Elongating the back of the thighs still further upwards, place the hands and head in between the feet on the earth. The hands are at shoulder width and the fingers point straight forwards. The elbows are in line with the hands and armpits.
- The distance between the feet should be such that the head barely touches the earth. If the distance is too short, the back will bend.
- Hold for one minute and then proceed to 20c.

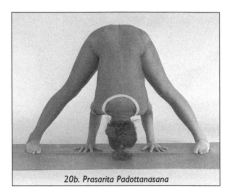

20b. Prasarita Padottanasana

20c. *Holding the ankles with the hands, keeping the head on the earth in between feet*

- Hold the outer ankles with the hands, keeping the hips in line with the feet and the head on the earth in between the feet.
- Hold for one minute and then proceed to 20d.

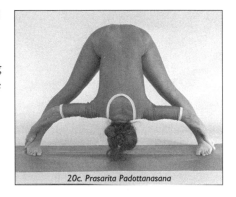

20c. Prasarita Padottanasana

20d. *Namasté II, the head on the earth in between the feet*

- On an inhalation raise the head and trunk. Join the palms on the back in Namasté II and press the knuckles of the index fingers together by taking the elbows back.
- On the exhalation take the head down again in between the feet. Keep the elbows up towards the sky and the palms of the hands firmly pressed together.
- Hold for one minute and then come up on an inhalation.

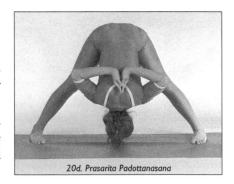

20d. Prasarita Padottanasana

21. Padangusthasana

padangustha=big toe

21a. The head up

- Stand in Tadasana.
- On a Mula Bandha inhalation elongate the legs and lift the trunk and pelvis up from the femur heads. On the exhalation rotate the pelvis forward and hold the big toes with the index and middle fingers of both hands.
- On each inhalation lift the head and chest further up, so that the arms are straight and the spine is elongated.
- Hold for one minute and then proceed to 21b.

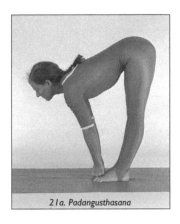

21a. Padangusthasana

21b. The head on the shins

- On an exhalation bend the arms and rest the head on the shins.
- Hold for one minute and then come up on an inhalation.

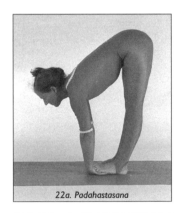

21b. Padangusthasana

22. Padahastasana

pada=leg, foot; hasta=hand

22a. The head up

- Stand in Tadasana.
- On a Mula Bandha inhalation elongate the legs and lift the trunk and pelvis up from the femur heads. On the exhalation rotate the pelvis forward and place the hands underneath the soles of the feet.
- On each inhalation lift the head and chest further up, so that the arms are straight and the spine is elongated.
- Hold for one minute and then proceed to 22b.

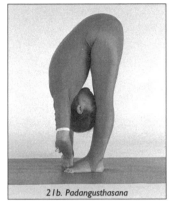

22a. Padahastasana

22b. The head on the shins

- On an exhalation bend the arms and rest the head on the shins.
- Hold for one minute and then come up on an inhalation.

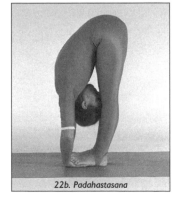

22b. Padahastasana

23. Uttanasana

uttana=intense stretch

23a. The hands on the earth, the head up

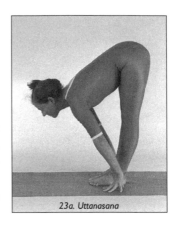

23a. Uttanasana

- Stand in Tadasana.
- On a Mula Bandha inhalation elongate the legs and lift the trunk and pelvis up from the femur heads. On the exhalation rotate the pelvis forward and place the hands next to the feet on the earth.
- On each inhalation lift the head and chest further up so that the arms are straight and the spine is elongated.
- Hold for one minute and then proceed to 23b.

23b. The hands on the earth, the head on the shins

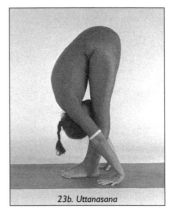

23b. Uttanasana

- On an exhalation take the hands further back and rest the head on the shins.
- Hold for one minute and then proceed to 23c.

23c. Holding the ankles, the head on the shins

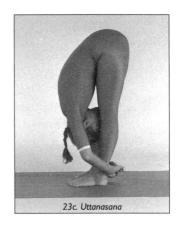

23c. Uttanasana

- On an exhalation hold the hands behind the ankles.
- Hold for one minute and then come up on an inhalation.

4.4 Sitting Poses

Sitting Poses

a. *Padmasana cycle*
b. *Vajrasana cycle*
c. *Virasana cycle*
d. *Baddha Konasana cycle*

Introduction to Padmasana
padma=lotus

Padmasana or the *Lotus Pose* is the most classic of all yoga poses, and is much praised in the Hatha Yoga texts. It is also the pose in which Pranayama (breathing) is usually practiced. Therefore it is described in detail, before proceeding to its variations.

In the "Hatha Yoga Pradipika", *Padmasana* is explained in Chapter I, sutras 46-51, in the following way:
* "Place the right foot on the left thigh and the left foot on the right thigh, and grasp the toes with the hands crossed over the back. Press the chin against the chest and gaze on the tip of the nose. This is called Padmasana, the destroyer of the diseases of the Yamis." (sutra 46)
* "Place the feet on the thighs, with the soles upwards, and place the hands on the thighs, with the palms upwards." (sutra 47)
* "Gaze on the tip of the nose, keeping the tongue pressed against the root of the teeth of the upper jaw, and the chin against the chest, and raise the air up slowly, i.e. pull the Apana-vayu gently upwards." (sutra 48)
* "This is called Padmasana, the destroyer of all diseases. It is difficult of attainment by everybody, but can be learned by intelligent people in this world." (sutra 49)
* "Having kept both the hands together in the lap, performing Padmasana firmly, keeping the chin fixed to the chest and contemplating on Him in the mind, by drawing the Apana-vayu up (performing Mula Bandha) and pushing down the air after inhaling it, joining thus the Prana and Apana in the navel, one gets the highest intelligence by awakening the Shakti (Kundalini) thus." (sutra 50)
* "The Yogi who, sitting with Padmasana, can control breathing, there is no doubt, is free from bondage." (sutra 51)

The "Gheranda Samhita" describes *Padmasana* in the Second Lesson, sutra 8, in the following way:
* "Place the right foot on the left thigh and similarly the left one on the right thigh, also cross the hands behind the back and firmly get hold of the big toes of the feet so crossed. Place the chin on the chest and fix the gaze on the tip of the nose. This posture is called Padmasana. This posture destroys all diseases."

The "Shiva Samhita" describes *Padmasana* in Chapter III, sutras 88-91, in the following way:

- "I describe now Padmasana which cures all diseases. Having crossed the legs, carefully place the feet on the opposite thighs, cross both the hands and place them similarly on the thighs. Fix the sight on the tip of the nose, pressing the tongue against the root of the teeth, the chin should be elevated, the chest expanded. Then draw the air slowly, fill the chest with all your might, and expel it slowly, in an unobstructed stream." (sutra 88)
- "It cannot be practiced by everybody, only the wise attains success in it." (sutra 89)
- "By performing and practicing the posture, undoubtedly the vital airs of the practitioner at once become completely equable, and flow harmoniously through the body." (sutra 90)
- "Sitting in the Padmasana posture, and knowing the action of the Prana and Apana, when the yogi performs the regulation of the breath, he is emancipated. I tell you the truth. Verily, I tell you the truth." (sutra 91)

Technique

Do not try to do the full position right away, but work through the intermediate poses Sukhasana and Siddhasana. Many people damage their knees in this pose, because they force them. The knees are one of the most delicate joints of the body, and if they are damaged, it is usually for life, not temporarily as with other parts of the body. So work slowly, without force; pain, especially here, is a danger signal.

The legs

Sit with your legs cross-legged. This position is called **Sukhasana** or the *Easy Pose.* Take the right foot in both hands, holding it from underneath, and lift it as high as you can (picture 5a (1)). The right hand supports the ankle and the left hand the arch. Turn the sole of the foot towards your face, at face level, and rotate the knee forwards as much as you can. Keeping the head

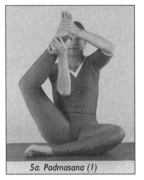
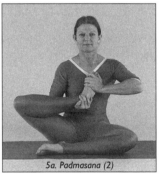

5a. Padmasana (1)   *5a. Padmasana (2)*

up and the back as straight as possible, bring the arch of the foot to the forehead, rotating the leg in the hip joint, *not* in the knee. Turn the sole of the foot towards you as if you want to read it: the more you turn it, the more the leg rotates in the right hip joint. At the same time rotate the right knee forward.

After touching the forehead, lower the foot and place the sole lengthwise on the sternum (picture 5a (2)); then lower it completely and place it in the left groin. The right knee rests on the left foot. This position is called **Siddhasana** or the *Pose of the Siddha* (an accomplished yogi).

If the right knee does not reach the left foot, practice bringing it down, until it rests on it with ease. Then proceed. Before lifting the left leg to cross it over the right, lean the body backwards, till you are balancing on the back of the buttock bones. Then lift the left foot up in the same way as the right one, holding the hands underneath the foot, with the left hand supporting the ankle and the right hand the arch (picture 5a (3)). Lift the foot up to face level and turn the sole of the foot towards you. Then place it lengthwise on the sternum, so that the leg rotates in the left hip rather than in the knee. Finally, lower the foot and place it in the right groin (picture 5a (4)). Then bring the body forward

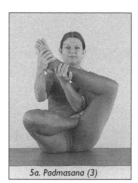

5a. Padmasana (3)

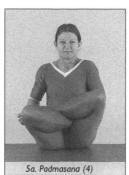

5a. Padmasana (4)

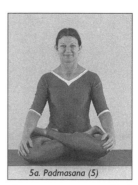

5a. Padmasana (5)

again so that the knees come down to the earth (picture 5a (5)). This position is called ***Padmasana*** or the *Lotus Pose*. Both knees point forward at an angle of about forty-five degrees, and the left shin is crossed over the right. Try to bring the left knee down as well.

The pelvis

Pull the buttock muscles sideways and backwards with the hands, so that you sit on the points of the buttock bones, not on the flesh. The weight of the trunk is evenly distributed between the buttock bones, so that the pelvis is straight, not tilted to one side. Check the two frontal hip bones with your fingers: they should be equally high and evenly forward. The shoulder joints are in line with the hip joints, so that the trunk is at right angles to the earth; thus the weight of the trunk is transmitted to the buttock bones in a straight line. The body balances finely tuned on the gravitational line in order to sit with lightness and ease, it should not lean forward nor backward. If the body leans backward, it hangs from the frontal muscles in order not to fall over backwards; if the body leans forward, the muscles in the back are tensed in order to keep the body from falling forwards. With the spine aligned on the gravitational line, the body does not need much effort to keep straight. This means that the frontal side and the backside of the body are parallel to each other.

Keeping these joints in line, the next step, as in Tadasana, is to assess the position of the pelvis. Here too, the pelvis can assume three positions. The correct one is the neutral position, in which the pelvis is vertical: the trunk rests on the points of the buttock bones, making an angle of ninety degrees with the thighs in the hip joints, and the two frontal hip bones are in vertical alignment with the groins. This position is quite rare. With most people the pelvis is rotated backwards and the trunk rests on the back of the buttock bones, or even on the coccyx.

This causes the whole back to bend, forcing the spinal vertebrae out of alignment, so that neither the spine nor the pelvis makes an angle of ninety degrees with the thighs in the hip joints. With some over-supple people, on the other hand, one sees the opposite: the pelvis is rotated too far forward, with the result that the lumbar spine curves in too much. In this case the pelvis makes an angle of less than ninety degrees with the thighs in the hip joints, and the muscles of the abdomen lose their tone; at the same time, as the coccyx is tipped back and up in the direction of the lumbar spine, the muscles in the lower back become short, narrow and tight.

You can check the position of the pelvis in the following way. Choose an outer corner where two walls meet, and sit with the back against it, resting the sacrum and the back of the head against it. If the lumbar and thoracic spine touch the corner, instead of the sacrum, the pelvis is rotated backwards: this causes the whole spinal column to bend. If, on the other hand, only the sacrum is in contact with the corner and there is a wide gap in the small of the back, between the waist and the corner, the pelvis is rotated too far forwards: this causes the lumbar spine to curve in too much. In both cases the pelvis has to be brought to a vertical position. When the pelvis is vertical, the trunk rests on the points of the buttock bones and the two frontal hip bones are in line with the groins; the spine is aligned on the corner and leaves only a space of about one inch between the lumbar spine and the corner.

Then, action has to be brought into the sacro-iliac joints. Constrict the tensor fascia lata and the adductors of the thighs slightly inwards towards each other, keep the two frontal hip bones in line with the groins and lift them *up* towards the ribs, so that they move forward into the arches of the feet. At the same time, root the coccyx by making the movement of counter-nutation of the sacrum and coccyx in relation to the pelvis: the coccyx roots down into the earth and moves forwards towards the pubic bone; simultaneously the upper rim of the sacrum moves also forwards. As a result of these movements, the sacro-iliac joints open, the sacrum becomes vertical, and moves forwards into the space between the two ilea, thus wedging them slightly apart. The entire pelvis widens laterally, moves vertically forwards against the femur heads and lifts up from the femur heads. As the distance between the two frontal hip bones widens, the lower abdomen moves in and up towards the navel; this tones the muscles of the lower abdomen and strengthens the internal organs. At the same time, the lumbar spine moves back to come almost in line with the, now vertical, sacrum.

As described in Tadasana, the result of these movements is that the body is centered in the center of gravity (in the pelvis); do not collapse the chest or the abdominal area between the navel and the lower ribs. Keeping the shoulder joints in line with the hip joints, root the buttock bones and on each Mula Bandha inhalation, elongate the spinal column upwards, and on each exhalation maintain the height of the body. Do not bend the spine in the thoracic and lumbar area: the groove of the spine should be even, from base to top, and run straight upwards.

In the action of rebouncing, something has to go down for something else to go up. For example, when you jump, the feet push down onto the earth; they go down heavily with the force of gravity, so that the rest of the body can move up against gravity (the Normal Force of Newton). To get the rebounce action in the pelvis, the outer hips and inner thighs have to constrict inwards towards each other, and the buttock bones and coccyx have to root into the earth, going down with the force of gravity. Thus the rest of the pelvis, the lower abdomen and the trunk can move up against gravity, rebouncing the weight of the body back up. The only muscles that are actively used are the tensor fascia lata, the adductors and the muscles in the lower abdomen. The rest of the body - the solar plexus, chest and shoulders - are relaxed.

Most of us live from the waist up, while the trunk, from the waist down, is forgotten. The area below the navel should be full, and the trunk from the navel upwards should be empty. When the pelvis rebounces the weight of the body back upwards, the spinal vertebrae continue that movement, the trunk should not sag into the pelvis. Negating gravity, the spine elongates upwards, so that the trunk is light.

When you practice this on an outer corner between two walls, the sacrum and back of the head are in contact with the corner, but not the thoracic vertebrae. Without pushing the chest forward, you have to move the thoracic vertebrae into the body.

To open the upper part of the chest, do as follows:
a.   Keep the ears in line with the shoulder and hip joints.
b.   Keep the lower ribs down and in.
c.   Elongate the neck up, as if balancing a book on the head. Keep the face vertical, do not tilt the chin up.

As described in Tadasana, the spine should show an even groove, from the sacrum to the first thoracic vertebra, and should be straight: draw the spine upwards, out of the muscular periphery of the body, like drawing a sword out of its scabbard. Keep the hands loosely folded in front of the lower abdomen on the shins, or, palms facing up, on the knees, without putting any weight on them. The arms hang passively from the shoulder joints, and the shoulders and shoulder blades widen laterally and move down towards the waist. The head balances evenly on the spinal column: if it moves too far forward, the muscles at the back of the upper trunk and neck will be tense to prevent it from falling forwards. Keep the ears in line with the shoulder joints and hip joints, and the face vertical; do not push the chin up, but do not pull it in too much either. The cervical spine also follows the gravitational line, so that the neck elongates upwards. Change the crossing of the legs; then repeat the pose on the other side.

The above description is the physically technical description of how to sit straight, holding the body lightly up from the center of gravity, with the spine erect. The beauty of the body is when it is light. Everybody knows how to be heavy, but find out how light the body can be. This lightness depends only on the skeleton, not on the muscles. The body is light when the skeletal frame lifts up, and the muscles hang loosely from this frame: keeping the spine on the central gravitational line of the body, the muscular system has to relax: muscles relaxed, skeleton firm. Shift the weight of your awareness onto the back of the body - not the physical weight of your body, but the internal weight of your awareness. People do not realize that awareness, consciousness, has bulk and weight. It can move around and throw light on different areas of the body. Usually the internal weight of the awareness is on the frontal side of the body, on the face, the throat, the sternum, the solar plexus, creating tensions. This is where we feel most at home, and thus the neck and shoulders are pulled forwards chronically, and the back stoops. Moving the internal weight backwards automatically straightens and elongates the body, and releases the tensions at the frontal side of the body. This does not mean, however, that the spine bends backwards; rather, the spine is straight, and the internal weight 'leans' against the spine. This automatically broadens the whole back, and this, in turn, allows the spine to elongate upwards. In this action there is no muscular effort involved.

You can do the same thing in the region of the head and neck. Here too we usually keep all the tensions on the frontal side, especially on the face. This drags the head and neck forward. Moving the internal weight backwards, from the face into the back of the head and neck, will bring the head automatically in alignment with the chest. The neck broadens and elongates, without any muscular effort, so that the head comes out of the trunk like a turtle drawing its head out of its shell; when the turtle pulls its head out, the shell stays where it is. So here too, the chest stays where it is when the head elongates upwards through internal weight shifting.

Try to experiment with the feeling of making an 'X-ray' of your body, keeping the skeletal structure sharply outlined, but both the muscular structure and the skin in a semi-transparent state. Then, in that semi-transparent state, carefully and deliberately expand the Energy Body, the Body of Light, till it transcends the skin.

4.4a   Padmasana cycle

These positions can be done in <u>four different modes</u>:

a.   Performing each position separately and holding it for one minute. To release the knees, you can do one minute of Paschimottanasana in between poses.

b.   Vinyasa
Connecting two or more positions by flowing from one into the other, using the breathing.

c.   Mala
Connecting all the positions through Surya Namaskar, using the breathing, and holding each of the Padmasana Poses for the duration of three breaths.

d.   Taking only a few positions and holding them for *five minutes* each. Here too you can release the knees by doing one minute of Paschimottanasana in between poses.

Padmasana cycle

1. Sukhasana
2. Lolasana
3. Swastikasana
4. Siddhasana
5. Padmasana
   a. Padmasana
   b. Parvatasana
   c. Gomukhasana
   d. Namasté II
6. Yoga Mudrasana I
   a. Supta Parvatasana
   b. Supta Gomukhasana
   c. Supta Namasté II
7. Supta Padmasana

8. Matsyasana I
   a. Matsyasana I
   b. Paryankasana I
   c. Paryankasana II
9. Matsyasana II
   a. Adhomukha Matsyasana II
   b. Urdhvamukha Matsyasana II
10. Parivrtta Padmasana
11. Tolasana
12. Kukkutasana
13. Garbha Pindasana
14. Goraksasana
15. Baddha Padmasana
16. Yoga Mudrasana II

1. Sukhasana

sukha=easy

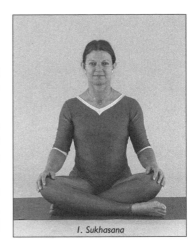

1. Sukhasana

- Sit on a blanket with the legs crossed. In all the following positions the thighs are in an exorotation position in the hip joints.
- Pull the buttock muscles backwards with the hands, so that you are sitting on the buttock bones, not on the flesh. The body weight is divided evenly between the buttock bones.
- The pelvis is in a vertical position, with the two frontal hip bones in vertical alignment above the groins. The groove of the spine is even from base to top, and runs straight upwards. Place the hands on the thighs.
- Root the two buttock bones, the coccyx and the pubic bone into the earth with the support of the Pada Bandha.
- On each Mula Bandha inhalation, elongate the spinal column upwards. On each exhalation, maintain the height of the body.
- Hold for one minute; then change the crossing of the legs.

2. Lolasana

lola=dangling

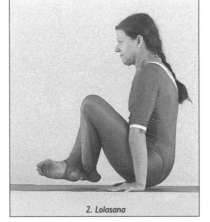

2. Lolasana

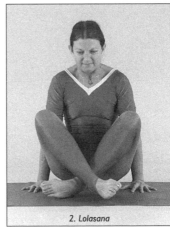

2. Lolasana

- Sit in Sukhasana (1) and then proceed:
- Place the hands next to the hips on the blanket, with the fingers pointing forwards.
- On an exhalation, lift the whole body up, supporting yourself only on the hands, till the arms are straight.
- Root the hands into the earth, and perform Hasta Bandha to elongate the arms. Pull the knees up towards the abdomen and look straight forward.
- Hold for ten seconds; then change the crossing of the legs.

3. Swastikasana

swastika=auspicious

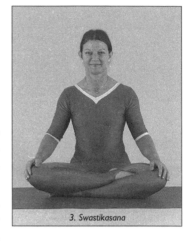

3. Swastikasana

- Sit in Sukhasana (1) and then proceed:
- Widen the knees and lift one foot up. Insert the toes, pointing downwards, between the calf and biceps muscle of the other leg, turning the heel upwards.
- Pull the buttock muscles backwards with the hands, so that you are sitting on the buttock bones, not on the flesh. The body weight is divided evenly between the buttock bones.
- The pelvis is in a vertical position, with the two frontal hip bones in vertical alignment above the groins. The groove of the spine is even from base to top, and runs straight upwards. Place the hands on the thighs.
- On each Mula Bandha inhalation, root the buttock bones, the coccyx and the pubic bone into the earth, with the support of the Pada Bandha, and elongate the spinal column upwards. On each exhalation, maintain the height of the body.
- Hold for one minute; then change the crossing of the legs.

4. Siddhasana

siddha=sage

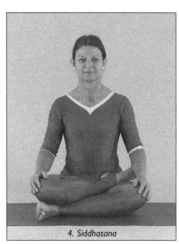

4. Siddhasana

- Sit in Sukhasana (1) and then proceed:
- Lift the right foot up as described in Padmasana (see page 77) and place it in the groin of the left leg, turning the sole of the foot upwards. In this pose the knees are closer together than in the previous one, and the right knee rests on the left foot.
- Pull the buttock muscles backwards with the hands, so that you are sitting on the buttock bones, not on the flesh. The body weight is divided evenly between the buttock bones.
- The pelvis is in a vertical position, with the two frontal hip bones in vertical alignment above the groins. The groove of the spine is even from base to top, and runs straight upwards. Place the hands on the thighs.
- Root the two buttock bones, the coccyx and the pubic bone into the earth with the support of the Pada Bandha.
- On each Mula Bandha inhalation, elongate the spinal column upwards. On each exhalation, maintain the height of the body.
- Hold for one minute; then change the crossing of the legs.

5. Padmasana

padma=lotus

5a. Padmasana

- For a complete explanation of this pose, see page 77.

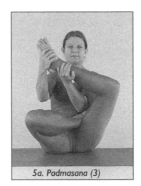 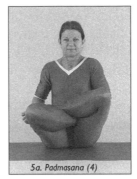 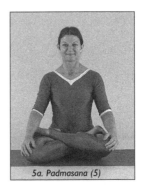

5a. Padmasana (3)   *5a. Padmasana (4)*   *5a. Padmasana (5)*

5b. Parvatasana

parvata=mountain

- Sit in Siddhasana (4) or Padmasana (5) and then proceed:
- On a Mula Bandha inhalation, raise the arms over the head. Rooting the buttock bones, the coccyx and the pubic bone into the earth with the support of the Pada Bandha, constrict the outer hips and inner thighs inwards towards each other, and lift the pelvis and trunk up from the femur heads (Mula Bandha).
- Keep the front and back of the trunk parallel to each other, and the hands, shoulder joints and hip joints in vertical alignment.
- Clasp the hands over the head and turn the palms facing upwards, extending the knuckles of the fingers up to the sky.
- Hold for one minute; then change the crossing of the feet and the interlock of the hands.

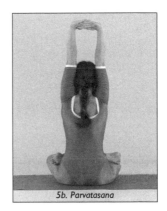

5b. Parvatasana

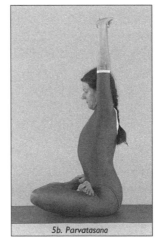 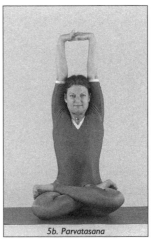

5b. Parvatasana   *5b. Parvatasana*

5c.   *Gomukhasana*

go=cow; mukha=face

- Sit in Siddhasana (4) or Padmasana (5) and then proceed:
- Elongate the left arm sideways and bring the hand onto the back in a circular movement. With the thumb and index finger of the right hand clasp the left wrist, push the left hand away from the back, and then up in between the shoulder blades, so that the knuckle of the little finger of the left hand rests on the spine.
- On a Mula Bandha inhalation, elongate the right arm up over the head, out of the right hip joint. On the exhalation, bend the elbow and clasp the left hand on the back. Keep the inner upper arm next to the ear. On each inhalation, elongate the right elbow further up, so that the hand can go further down.
- Take the left elbow back, but do not push the ribs forward. Keep the frontal ribs down and in, and the lower abdomen in and up.
- Hold for one minute; then change hands and the crossing of the feet.

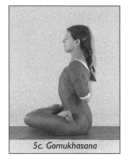

5c. Gomukhasana

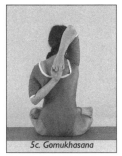

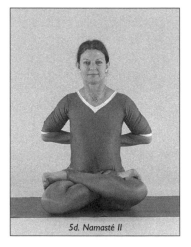

5c. Gomukhasana   5c. Gomukhasana

5d.   *Namasté II*

- Sit in Siddhasana (4) or Padmasana (5) and then proceed:
- Elongate both arms forward, and then take them back in a circular movement to join the palms at the back. Bend the elbows, turn the fingers so that they point to the spine, and then turn them upwards. Slide the edge of the little fingers up on the spine, till the hands are in between the shoulder blades. Join the palms of the hands firmly together by taking the elbows back.
- Roll the shoulders and upper arms back, so that the shoulder blades go down and the knuckles of the index fingers are pressed together.
- Do not push the ribs forward, but keep the frontal ribs down and in, and the lower abdomen in and up.
- Hold for one minute; then release the arms and change the crossing of the feet.

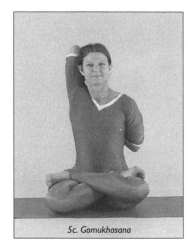

5d. Namasté II

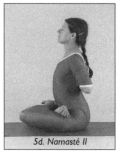

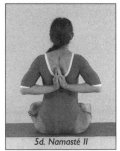

5d. Namasté II   5d. Namasté II

6. Yoga Mudrasana I

mudra=closing, sealing

In poses 6 and 7 and their variations, the pelvis is rotated forward around the femur heads as in Forward Bendings.

6a. Supta Parvatasana

supta=lying down; parvata=mountain

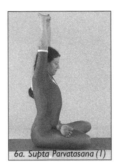
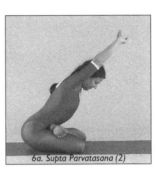

6a. Supta Parvatasana (1) *6a. Supta Parvatasana (2)*

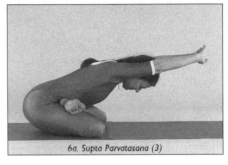

6a. Supta Parvatasana (3)

- Sit in Parvatasana (5b) and then proceed:
- On a Mula Bandha inhalation, lift the pelvis and trunk up from the femur heads, rooting the buttock bones into the earth with the support of the Pada Bandha. On the exhalation, bend forward till the whole trunk, from the groins to the sternum, rests on the crossed legs, and the head and hands rest on the blanket.
- The trunk arrives on the legs before the head and hands arrive on the blanket. Do not lift the buttock bones up, but extend them backwards, spreading them at the same time so that the lumbar spine moves in.
- On each inhalation, extend the groins, the buttock bones and the back of the thighs further backwards. At the same time, elongate the lower abdomen, rib cage, spine, head and hands further forwards.
- On each exhalation, lower the trunk and head further with gravity onto the legs and earth.
- Hold for one minute; then come up on an inhalation, and change the crossing of the legs.

6b. Supta Gomukhasana

supta=lying down; go=cow; mukha=face

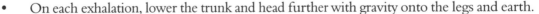

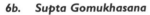

6b. Supta Gomukhasana

- Sit in Gomukhasana (5c) and then proceed:
- On a Mula Bandha inhalation, lift the pelvis and trunk up from the femur heads, rooting the buttock bones into the earth with the support of the Pada Bandha. On the exhalation, bend forward till the whole trunk, from the groins to the sternum, rests on the crossed legs and the head rests on the blanket.
- The trunk arrives on the legs before the head arrives on the blanket. Do not lift the buttock bones up, but extend them backwards, spreading them at the same time, so that the lumbar spine moves in.

- On each inhalation, extend the groins, the buttock bones and the back of the thighs further backwards. At the same time elongate the lower abdomen, rib cage, spine and head further forwards.
- On each exhalation, lower the trunk and head further with gravity onto the legs and earth, keeping both elbows up towards the sky.
- Hold for one minute. Then come up on an inhalation, raising first the head, then the chest, and then the abdomen. Change hands and the crossing of the legs.

6c. *Supta Namasté II*
supta=lying down

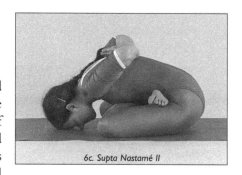

6c. Supta Nastamé II

- Sit in Namasté II (5d) and then proceed:
- On a Mula Bandha inhalation, lift the pelvis and trunk up from the femur heads, rooting the buttock bones into the earth with the support of the Pada Bandha. On the exhalation, bend forward till the whole trunk, from the groins to the sternum, rests on the crossed legs, and the head rests on the blanket.
- The trunk arrives on the legs before the head arrives on the blanket. Do not lift the buttock bones up, but extend them backwards, spreading them at the same time so that the lumbar spine moves in.
- On each inhalation, extend the groins, the buttock bones and the back of the thighs further backwards. At the same time, elongate the lower abdomen, rib cage, spine and head further forwards.
- On each exhalation, lower the trunk and head further with gravity onto the legs and earth, keeping the elbows up towards the sky.
- Hold for one minute. Then come up on an inhalation, raising first the head, then the chest, and then the abdomen. Change the crossing of the legs.

7. **Supta Padmasana**
supta=lying down; padma=lotus

This is Yoga Mudrasana I (6) performed while lying on the back, so the same rules apply.

- Sit in Siddhasana (4) or Padmasana (5) and then proceed:
- Keep the hands behind you on the blanket and, lifting the pelvis, so that you are standing on the knees, rotate it backwards, so that the coccyx rolls towards the pubic bone and the two frontal hip bones move up towards the ribs. Then lower yourself onto the elbows, and finally onto the blanket.
- Bring the knees to the chest and clasp the arms around the crossed knees.

7. Supta Padmasana

- On each Mula Bandha inhalation, elongate the groins, the buttock bones and the back of the thighs backwards, away from the trunk, and the lower abdomen and rib cage forwards towards the head.
- The Mula Bandha inhalation always starts in the lower abdomen. Zigzagging along the spinal column through the kidney region (widening that region) and the upper chest (lifting the upper ribs), it ends up in the back of the head. Thus the back of the head is elongated away from the shoulders, and the groins are elongated away from the lower abdomen. The whole back rests evenly on the blanket, and the sacro-iliac joints, kidneys and shoulder blades are widened.
- Roll the shoulders back to the earth. On each inhalation, elongate the spinal column further, and on each exhalation, flatten the back further onto the blanket.
- Hold for one minute; then change the crossing of the legs.

8. Matsyasana I
matsya=fish

In poses 8 and 9 and their variations, the pelvis is rotated backwards around the femur heads as in Back Bendings.

8a. Matsyasana I

- Sit in Siddhasana (4) or Padmasana (5) and then proceed:
- Keep the hands behind you on the blanket and, lifting the pelvis, so that you are standing on the knees, rotate it backwards, so that the coccyx rolls towards the pubic bone and the two frontal hip bones move up towards the ribs. Then lower yourself onto the elbows, and finally onto the blanket. Keep the knees down.

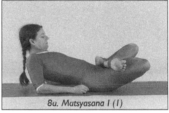
8a. Matsyasana I (1)

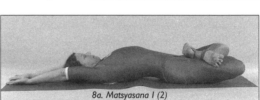
8a. Matsyasana I (2)

- Keep the backward rotation of the pelvis, so that the lower abdomen moves in the direction of the ribs, and slide the back of the chest up in the direction of the head. In this way the whole lumbar region is elongated and brought down onto the blanket.

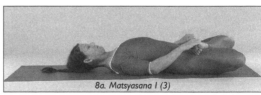
8a. Matsyasana I (3)

- Extend the thighs out of the groins, and pull the two frontal hip bones up towards the ribs: double action, down and up, so that the groins in the middle are opened.
- On a Mula Bandha inhalation, extend the arms over the head on the blanket, without curving the lumbar up.
- On each inhalation, extend the thighs further downwards, out of the hip joints, and the spine and arms further upwards.
- On each exhalation, press the lumbar further onto the blanket, maintaining the length of the body.
- Hold for one minute; then proceed to 8b.

8b.   *Paryankasana I*
paryanka=couch

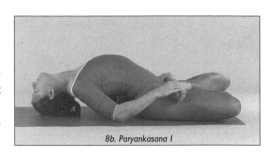

8b. Paryankasana I

- Place the elbows next to the trunk on the blanket and hold the arches of the feet with the hands.
- Arch the back and chest, and rest the crown of the head on the blanket.
- Hold for thirty seconds; then proceed to 8c.

8c.   *Paryankasana II*

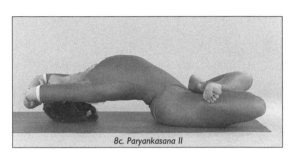

8c. Paryankasana II

- Clasp the elbows over the head and elongate the upper arms out of the shoulders, so that the elbows go further down to the earth.
- Hold for thirty seconds; then change the crossing of the legs and repeat 8a, b and c.

9.   Matsyasana II
matsya=fish

9a.   *Adhomukha Matsyasana II*
adho=downwards;
mukha=face; matsya=fish

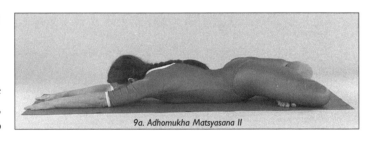

9a. Adhomukha Matsyasana II

This is basically the same position as Matsyasana I (8a), performed upside down, so the same rules apply.

- Sit in Padmasana (5) and then proceed:
- Stand up on your knees then and lower yourself forward onto the stomach. Pull the two frontal hip bones up towards the rib cage, so that the lumbar spine elongates, and extend the thighs backwards out of the groins: double action forwards and backwards, so that the groins in the middle are opened.
- Keep the backward rotation of the pelvis, so that the lower abdomen moves in the direction of the ribs, and pull the chest in the direction of the head.
- Extend the arms over the head on the blanket and rest on the forehead.
- Hold for one minute; then proceed to 9b.

9b. *Urdhvamukha Matsyasana II*
urdhva=upwards; mukha=face;
matsya=fish

- Bend the arms. Place the hands and lower arms next to the head on the blanket, and raise the head and chest till you are resting on the bent elbows.
- On each Mula Bandha inhalation, pull the lower abdomen further forwards towards the rib cage, and the ribs towards the head. The back is arched as in Bhujangasana I (see page 215).
- Hold for one minute; then change the crossing of the legs and repeat 9a and b.

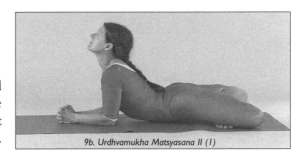

9b. Urdhvamukha Matsyasana II (1)

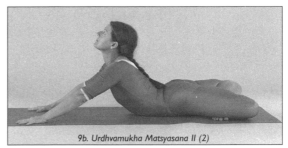

9b. Urdhvamukha Matsyasana II (2)

10. Parivrtta Padmasana
parivrtta=turned around; padma=lotus

- Sit in Padmasana (5) with the right foot crossed over the left. The knees should be fairly close together, so that both feet stick out on the sides of the thighs.
- On a Mula Bandha inhalation, elongate the right arm up to the sky. Lift the pelvis up from the femur heads and elongate the whole body upwards, rooting the buttock bones and the knees into the earth.
- On the exhalation, rotate the trunk towards the right, swing the right arm around the back and hold the right foot. Curl the toes of the foot around the fingers, so that the foot holds the hand as much as the hand the foot.
- Place the left hand on the right knee and turn the head towards the right.
- On each Mula Bandha inhalation, elongate the spinal column further upwards, rooting the buttock bones and the knees.
- On each exhalation, rotate the trunk, chest, shoulders and head further towards the right, till the chest and shoulders are perpendicular to the line between the knees.
- Hold for one minute; then change the crossing of the legs.

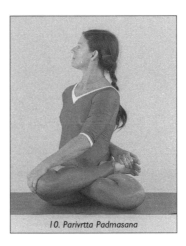

10. Parivrtta Padmasana

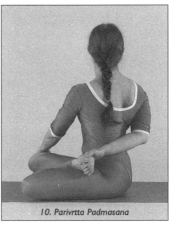

10. Parivrtta Padmasana

11. Tolasana

tola=a pair of scales

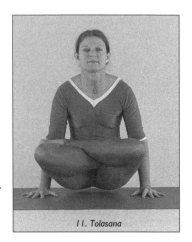

11. Tolasana

- Sit in Padmasana (5).
- Place the hands next to the thighs on the blanket, with the fingers pointing forwards.
- On an exhalation, lift the whole body up from the blanket, supporting yourself only on the hands, till the arms are straight. Root the hands into the earth, performing Hasta Bandha to elongate the arms.
- Pull the knees up towards the ribs with the support of the Pada Bandha, and look straight forward.
- Hold for ten seconds; then change the crossing of the legs.

12. Kukkutasana

kukkuta=cock

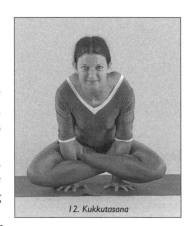

12. Kukkutasana

- Sit in Padmasana (5).
- Lift the knees up and insert the lower arms in the triangular spaces between the dorsal side of the feet, the calf muscles and the thigh muscles. Place the hands on the blanket, with the fingers pointing forwards.
- On an exhalation, lift the whole body up from the blanket, supporting yourself only on the hands, till the arms are straight. Root the hands into the earth, performing Hasta Bandha to elongate the arms.
- Pull the knees up towards the ribs with the support of the Pada Bandha, and look straight forward.
- Hold for ten seconds; then proceed to 13.

13. Garbha Pindasana

garbha=womb; pinda=embryo

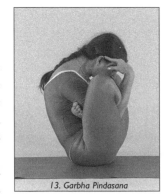

13. Garbha Pindasana

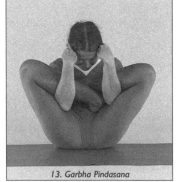

13. Garbha Pindasana

- Lower the buttock bones onto the earth again. Lift the crossed knees, and slide the arms still further through the legs so that the elbows also go through.
- Then bend the elbows and bring the hands to the ears, balancing the body only on the buttock bones. The spine is bent and the head is brought forward to the knees.
- Hold for ten seconds; then change the crossing of the legs and repeat 12 and 13.

14. Goraksasana

Goraksa=cowherd

This is basically the same pose as Matsyasana I (8a), so the same
rules apply.
- Sit in Padmasana (5).
- Push up till you are standing on the knees.
- Lift the hands up from the blanket, till the thighs and trunk
  are vertical and you are balancing only on the knees.
- Join the palms of the hands in front of the sternum in
  Namasté I and look straight forward.
- Hold for ten seconds; then change the crossing of the legs.

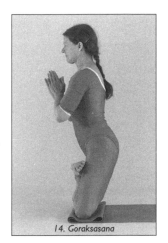

14. Goraksasana

15. Baddha Padmasana

baddha=bound; padma=lotus

- Sit in Padmasana (5). To perform this pose,
  the knees have to be very close together.
- Wrap the arms around the back and hold
  the feet, the right hand holding the right
  foot and the left hand holding the left
  foot. Hold the top (left) foot first and then
  the bottom (right) one.
- Hold for thirty seconds; then proceed to 16.

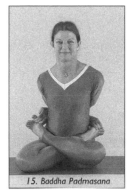

15. Baddha Padmasana

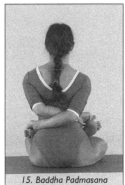

15. Baddha Padmasana

16. Yoga Mudrasana II

mudra=closing, sealing

- On a Mula Bandha inhalation, lift the pelvis
  and trunk up from the femur heads, rooting
  the buttock bones into the earth with the
  support of the Pada Bandha. On the exhalation,
  bend forward till the whole trunk, from the
  groins to the sternum, rests on the crossed legs
  and the head rests on the blanket.

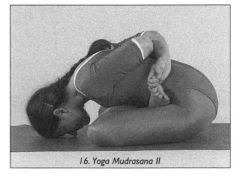

16. Yoga Mudrasana II

- The trunk arrives on the legs before the head arrives on the blanket. Do not lift the
  buttock bones up, but extend them backwards, spreading them at the same time, so that
  the lumbar spine moves in.
- On each inhalation, extend the groins, the buttock bones and the back of the thighs
  further backwards. At the same time, elongate the lower abdomen, rib cage, spine and
  head further forwards.
- On each exhalation, lower the trunk and head further with gravity onto the legs and earth.
- Hold for thirty seconds. Then come up on an inhalation, raising first the head, then
  the chest, and then the abdomen. Change the crossing of the legs and the arms and
  repeat 15 and 16.

4.4b   Vajrasana cycle

These positions can be done in <u>four different modes</u>:

•   **Performing each position separately** and holding it for one minute. To release the knees, you can do one minute of Paschimottanasana in between poses.

•   **Vinyasa**
Connecting two or more positions by flowing from one into the other, using the breathing.

•   **Mala**
Connecting all the positions through Surya Namaskar, using the breathing, and holding each of the Vajrasana Poses for the duration of three breaths.

•   **Taking only a few positions** and holding them for *five minutes* each. Here too you can release the knees by doing one minute of Paschimottanasana in between poses:

Vajrasana cycle

1. Vajrasana I
    a.   Vajrasana I
    b.   Parvatasana
    c.   Gomukhasana
    d.   Namasté II
2. Vajrasana II
    a.   Vajrasana II
    b.   Supta Parvatasana
    c.   Supta Gomukhasana
    d.   Supta Namasté II

3. Supta Vajrasana
    a.   Dvipada Supta Vajrasana
    b.   Ekapada Supta Vajrasana
4. Utkatasana II

I. Vajrasana I

vajra=thunderbolt, the weapon on Indra

Ia. Vajrasana I

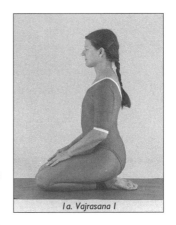

Ia. Vajrasana I

- Kneel on a blanket with the knees and feet together, and then sit down on the heels, keeping the heels united. This is a neutral position of the thighs in the hip joints. Make sure that the feet and knees are even.
- Pull the buttock muscles backwards with the hands, so that the buttock bones are above the arches, not on the heels. The body weight is divided evenly between the heels.
- The pelvis is in a vertical position, with the two frontal hip bones in vertical alignment above the groins. The groove of the spine is even from base to top, and runs straight upwards. Place the hands on the thighs.
- On each Mula Bandha inhalation, root the shins and the back of the feet into the earth, with the support of the Pada Bandha, and elongate the spinal column upwards. On each exhalation, maintain the height of the body.
- Hold for one minute.

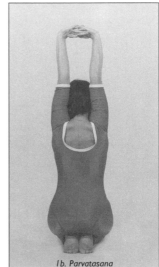

Ia. Vajrasana I

Ib. Parvatasana

parvata=mountain

- Sit in Vajrasana I (1a) and then proceed:
- On a Mula Bandha inhalation, raise the arms over the head. Rooting the shins and the back of the feet into the earth with the support of the Pada Bandha, and the buttock bones into the heels, constrict the outer hips and inner thighs inwards towards each other, and lift the pelvis and trunk up from the femur heads (Mula Bandha).

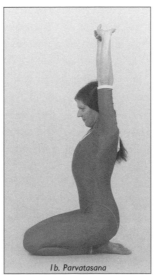

Ib. Parvatasana

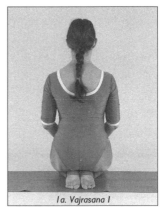

Ib. Parvatasana

- Keep the front and back of the trunk parallel to each other, and the hands, shoulder joints and hip joints in vertical alignment.
- Clasp the hands over the head and turn the palms facing upwards, extending the knuckles of the fingers up to the sky.
- Hold for one minute; then change the interlock of the hands.

Ic. *Gomukhasana*
go=cow; mukha=face

- Sit in Vajrasana I (1a) and then proceed:
- Elongate the left arm sideways and bring the hand onto the back in a circular movement. With the thumb and index finger of the right hand clasp the left wrist, push the left hand away from the back, and then up in between the shoulder blades, so that the knuckle of the little finger of the left hand rests on the spine.
- On a Mula Bandha inhalation, elongate the right arm up over the head, out of the right hip joint. On the exhalation, bend the elbow and clasp the left hand on the back. Keep the inner upper arm next to the ear. On each inhalation, elongate the right elbow further up, so that the hand can go further down.
- Take the left elbow back, but do not push the ribs forward. Keep the frontal ribs down and in, and the lower abdomen in and up.
- Hold for one minute; then change hands.

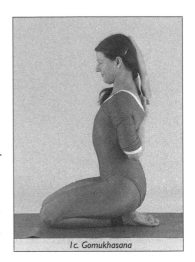

Ic. Gomukhasana

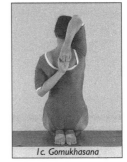

Ic. Gomukhasana

Id. *Namasté II*

- Sit in Vajrasana I (1a) and then proceed:
- Elongate both arms forward, and then take them back in a circular movement to join the palms at the back. Bend the elbows, turn the fingers so that they point to the spine, and then turn them upwards. Slide the edge of the little fingers up on the spine, till the hands are in between the shoulder blades. Join the palms of the hands firmly together by taking the elbows back.
- Roll the shoulders and upper arms back, so that the shoulder blades go down, and the knuckles of the index fingers are pressed together.
- Do not push the ribs forward, but keep the frontal ribs down and in, and the lower abdomen in and up.
- Hold for one minute; then release the arms.

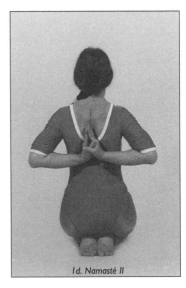

Id. Namasté II

2. Vajrasana II

In poses 2 through 4 and their variations, the pelvis is rotated forward around the femur heads as in Forward Bendings.

2a. Vajrasana II

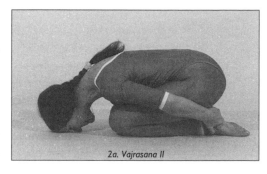

2a. Vajrasana II

- Sit in Vajrasana I (1a), hold the heels with the hands, and then proceed:
- On a Mula Bandha inhalation, lift the pelvis and trunk up from the femur heads, rooting the buttock bones into the heels, and the shins and the back of the feet into the earth with the support of the Pada Bandha. On the exhalation, bend forward till the whole trunk, from the groins to the sternum, rests on the thighs, and the head rests on the blanket.
- The trunk arrives on the thighs before the head arrives on the blanket. Do not lift the buttock bones up from the heels, but extend them backwards, spreading them at the same time so that the lumbar spine moves in.
- On each inhalation, extend the buttock bones and the back of the thighs further backwards. At the same time elongate the lower abdomen, rib cage, spine and head further forwards.
- On each exhalation, lower the trunk and head further with gravity onto the thighs and earth.
- Hold for one minute; then come up on an inhalation, raising first the head, then the chest, and then the abdomen.

2b. Supta Parvatasana
supta=lying down; parvata=mountain

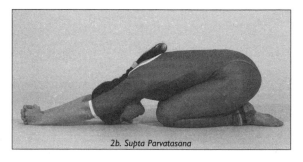

2b. Supta Parvatasana

- Sit in Parvatasana (1b) and then proceed:
- On a Mula Bandha inhalation, lift the pelvis and trunk up from the femur heads, rooting the buttock bones into the heels, and the shins and the back of the feet into the earth with the support of the Pada Bandha. On the exhalation, bend forward till the whole trunk, from the groins to the sternum, rests on the thighs, and the head and hands rest on the blanket.
- The trunk arrives on the thighs before the head and hands arrive on the blanket. Do not lift the buttock bones up from the heels, but extend them backwards, spreading them at the same time so that the lumbar spine moves in.
- On each inhalation, extend the buttock bones and the back of the thighs further backwards. At the same time elongate the lower abdomen, rib cage, spine, head and hands further forwards.
- On each exhalation, lower the trunk and head further with gravity onto the thighs and earth.
- Hold for one minute; then come up on an inhalation.

2c.   Supta Gomukhasana

supta=lying down; go=cow; mukha=face

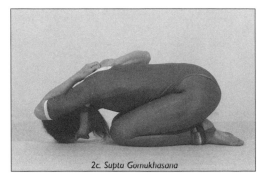

2c. Supta Gomukhasana

- Sit in Gomukhasana (1c) and then proceed:
- On a Mula Bandha inhalation, lift the pelvis and trunk up from the femur heads, rooting the buttock bones into the heels, and the shins and the back of the feet into the earth with the support of the Pada Bandha. On the exhalation, bend forward till the whole trunk, from the groins to the sternum, rests on the thighs and the head rests on the blanket.
- The trunk arrives on the thighs before the head arrives on the blanket. Do not lift the buttock bones up from the heels, but extend them backwards, spreading them at the same time, so that the lumbar spine moves in.
- On each inhalation, extend the buttock bones and the back of the thighs further backwards. At the same time elongate the lower abdomen, rib cage, spine and head further forwards.
- On each exhalation, lower the trunk and head further with gravity onto the thighs and earth, keeping both elbows up towards the sky.
- Hold for one minute. Then come up on an inhalation, raising first the head, then the chest and then the abdomen. Change hands.

2d.   Supta Namasté II

supta=lying down

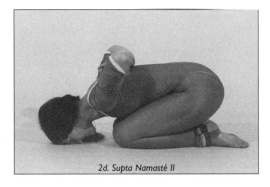

2d. Supta Namasté II

- Sit in Namasté II (1d) and then proceed:
- On a Mula Bandha inhalation, lift the pelvis and trunk up from the femur heads, rooting the buttock bones into the heels, and the shins and the back of the feet into the earth with the support of the Pada Bandha. On the exhalation, bend forward till the whole trunk, from the groins to the sternum, rests on the thighs and the head rests on the blanket.
- The trunk arrives on the thighs before the head arrives on the blanket. Do not lift the buttock bones up from the heels, but extend them backwards, spreading them at the same time so that the lumbar spine moves in.
- On each inhalation, extend the buttock bones and the back of the thighs further backwards. At the same time elongate the lower abdomen, rib cage, spine and head further forwards.
- On each exhalation, lower the trunk and head further with gravity onto the thighs and earth, keeping the elbows up towards the sky.
- Hold for one minute; then come up on an inhalation, raising first the head, then the chest, and then the abdomen.

3. Supta Vajrasana

supta=lying down

3a. Dvipada Supta Vajrasana

*dvi=two; pada=leg,foot; supta=lying down;
vajra=thunderbolt,the weapon on Indra*

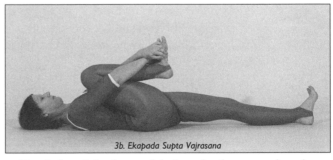

This is Vajrasana II (2a) performed while lying
on the back, so the same rules apply.

*   Lie on the back on the blanket. Bend the
    legs and bring the knees to the chest.
*   Clasp the knees between the crossed arms

3a. Dvipada Supta Vajrasana

    and hold the feet, the right hand holding the outer edge of the left foot and the left hand
    the outer edge of the right foot.
*   On each Mula Bandha inhalation, elongate the groins, the buttock bones and the back
    of the thighs backwards, away from the trunk, and the lower abdomen and rib cage
    forwards towards the head.
*   The Mula Bandha inhalation always starts in the lower abdomen. Zigzagging along the
    spinal column through the kidney region (widening that region) and the upper chest
    (lifting the upper ribs), it ends up in the back of the head. Thus the back of the head is
    elongated away from the shoulders, and the groins are elongated away from the lower
    abdomen. The whole back rests evenly on the blanket, and the sacro-iliac joints, kidneys
    and shoulder blades are widened.
*   Roll the shoulders back to the earth. On each inhalation, elongate the spinal column
    further, and on each exhalation, flatten the back further onto the blanket.
*   Hold for one minute; then change the crossing of the arms.

3b. Ekapada Supta Vajrasana

*eka=one; pada=leg, foot; supta=
lying down; vajra=thunderbolt,
the weapon on Indra*

This is basically the same position
as the previous one, performed
with one leg only, so the same
rules apply.

3b. Ekapada Supta Vajrasana

*   Lie on the back on the blanket. Bend the right leg and bring the knee to the chest,
    keeping the left leg straight on the blanket.
*   Clasp the right knee between the crossed arms and hold the foot: the right hand holding
    the inner arch and the left hand, crossing over the right, holding the outer edge of the foot.
*   On each Mula Bandha inhalation, elongate the right groin, the right buttock bone and
    the back of the right thigh backwards, away from the trunk, and the lower abdomen
    and rib cage forwards towards the head.
*   The Mula Bandha inhalation always starts in the lower abdomen. Zigzagging along the
    spinal column through the kidney region (widening that region) and the upper chest

(lifting the upper ribs), it ends up in the back of the head. Thus the back of the head is elongated away from the shoulders, and the right groin is elongated away from the lower abdomen. The whole back rests evenly on the blanket, and the sacro-iliac joints, kidneys and shoulder blades are widened.

- Roll the shoulders back to the earth. On each inhalation, elongate the spinal column further, and on each exhalation, flatten the back further onto the blanket.
- Hold for one minute; then change legs and the crossing of the arms.

4. Utkatasana II

utkata=powerful, fierce

This is basically the same position as Supta Parvatasana (2b) performed while squatting, so the same rules apply.
- Stand in Tadasana.
- On a Mula Bandha inhalation, elongate the arms up over the head. On the exhalation, proceed to Utkatasana I (see page 62), inclining the trunk forwards at an angle of about thirty degrees.
- Inhale, and on the next exhalation bend the knees completely and squat down. Keep the inner knees together, and the heels on the earth. The arms form one continuous line with the chest and pelvis, and the trunk is now inclined forwards at an angle of forty-five degrees.
- Root the feet into the earth and perform Pada Bandha to support the action in the pelvis.
- On each Mula Bandha inhalation, elongate the buttock bones and the back of the thighs backwards, away from the trunk, and at the same time the lower abdomen, rib cage, spine, head and hands up towards the sky.
- On each exhalation, maintain that height.
- Hold for one minute; then stand up again.

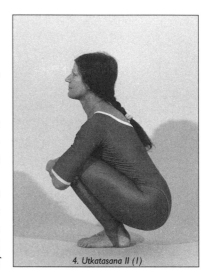

4. Utkatasana II (1)

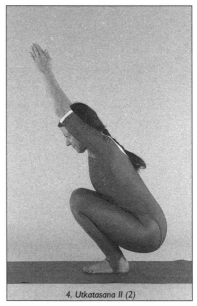

4. Utkatasana II (2)

4.4c Virasana cycle

These positions can be done in <u>four different modes</u>:

a. **Performing each position separately** and holding it for one minute. To release the knees, you can do one minute of Paschimottanasana in between poses.

b. **Vinyasa**
Connecting two or more positions by flowing from one into the other, using the breathing.

c. **Mala**
Connecting all the positions through Surya Namaskar, using the breathing, and holding each of the Virasana Poses for the duration of three breaths.

d. **Taking only a few positions** and holding them for *five minutes* each. Here too you can release the knees by doing one minute of Paschimottanasana in between poses.

Virasana cycle

1. Virasana I
   a. Virasana I
   b. Parvatasana
   c. Gomukhasana
   d. Namasté II
   e. Upavistha Virasana I
2. Virasana II
   a. Virasana II
   b. Supta Parvatasana
   c. Supta Gomukhasana
   d. Supta Namasté II
   e. Upavistha Virasana II

3. Supta Virasana
   a. Dvipada Supta Virasana
   b. Ekapada Supta Virasana
   c. Paryankasana I
   d. Paryankasana II
4. Bhekasana

1. Virasana I
vira=hero

1a. Virasana I

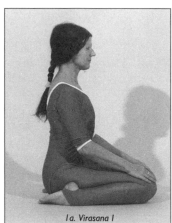

1a. Virasana I

- Kneel down on a blanket with the knees together and the feet spread. Sit down in between the feet, turning the calf muscles out: this is an endorotation of the thighs in the hip joints. Make sure that the feet and knees are even.
- With the fingers, turn the toes one by one towards the coccyx, so that the inner (big) arches of the feet follow the outer contours of the hips, and the big toes form a continuous line with the curve of the arches.
- Pull the buttock muscles backwards with the hands, so that you are sitting on the buttock bones, not on the flesh. The body weight is divided evenly between the buttock bones.
- The pelvis is in a vertical position, with the two frontal hip bones in vertical alignment above the groins. The groove of the spine is even, from base to top, and runs straight upwards. Place the hands on the thighs.
- On each Mula Bandha inhalation, root the buttock bones, the shins and the back of the feet into the earth, with the support of the Pada Bandha, and elongate the spinal column upwards. On each exhalation, maintain the height of the body.
- Hold for one minute.

1b. Parvatasana
parvata=mountain

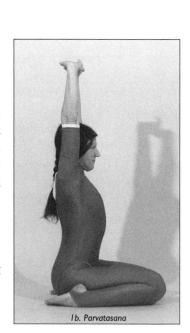

1b. Parvatasana

- Sit in Virasana I (1a) and then proceed:
- On a Mula Bandha inhalation, raise the arms over the head. Rooting the buttock bones, the shins and the back of the feet into the earth with the support of the Pada Bandha, constrict the outer hips and inner thighs inwards towards each other, and lift the pelvis and trunk up from the femur heads (Mula Bandha).
- Keep the front and back of the trunk parallel to each other, and the hands, shoulder joints and hip joints in vertical alignment.
- Clasp the hands over the head and turn the palms facing upwards extending the knuckles of the fingers up to the sky.
- Hold for one minute; then change the interlock of the hands.

Ic. *Gomukhasana*
go=cow; mukha=face

- Sit in Virasana I (1a) and then proceed:
- Elongate the left arm sideways and bring the hand onto the back in a circular movement. With the thumb and index finger of the right hand clasp the left wrist, push the left hand away from the back, and then up in between the shoulder blades, so that the knuckle of the little finger of the left hand rests on the spine.
- On a Mula Bandha inhalation, elongate the right arm up over the head, out of the right hip joint. On the exhalation, bend the elbow and clasp the left hand on the back. Keep the inner upper arm next to the ear.

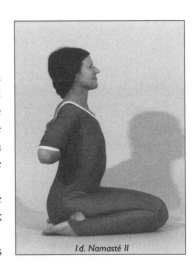

Ic. Gomukhasana

On each inhalation, elongate the right elbow further up, so that the hand can go further down.
- Take the left elbow back, but do not push the ribs forward. Keep the frontal ribs down and in, and the lower abdomen in and up.
- Hold for one minute; then change hands.

Id. *Namasté II*

- Sit in Virasana I (1a) and then proceed:
- Elongate both arms forward, and then take them back in a circular movement to join the palms at the back. Bend the elbows, turn the fingers so that they point to the spine, and then turn them upwards. Slide the edge of the little fingers up on the spine, till the hands are in between the shoulder blades. Join the palms of the hands firmly together by taking the elbows back.
- Roll the shoulders and upper arms back, so that the shoulder blades go down and the knuckles of the index fingers are pressed together.
- Do not push the ribs forward, but keep the frontal ribs down and in, and the lower abdomen in and up.
- Hold for one minute; then release the arms.

Id. Namasté II

1e.   *Upavistha Virasana I*
upavistha=seated; vira=hero

This is a variation of Virasana I (1a). In this pose the knees are spread and the tips of the big toes touch each other at the back, close to the coccyx. The inner arches of the feet adhere to the backside of the buttocks, and the big toes form a continuous line with the curve of the arches. Do not sit on the heels, but in front of them on the earth. For the rest follow the instructions given for Virasana I (1a).

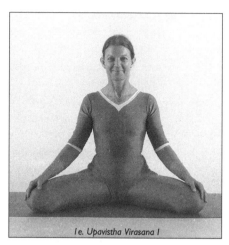
1e. Upavistha Virasana I

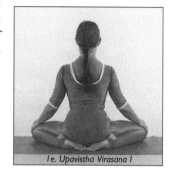
1e. Upavistha Virasana I

2.   **Virasana II**

In pose 2 and its variations, the pelvis is rotated forward around the femur heads as in Forward Bendings.

2a.   *Virasana II*

- Sit in Virasana I (1a), hold the heels with the hands, and then proceed:
- On a Mula Bandha inhalation, lift the pelvis and trunk up from the femur heads, rooting the buttock bones, the shins and the back of the feet into the earth with the support of the Pada Bandha. On the exhalation, bend forward till the whole trunk, from the groins to the sternum, rests on the thighs, and the head rests on the blanket.

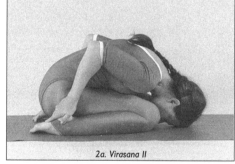
2a. Virasana II

- The trunk arrives on the thighs before the head arrives on the blanket. Do not lift the buttock bones up, but extend them backwards, spreading them at the same time so that the lumbar spine moves in.
- On each inhalation, extend the groins, the buttock bones and the back of the thighs further backwards. At the same time elongate the lower abdomen, rib cage, spine and head further forwards.
- On each exhalation, lower the trunk and head further with gravity onto the thighs and earth.
- Hold for one minute; then come up on an inhalation, raising first the head, then the chest, and then the abdomen.

2b. **Supta Parvatasana**

supta=lying down; parvata=mountain

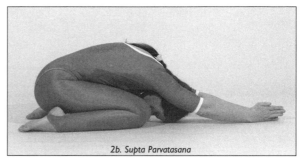

2b. Supta Parvatasana

- Sit in Parvatasana (1b) and then proceed:
- On a Mula Bandha inhalation, lift the pelvis and trunk up from the femur heads, rooting the buttock bones, the shins and the back of the feet into the earth with the support of the Pada Bandha. On the exhalation, bend forward till the whole trunk, from the groins to the sternum, rests on the thighs, and the head and hands rest on the blanket.
- The trunk arrives on the thighs before the head and hands arrive on the blanket. Do not lift the buttock bones up, but extend them backwards, spreading them at the same time so that the lumbar spine moves in.
- On each inhalation, extend the groins, the buttock bones and the back of the thighs further backwards. At the same time elongate the lower abdomen, rib cage, spine, head and hands further forwards.
- On each exhalation, lower the trunk and head further with gravity onto the thighs and earth.
- Hold for one minute; then come up on an inhalation.

2c. **Supta Gomukhasana**

supta=lying down; go=cow; mukha=face

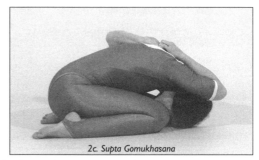

2c. Supta Gomukhasana

- Sit in Gomukhasana (1c) and then proceed:
- On a Mula Bandha inhalation, lift the pelvis and trunk up from the femur heads, rooting the buttock bones, the shins and the back of the feet into the earth with the support of the Pada Bandha. On the exhalation, bend forward till the whole trunk, from the groins to the sternum, rests on the thighs, and the head rests on the blanket.
- The trunk arrives on the thighs before the head arrives on the blanket. Do not lift the buttock bones up, but extend them backwards, spreading them at the same time, so that the lumbar spine moves in.
- On each inhalation, extend the groins, the buttock bones and the back of the thighs further backwards. At the same time elongate the lower abdomen, rib cage, spine and head further forwards.
- On each exhalation, lower the trunk and head further with gravity onto the thighs and earth, keeping both elbows up towards the sky.
- Hold for one minute. Then come up on an inhalation, raising first the head, then the chest, and then the abdomen. Change hands.

2d. Supta Namasté II
supta=lying down

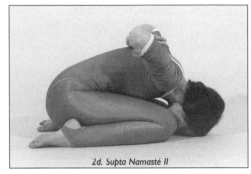

2d. Supta Namasté II

- Sit in Namasté II (1d) and then proceed:
- On a Mula Bandha inhalation, lift the pelvis and trunk up from the femur heads, rooting the buttock bones, the shins and the back of the feet into the earth with the support of the Pada Bandha. On the exhalation, bend forward till the whole trunk, from the groins to the sternum, rests on the thighs, and the head rests on the blanket.
- The trunk arrives on the thighs before the head arrives on the blanket. Do not lift the buttock bones up, but extend them backwards, spreading them at the same time so that the lumbar spine moves in.
- On each inhalation, extend the groins, the buttock bones and the back of the thighs further backwards. At the same time elongate the lower abdomen, rib cage, spine and head further forwards.
- On each exhalation, lower the trunk and head further with gravity onto the thighs and earth, keeping the elbows up towards the sky.
- Hold for one minute; then come up on an inhalation, raising first the head, then the chest, and then the abdomen.

2e. Upavistha Virasana II
upavistha=seated; vira=hero

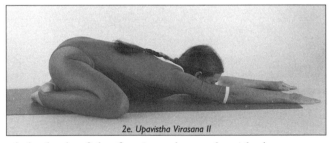

2e. Upavistha Virasana II

- Sit in Upavistha Virasana I (1e) and proceed:
- On a Mula Bandha inhalation, lift the pelvis and trunk up from the femur heads, rooting the buttock bones, the shins and the back of the feet into the earth with the support of the Pada Bandha. On the exhalation, bend forward till the chest and head rest on the blanket in between the thighs. Extend the arms forwards on the blanket.
- Do not lift the buttock bones up, but extend them backwards, spreading them at the same time so that the lumbar spine moves in.
- On each inhalation, extend the groins and buttock bones further backwards. At the same time elongate the lower abdomen, rib cage, spine, head and arms further forwards.
- On each exhalation, lower the trunk and head further with gravity onto the earth.
- Hold for one minute; then come up on an inhalation.

3. Supta Virasana

In pose 3 and its variations, the pelvis is rotated backwards around the femur heads as in Back Bendings.

3a. *Dvipada Supta Virasana*
supta=lying down; vira=hero

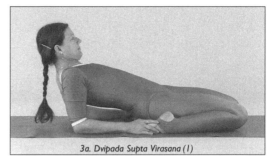

3a. Dvipada Supta Virasana (1)

- Sit in Virasana I (1a) and then proceed:
- Keep the hands behind you on the blanket and, lifting the pelvis so that you are standing on the shins, rotate the pelvis backwards, so that the coccyx rolls towards the pubic bone and the two frontal hip bones move up towards the ribs. Then lower yourself onto the elbows, and finally onto the blanket. Keep the knees together and down.
- Keep the backward rotation of the pelvis, so that the lower abdomen moves in the direction of the ribs, and slide the back of the chest upwards in the direction of the head. In this way the whole lumbar region is elongated and brought down onto the blanket.
- Extend the thighs out of the groins and pull the two frontal hip bones up towards the ribs: double action down and up, so that the groins in the middle are opened.

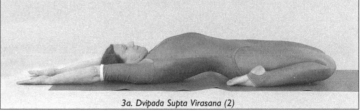

3a. Dvipada Supta Virasana (2)

- On a Mula Bandha inhalation, extend the arms over the head on the blanket, without curving the lumbar up.
- On each inhalation, extend the thighs further downwards out of the hip joints, and the spine and arms further upwards.
- On each exhalation, press the lumbar further onto the blanket, maintaining the length of the body.
- Hold for one minute; then proceed to 3b.

3b. *Ekapada Supta Virasana*
eka=one; pada=leg, foot; supta=lying down; vira=hero

- Unfold the right leg and extend it up to the sky, holding it with both hands.
- Hold for thirty seconds; then change legs.

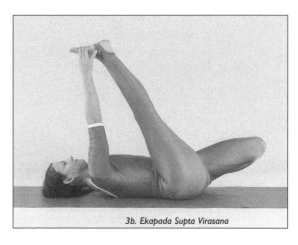

3b. Ekapada Supta Virasana

3c. *Paryankasana I*
paryanka=couch

- Lie down in Supta Virasana (3a) and then proceed:
- Place the elbows next to the trunk on the blanket, and hold the arches of the feet with the hands.
- Arch the back and chest and rest the crown of the head on the blanket.
- Hold for thirty seconds; then proceed to 3d.

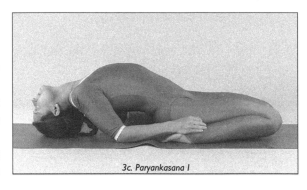
3c. Paryankasana I

3d. *Paryankasana II*

- Clasp the elbows over the head and elongate the upper arms out of the shoulders, so that the elbows go further down to the earth.
- Hold for thirty seconds.

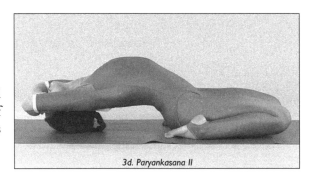
3d. Paryankasana II

4. Bhekasana
bheka=frog

This is Paryankasana I (3c) performed while lying on the stomach.
- Lie down on the stomach on the blanket and fold the legs as in Virasana I (1a)
- Place the hands on the dorsal side of the feet, with the fingers pointing

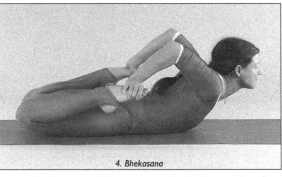
4. Bhekasana

forward and the elbows pointing up towards the sky (like locust legs). Push the feet down and raise the head and chest up.
- Hold for a few seconds.

4.4d   **Baddha Konasana cycle**

These positions can be done in <u>four different modes</u>:

a.   Performing each position separately and holding it for one minute. To release the knees, you can do one minute of Paschimottanasana in between poses.

b.   Vinyasa
Connecting two or more positions by flowing from one into the other, using the breathing.

c.   Mala
Connecting all the positions through Surya Namaskar, using the breathing, and holding each of the Baddha Konasana poses for the duration of three breaths.

d.   Taking only a few positions and holding them for *five minutes* each. Here too you can release the knees by doing one minute of Paschimottanasana in between poses

---

Baddha Konasana cycle

1.   Baddha Konasana I
     a. Baddha Konasana I
     b. Parvatasana
     c. Gomukhasana
     d. Namasté II
2.   Baddha Konasana II
     a. Baddha Konasana II
     b. Supta Parvatasana
     c. Supta Gomukhasana
     d. Supta Namasté II

3.   Kandasana
4.   Mulabandhasana
5.   Supta Baddha Konasana

I. Baddha Konasana I

baddha=bound; kona=angle

In all the following positions the thighs are in an exorotation position in the hip joints.

Ia. Baddha Konasana I

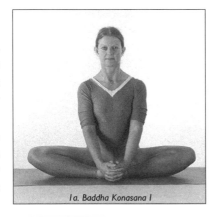

Ia. Baddha Konasana I

- Sit on a blanket with the knees spread sideways and the soles of the feet united. Hold the feet with the hands and pull the heels as close to the pubic bone as possible. Bring the knees down to the blanket by extending the thighs sideways out of the hip joints.
- Pull the buttock muscles backwards with the hands, so that you are sitting on the buttock bones, not on the flesh. The body weight is divided evenly between the buttock bones. Then hold the feet with the hands again.
- The pelvis is in a vertical position, with the two frontal hip bones in vertical alignment above the groins. The groove of the spine is even from base to top and runs straight upwards. On each Mula Bandha inhalation, root the buttock bones and the outer edges of the feet into the earth with the support of the Pada Bandha, and elongate the spinal column upwards. On each exhalation, maintain the height of the body.
- Hold for one minute.

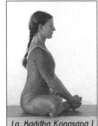

Ia. Baddha Konasana I

Ib. Parvatasana

parvata=mountain

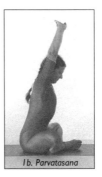

Ib. Parvatasana

- Sit in Baddha Konasana I (Ia) and then proceed:
- On a Mula Bandha inhalation, raise the arms over the head. Rooting the buttock bones and the outer edges of the feet into the earth with the support of the Pada Bandha, constrict the outer hips inwards towards each other, extend the thighs and knees sideways out of the hip joints, and lift the pelvis and trunk up from the femur heads (Mula Bandha).
- Keep the front and back of the trunk parallel to each other, and the hands, shoulder joints and hip joints in vertical alignment.
- Clasp the hands over the head and turn the palms facing upwards, extending the knuckles of the fingers up to the sky.
- Hold for one minute; then change the hands interlock.

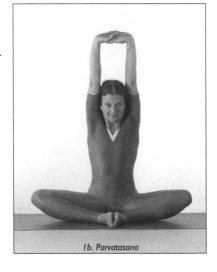

Ib. Parvatasana

1c. *Gomukhasana*
go=cow; mukha=face

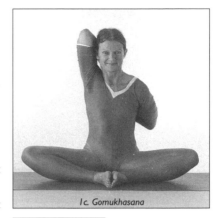
1c. Gomukhasana

- Sit in Baddha Konasana I (1a) and then proceed:
- Elongate the left arm sideways and bring the hand onto the back in a circular movement. With the thumb and index finger of the right hand clasp the left wrist, push the left hand away from the back, and then up, in between the shoulder blades, so that the knuckle of the little finger of the left hand rests on the spine.
- On a Mula Bandha inhalation, elongate the right arm up over the head, out of the right hip joint. On the exhalation, bend the elbow and clasp the left hand on the back. Keep the inner upper arm next to the ear. On each inhalation, elongate the right elbow further up, so that the hand can go further down.
- Take the left elbow back, but do not push the ribs forward. Keep the frontal ribs down and in, and the lower abdomen in and up.
- Hold for one minute; then change hands.

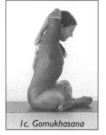
1c. Gomukhasana

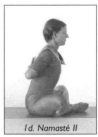
1d. Namasté II

1d. *Namasté II*

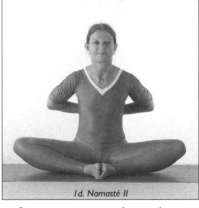
1d. Namasté II

- Sit in Baddha Konasana I (1a) and then proceed:
- Elongate both arms sideways and then take them back in a circular movement to join the palms at the back. Bend the elbows, turn the fingers so that they point to the spine, and then turn them upwards. Slide the edge of the little fingers up on the spine, till the hands are in between the shoulder blades. Join the palms of the hands firmly together by taking the elbows back.
- Roll the shoulders and upper arms back, so that the shoulder blades go down and the knuckles of the index fingers are pressed together.
- Do not push the ribs forward, but keep the frontal ribs down and in, and the lower abdomen in and up.
- Hold for one minute; then release the arms.

2. Baddha Konasana II

In pose 2 and its variations, the pelvis is rotated forward around the femur heads as in Forward Bendings.

2a. Baddha Konasana II

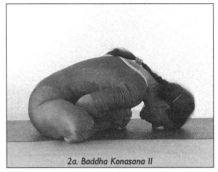

2a. Baddha Konasana II

- Sit in Baddha Konasana I (1a), hold the feet with the hands, and then proceed:
- On a Mula Bandha inhalation, lift the pelvis and trunk up from the femur heads, rooting the buttock bones and the outer edges of the feet into the earth with the support of the Pada Bandha,and elongating the thighs and knees sideways out of the hip joints. On the exhalation, bend forward till the sternum rests on the feet, and the head rests on the blanket. The sternum arrives on the feet before the head arrives on the blanket. Do not lift the buttock bones up, but extend them backwards, spreading them at the same time so that the lumbar spine moves in.
- On each inhalation, extend the groins and buttock bones further backwards and the thighs further sideways. At the same time elongate the lower abdomen, rib cage, spine and head further forwards.
- On each exhalation, lower the chest and head further with gravity onto the feet and earth.
- Hold for one minute; then come up on an inhalation, raising first the head, then the chest, and then the abdomen.

2b. Supta Parvatasana
supta=lying down; parvata=mountain

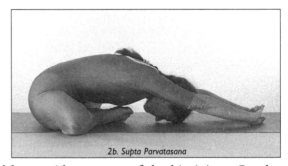

2b. Supta Parvatasana

- Sit in Parvatasana (1b) and then proceed:
- On a Mula Bandha inhalation, lift the pelvis and trunk up from the femur heads, rooting the buttock bones and the outer edges of the feet into the earth with the support of the Pada Bandha and elongating the thighs and knees sideways out of the hip joints. On the exhalation, bend forward till the sternum rests on the feet, and the head and hands rest on the blanket. The sternum arrives on the feet before the head and hands arrive on the blanket. Do not lift the buttock bones up, but extend them backwards, spreading them at the same time so that the lumbar spine moves in.
- On each inhalation, extend the groins and buttock bones further backwards and the thighs further sideways. At the same time elongate the lower abdomen, rib cage, spine, head and hands further forwards.
- On each exhalation, lower the chest and head further with gravity onto the feet and earth.
- Hold for one minute; then come up on an inhalation.

2c. Supta Gomukhasana

supta=lying down; go=cow; mukha=face

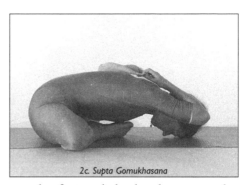

2c. Supta Gomukhasana

- Sit in Gomukhasana (1c) and then proceed:
- On a Mula Bandha inhalation, lift the pelvis and trunk up from the femur heads, rooting the buttock bones and the outer edges of the feet into the earth with the support of the Pada Bandha and elongating the thighs and knees sideways out of the hip joints. On the exhalation, bend forward till the sternum rests on the feet and the head rests on the blanket. The sternum arrives on the feet before the head arrives on the blanket. Do not lift the buttock bones up, but extend them backwards, spreading them at the same time, so that the lumbar spine moves in.
- On each inhalation, extend the groins and buttock bones further backwards and the thighs further sideways. At the same time elongate the lower abdomen, rib cage, spine and head further forwards.
- On each exhalation, lower the chest and head further with gravity onto the feet and earth, keeping both elbows up towards the sky.
- Hold for one minute. Then come up on an inhalation, raising first the head, then the chest, and then the abdomen. Change hands.

2d. Supta Namasté II

supta=lying down

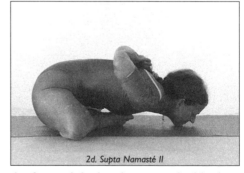

2d. Supta Namasté II

- Sit in Namasté II (1d) and then proceed:
- On a Mula Bandha inhalation, lift the pelvis and trunk up from the femur heads, rooting the buttock bones and the outer edges of the feet into the earth with the support of the Pada Bandha and elongating the thighs and knees sideways out of the hip joints. On the exhalation, bend forward till the sternum rests on the feet and the head rests on the blanket. The sternum arrives on the feet before the head arrives on the blanket. Do not lift the buttock bones up, but extend them backwards, spreading them at the same time so that the lumbar spine moves in.
- On each inhalation, extend the groins and buttock bones further backwards and the thighs further sideways. At the same time elongate the lower abdomen, rib cage, spine and head further forwards.
- On each exhalation, lower the chest and head further with gravity onto the feet and earth, keeping the elbows up towards the sky.
- Hold for one minute; then come up on an inhalation, raising first the head, then the chest, and then the abdomen.

3. Kandasana

kanda=root, base of the trunk

- Sit in Baddha Konasana I (1a) and then proceed:
- Hold the feet, keeping the thumbs on the inner arches, and the fingers covering the dorsal side of the feet.
- Lean the body backwards and lift the feet and legs till the feet are at the height of the sternum.
- Rotate the soles of the feet towards you and place them on the sternum.
- Rotate the knees forwards as much as you can, keeping the balance on the buttock bones.
- Hold for a few seconds.

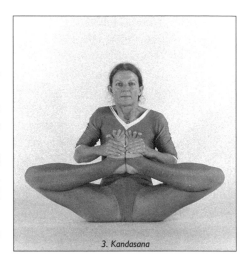

3. Kandasana

4. Mulabandhasana

mula=root, base, first chakra; bandha=fetter

- Sit in Baddha Konasana I (1a) and then proceed:
- Raise the heels, insert the arms underneath the ankles and clasp the fingers around the metatarsals of the big toes.
- Turn the heels further upwards and pull the toes under them, towards the pubic bone, till the feet rest vertically on the toes, close to the pubic bone.
- Hold for a few seconds.

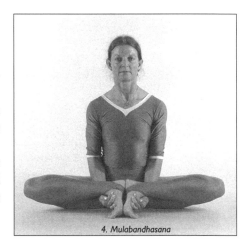

4. Mulabandhasana

5. Supta Baddha Konasana

supta=lying down;
baddha=bound; kona=angle

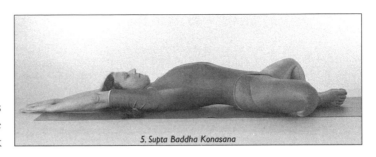

5. Supta Baddha Konasana

In this pose the pelvis is rotated backwards around the femur heads as in Back Bendings.

- Sit in Baddha Konasana I (1a) and then proceed:
- Keep the hands behind you on the blanket and, lifting the pelvis so that you are standing on the outer edges of the feet, rotate the pelvis backwards, so that the coccyx rolls towards the pubic bone and the two frontal hip bones move up towards the ribs. Then lower yourself onto the elbows, and finally onto the blanket. Keep the knees down.
- Keep the backward rotation of the pelvis, so that the lower abdomen moves in the direction of the ribs, and slide the back of the chest upwards in the direction of the head. In this way the whole lumbar region is elongated and brought down onto the blanket.
- Extend the thighs sideways out of the groins, and pull the two frontal hip bones up towards the ribs: double action, down and up, so that the groins in the middle are opened.
- On a Mula Bandha inhalation, extend the arms over the head on the blanket, without curving the lumbar up.
- On each inhalation, extend the thighs further sideways and downwards out of the hip joints, and the spine and arms further upwards.
- On each exhalation, press the lumbar further onto the blanket, maintaining the length of the body.
- Hold for one minute.

4.5 Navalama / Boat Poses

These positions are done in the *Vinyasa* mode, that is, going from one pose directly into the next one, using the breathing.

Navalama

....

1. *Dandasana*
2. *Paripurna Navasana*
3. *Ardha Navasana*
4. *Parvata Savasana*
5. *Supta Dandasana*

---

1. Dandasana
danda=staff

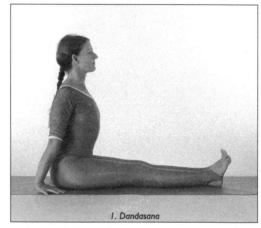

1. Dandasana

- Sit on a blanket with the legs extended straight in front of you as in Paschimotta-nasana (see page 127).
- Place the hands next to the hips on the blanket with the fingers pointing forwards towards the feet.
- On each Mula Bandha inhalation, root the buttock bones, the back of the legs and the hands into the earth, performing Hasta Bandha, and elongate the spinal column up towards the sky. Keep the feet together and the arches strong (Pada Bandha).
- Hold for three breaths. On an exhalation proceed to 2.

2. Paripurna Navasana

paripurna=entire, complete; nava=boat

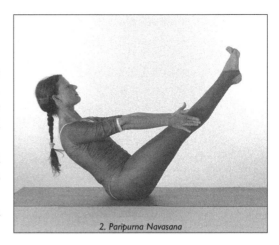
2. Paripurna Navasana

- Lean the trunk backwards and raise the legs up to an angle of forty-five degrees. Extend the arms forwards, parallel to the earth, with the palms of the hands parallel to the outer knees.
- Keep the back straight and the head and neck in line with the trunk. The trunk makes an angle of ninety degrees with the legs.
- Hold for three breaths. On an exhalation proceed to 3.

3. Ardha Navasana

ardha=half; nava=boat

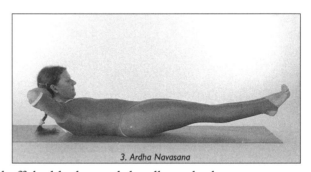
3. Ardha Navasana

- Clasp the hands behind the neck and lower the back and legs simultaneously, till the heels are about five inches above the blanket and the lumbar region and lower chest rest on the blanket. Keep the shoulder blades, shoulders and head off the blanket, and the elbows back.
- Hold for three breaths. On an exhalation proceed to 4.

4. Parvata Savasana

parvata=mountain;
sava=corpse

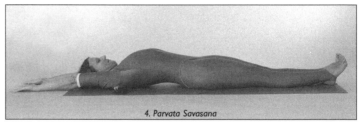
4. Parvata Savasana

- Lower the body completely onto the blanket and extend the arms over the head. Rest the back of the hands on the blanket, keeping the arms parallel to each other.
- On each Mula Bandha inhalation, elongate the arms out of the lower abdomen and sacro-iliac joints. On each exhalation, press the lumbar region more onto the blanket.
- Hold for three breaths. On an exhalation proceed to 5.

5. Supta Dandasana

supta=lying down; danda=staff

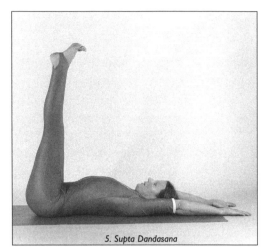

5. Supta Dandasana

- Raise the legs up to ninety degrees; keeping the knees straight and the arches strong.
- On each Mula Bandha inhalation, elongate the shoulders and arms further up towards the hands, and the groins further away from the lower abdomen, so that the sacrum remains flat on the blanket.
- Hold for three breaths. On an exhalation, return to Dandasana, bringing the legs down onto the blanket, and raising the trunk and arms in one smooth movement.

4.6 Leg Stretches

These positions are done in the *Vinyasa* mode, that is, going from one pose directly into the next one, using the breathing.

Leg Stretches

....

1. Urdhva Prasarita Padasana
2. Jathara Parivartanasana
3. Urdhvamukha Paschimottanasana II
4. Urdhvamukha Prasarita Padottanasana II
5. Supta Padangusthasana I
6. Supta Padangusthasana II
7. Supta Padangusthasana III
8. Anantasana
9. Hanumanasana
10. Samakonasana
11. Nakrasana

---

1. Urdhva Prasarita Padasana

urdhva=upwards; prasarita=extended;
pada=leg, foot

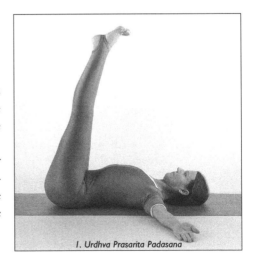

1. Urdhva Prasarita Padasana

- Lie on the back on a blanket with the legs together, extend the arms sideways at an angle of ninety degrees to the trunk and root the ulnar wrist points into the earth.
- On an exhalation, raise the legs to ninety degrees. Simultaneously extend the metatarsals of the big toes up towards the sky, the coccyx down towards the earth, and elongate the neck.
- Hold for one minute; then proceed to 2.

2. Jathara Parivartanasana

jathara=stomach; parivartana=turning, rolling

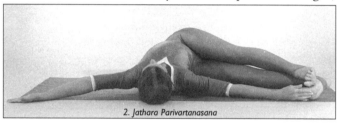

2. Jathara Parivartanasana

- On an exhalation, rotate the pelvis and bring the legs down to the right hand, keeping the knees straight and the feet together.
- Turn the head to the left and elongate the left arm, shoulder and shoulder blade away from the spine to the left, rooting the left ulnar wrist point, as a counter action to the legs going down towards the right.
- Inhale while the feet are on the right hand.
- On the exhalation lift the legs and take them over to the left hand, rotating the pelvis to the left and the head to the right.
- Elongate the right arm, shoulder and shoulder blade away from the spine to the right, rooting the right ulnar wrist point, as a counter action to the legs going down towards the left.
- Repeat three times; then return to Urdhva Prasarita Padasana (1) and proceed to 3.

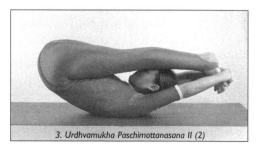

2. Jathara Parivartanasana

3. Urdhvamukha Paschimottanasana II

urdhva=upwards; mukha=face;
paschima=the West, the back of the body;
uttana=intense stretch

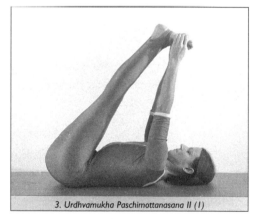

3. Urdhvamukha Paschimottanasana II (1)

3. Urdhvamukha Paschimottanasana II (2)

- On an exhalation hold the outer edges of the feet with the hands. Keep the knees straight and the back of the head and the sacrum on the blanket: elongate the back of the head upwards and the groins downwards, so that the whole spine is elongated.
- On an exhalation, raise the pelvis and bring the legs over the head, till they are parallel to the earth. Lift the head and bring the forehead to the shins.
- Hold for one minute; then lower the pelvis and head onto the blanket and proceed to 4.

4. Urdhvamukha Prasarita Padottanasana II

*urdhva=upwards; mukha=face;
prasarita=extended; pada=leg,foot;
uttana=intense stretch*

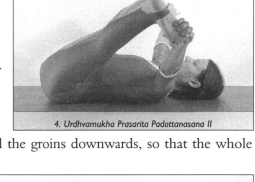

4. Urdhvamukha Prasarita Padottanasana II

- On an exhalation, hold the inner arches of the feet with the hands and spread the legs. Keep the knees straight and the back of the head and the sacrum on the blanket: elongate the back of the head upwards and the groins downwards, so that the whole spine is elongated.

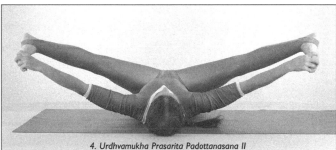

4. Urdhvamukha Prasarita Padottanasana II

- Turn the legs slightly outwards, elongate them out of the hip joints and lower the feet as much as you can, keeping the pelvis flat on the blanket.
- Hold for one minute; then return to Urdhva Prasarita Padasana (1) and proceed to 5.

5. Supta Padangusthasana I

supta=lying down; padangustha=big toe

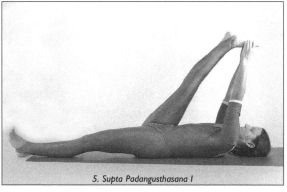

5. Supta Padangusthasana I

- On an exhalation, extend the left leg onto the blanket and hold the right foot with both hands. Keep both knees straight and the back of the head and the sacrum on the blanket: elongate the back of the head upwards and the groins downwards, so that the whole spine is elongated.
- On the next exhalation bring the right foot over the head, keeping the knee straight and the hips even; do not turn the right hip up.
- Keep the left foot strong (Pada Bandha) and the left knee straight; the back of the left leg and the left heel remain on the blanket.
- On each Mula Bandha inhalation, elongate the right groin away from the right ribs, and roll the right femur head backwards towards the left heel. On each exhalation, bring the right foot further over the head to the earth.
- Hold for one minute; then proceed to 6.

6. Supta Padangusthasana II
supta=lying down; padangustha=big toe

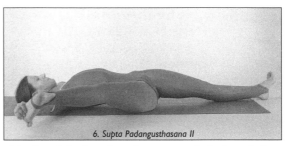
6. Supta Padangusthasana II

- Release the left hand and extend the left arm sideways on the blanket, at an angle of ninety degrees with the chest. Root the left ulnar wrist point into the blanket.

- Hold the inner arch of the right foot with the right hand and, on an exhalation, bring the foot down to the right side. Keep the left hip and heel down on the blanket and the left leg straight, performing Pada Bandha on the left foot to support the action in the pelvis.

- On each Mula Bandha inhalation, elongate the left leg and the spinal column, and on each exhalation take the right foot further down to the side.

- Turn the head to the left and elongate the left arm, shoulder and shoulder blade away from the spine to the left, rooting the left ulnar wrist point, as a counter action to the right leg going down towards the right.

- Hold for one minute; then proceed to 7.

7. Supta Padangusthasana III
supta=lying down; padangustha=big toe

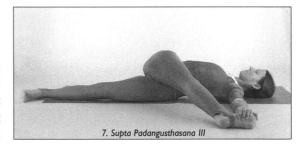
7. Supta Padangusthasana III

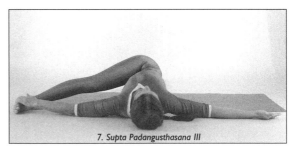
7. Supta Padangusthasana III

- On an exhalation lift the right leg up again. Release the right hand and hold the outer edge of the right foot with the left hand. Extend the right arm sideways on the blanket, at an angle of ninety degrees to the chest, and root the ulnar wrist point into the blanket.

- On the next exhalation take the right foot down to the left, rolling the hips to the left, so that you are resting on the left hip and the outer side of the left leg and foot. Keep the left foot strong (Pada Bandha) and the left knee straight.

- Turn the head to the right and elongate the right arm, shoulder and shoulder blade away from the spine to the right, rooting the right ulnar wrist point, as a counter action to the right leg going down towards the left.

- On each Mula Bandha inhalation, elongate the right groin away from the right ribs and roll the right femur backwards towards the left heel.

- Hold for one minute; then repeat 5, 6 and 7 with the left leg.

8. Anantasana

ananta=infinite

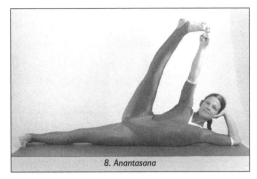

8. Anantasana

- Lie down on the left side of the trunk and the left leg. Extend the left arm in line with the side of the chest, so that the whole body makes one line, from the fingers of the left hand to the outer arch of the left foot. Bend the left arm and rest the left ear on the palm of the left hand.
- Bend the right leg. With the index and middle fingers of the right hand hold the big toe of the right foot and extend the leg up to the sky.
- Keep the body in alignment and stay on the side of the left hip; do not roll onto the backside of the pelvis.
- Rooting the whole left side of the body, especially the outer edge of the left foot (Pada Bandha) and the left ankle to keep the balance and lightness of the body, elongate the right leg up to the sky, out of the right hip joint.
- Hold for one minute.

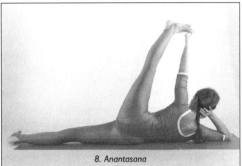

8. Anantasana

9. Hanumanasana

Hanuman is the monkey god. This pose is the Western 'split'.

9a. Hanumanasana

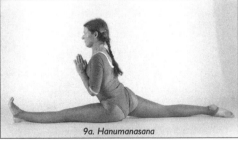

9a. Hanumanasana

- Kneel on hands and knees on a blanket, and then proceed:
- Bring the right leg forward between the hands, pointing the toes of the right foot up. Slide the right heel forward on the blanket, till the knee is straight and the calf muscle and thigh rest on the blanket. At the same time, lift the left knee and slide the left foot backwards on the blanket, till the left knee is straight and the shin bone and quadriceps muscle are resting on the blanket.
- Do not turn the left hip back, but roll it forwards, so that the left knee rests on the center of the knee on the blanket. The foot too should rest on the center of the dorsal side.
- Keep the pelvis and trunk as vertical as possible and the head, chest and pelvis facing in the direction of the right foot. Join the palms in front of the sternum in Namasté I and look straight forward.
- Hold for one minute; then proceed to 9b.

9b. ***Hanumanasana, arms upwards***

- On a Mula Bandha inhalation, elongate the arms up over the head and join the palms. Then proceed to 9c.

9c. ***Hanumanasana, bending forward***

- On the exhalation, bend forward and clasp the hands beyond the right foot as in Janu Sirsasana (see page 129). As in all Forward Bendings, it is the hand on the side of the straight (forward) leg which holds the opposite hand.
- Rest the head on the shin. On each inhalation, slide the head further forwards towards the right foot. On each exhalation, lower the trunk and head further with gravity onto the leg, keeping the back of the chest and the shoulder blades parallel to the earth.
- Hold for a few seconds; then repeat 9a and b on the other side.

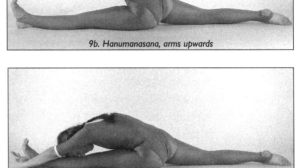

9b. Hanumanasana, arms upwards

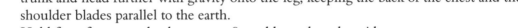

9c. Hanumanasana, bending forward

10. Samakonasana

sama=even, same; kona=angle

- Sit on the blanket with the legs spread as in Dvipada Upavistha Konasana (see page 142), and then proceed:
- Keep the feet vertical with the toes pointing straight up to the sky, and place the hands next to the hips on the blanket, with the fingers pointing forwards. Lift the pelvis and, sliding the legs and heels sideways out of the hip joints, bring the pelvis forwards while elongating the legs sideways, so that the angle between the two thighs increases.
- Keep the pelvis and trunk vertical and the face looking straight forward.
- Repeat lifting the pelvis and bringing it forward while sliding the legs out, till the legs form one continuous line with each other sideways (the sideways 'split').
- Join the palms in front of the sternum in Namasté I.
- Hold for one minute; then proceed to 11.

10. Samakonasana

11. Nakrasana

nakra=crocodile

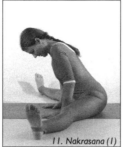
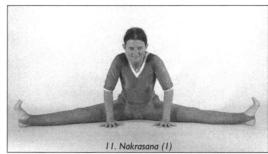

11. Nakrasana (1)   *11. Nakrasana (1)*

- Place the hands in front of you on the blanket with the fingers pointing forward.

- Rotate the pelvis forward and, shifting the weight of the body onto the hands, lift the pelvis and walk forwards on the hands while elongating the legs sideways, out of the hip joints, so that the heels slide away from the trunk. The legs will start to rotate inwards, till they slide backwards by themselves and you end up lying on the stomach with the legs extended backwards.

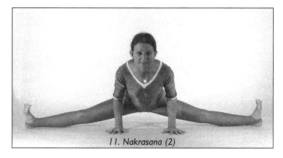

11. Nakrasana (2)

This position involves a complete rotation of the thighs in the hip joints. Do not attempt to do this pose until you have gained sufficient suppleness in Dvipada Upavistha Konasana (see page 142).

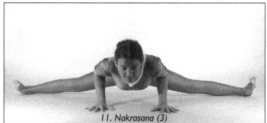

11. Nakrasana (3)

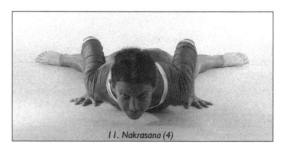

11. Nakrasana (4)

4.7 Forward Bendings

These positions can be done in <u>four different modes</u>:

a. **Performing each position separately** and holding it for one minute.

b. **Vinyasa**
Connecting two or more positions by flowing from one into the other, using the breathing.

c. **Mala**
Connecting all the positions through Surya Namaskar, using the breathing, and holding each of the Forward Bendings for the duration of three breaths.

d. **Taking only a few positions** and holding them for *five minutes* each.

Forward Bendings

1. Paschimottanasana
2. Parivrtta Paschimottanasana
3. Janu Sirsasana
   a. Maha Mudra
   b. Janu Sirsasana
4. Parivrtta Janu Sirsasana
5. Ardha Baddha Padma Paschimottanasana
6. Triangmukhaikapada Paschimottanasana I
7. Triangmukhaikapada Paschimottanasana II
8. Parivrtta Triangmukhaikapada Paschimottanasana II
9. Krounchasana
10. Akarna Dhanurasana
11. Marichyasana I
12. Marichyasana II
13. Ubhaya Padangusthasana
    a. Ubhaya Padangusthasana
    b. Urdhvamukha Prasarita Padottanasana I
14. Urdhvamukha Paschimottanasana I
15. Upavistha Konasana
    a. Dvipada Upavistha Konasana
    b. Ekapada Upavistha Konasana
    c. Parivrttaikapada Upavistha Konasana
16. Baddha Konasana II
17. Malasana
18. Kurmasana
19. Ekapada Sirsasana cycle
    a. Ekapada Sirsasana
    b. Kala Bhairavasana
    c. Bhairavasana
    d. Skandasana
    e. Chakorasana I
    f. Ruchikasana
    g. Durvasasana
20. Yoga Nidrasana
21. Dvipada Sirsasana
    a. Dvipada Sirsasana
    b. Chakorasana II

1. Paschimottanasana

paschima=the West, the back of the body;
uttana=intense stretch

Paschimottanasana is described in detail, as it forms the basic pose for all the following Forward Bending positions (see also Part Two: "Comparative Studies of Various Asanas", paragraph 4.13).

1. Paschimottanasana (1)

First part

- Sit on a blanket with the legs extended straight in front of you. Keep the knees straight with the knee caps facing the sky; do not turn the legs in or out. The back of the knees are in contact with the blanket.
- The feet are at equal distances from the trunk. Elongate the heels and big toe bones away from you, and pull the little toe bones towards you, so that the feet are vertical and all the toes are in line. Perform Pada Bandha in order to support the action in the pelvis.
- Pull the buttock muscles sideways and back with the hands, so that you sit on the buttock bones, not on the flesh. The weight of the trunk is evenly distributed between both buttock bones.
- The shoulder joints are in line with the hip joints and the back is vertical, so that the trunk is at a right angle to the legs. Thus the weight of the trunk is transmitted to the buttock bones in a straight line.
- The pelvis is vertical, so that the body rests on the points of the buttock bones, and is at right angles to the thighs in the hip joints, with the two frontal hip bones in line with the groins. Many people have the pelvis rotated backwards in Paschimottanasana, with the trunk resting on the back of the buttock bones or even on the coccyx, and this causes the back to bend, forcing the spinal vertebrae out of alignment. In this case one has to work at rotating the pelvis forward around the femur heads until it is vertical.
- With the pelvis in a vertical position, action has to be brought in the sacro-iliac joints. Constrict the outer hips and the adductor muscles on the inside of the thighs inwards towards each other and, keeping the two frontal hip bones in vertical alignment with the groins, lift them up and move them slightly forward, while rooting the buttock bones. The upper rim of the sacrum too is brought forward, together with the two frontal hip bones. At the same time, you have to also root the coccyx and move it forwards towards the pubic bone.
- As a result the entire pelvis widens laterally, is brought vertically forward towards the femur heads and lifted up from those femur heads, and the lower abdomen moves in and up towards the navel (Mula Bandha). This whole movement is the rebounce action: the coccyx and buttock bones root into the earth, going down with the force of gravity, so that the rest of the pelvis, the lower abdomen and the trunk elongate upwards against gravity.
- This whole movement is, of course, done on the Mula Bandha breathing, which creates the lightness in the spine that accompanies the anatomical movements.

Second part

- On an exhalation, rotate the pelvis forward to an angle of about forty-five degrees. Hold the outer edges of the feet with the hands, without moving the inner ankles apart and without bending the knees. Root the back of the thighs and the buttock bones into the earth without tightening the frontal part of the thighs.
- As the pelvis rotates forwards, do not draw the coccyx up towards the lumbar spine, but root it, elongating the back of the

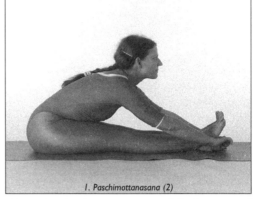

I. Paschimottanasana (2)

thighs, the buttock bones and the coccyx backwards. At the same time, lift the rest of the pelvis up from the femur heads and bring it forwards. Thus the pelvis is extended in opposite directions and widens at the back and the front: dual movement.
- One mistake is that the two frontal hip bones stay back when the body bends forwards, which means that the pelvis remains tilted backwards. This causes the body to bend in the lumbar vertebrae instead of in the groins. Another mistake is that the two frontal hip bones move forwards and *down*, which means that the whole pelvis, including the sacrum and the coccyx, is rotated forwards. Thus the coccyx is tipped back and up towards the lumbar spine, which collapses inward. This has a weakening effect on the lumbar spine.
- In the correct movement, the two frontal hip bones move forward and *up* as the pelvis rotates forwards. The abdomen below the navel moves forwards faster than the part above the navel, and the two frontal hip bones come to rest on the thighs before the ribs do.
- When the pelvis widens, the lower back widens too, and the lumbar spine elongates out of the pelvis by itself, giving the thrust for the entire spine to elongate forwards and up. No part of the trunk should aid the spine in elongating: the rib cage remains passive, and the spine and head are drawn out of the trunk like a sword out of its scabbard.
- When the lumbar spine elongates out of the pelvis, the thoracic spine continues that movement, so that the groove of the spine is visible from the sacrum up to the first thoracic vertebra, and has the same depth everywhere.

Third part

- When you have reached the maximum elongation from the sacrum to the back of the head, and from the pubic bone to the throat, place the head on the shins. The closer the forehead moves towards the feet, the better.
- Turn the palm of the right hand forward. With the thumb and the four fingers form a ring and place the dorsal side of the wrist

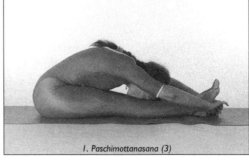

I. Paschimottanasana (3)

in the outer arch of the right foot. Turn the palm of the left hand forwards as well and insert the fingers of the left hand in the ring formed by the right hand. In this way there is the possibility of future elongation. Many people just clasp the fingers beyond the soles of the feet as in Head Balance, which means that there is no room for future elongation. In the way described above, the left hand can keep on sliding forward within the ring formed by the right hand, till the fingers of the right hand hold the left wrist, or even further. To maintain the evenness of the body, change hands every now and then.

- Many people pull the trunk forward with the hands, arms and shoulders. Thus they often pull only the chest, leaving the pelvis behind. The driving force for the trunk to elongate forwards lies in the pelvis: rubbing forwards on the buttock bones and rooting them, draw the two frontal hip bones forwards along the thighs towards the knees.
- The spinal column elongates forwards horizontally, but the chest remains passive: as the spine elongates forwards, the lower ribs too are drawn forwards along the thighs towards the knees as a result of the movement of pelvis and spine. Again, these movements should be done on the Mula Bandha breathing, elongating forwards on each inhalation, and lowering he trunk on each exhalation. Keep the shoulder blades, shoulders, arms and hands relaxed.
- Hold for one to ten minutes; then come up on an inhalation.

2. Parivrtta Paschimottanasana
parivrtta=turned around; paschima=the West, the back of the body; uttana=intense stretch

- Sit in Paschimottanasana (1).
- On an exhalation, turn to the right. Rotate the left arm as in Savasana (see page 286) and hold with the left hand the outer edge of the right foot. With the right hand hold the outer edge of the left foot. Turn the

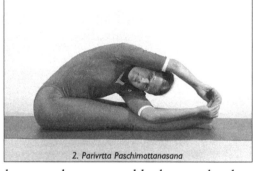

2. Parivrtta Paschimottanasana

trunk further to the right, insert the head in between the arms, and look up at the sky.
- Hold for one minute; then repeat on the other side .

3. Janu Sirsasana
janu=knee; sirsa=head

As Janu Sirsasana is one of the more complex positions in yoga, it is described here in great detail (see also Part Two: "Comparative Studies of Various Asanas: Front face - Back face", page 257).

3a. *Maha Mudra*
maha=great, noble; mudra=shutting, closing.

First part
- Sit on a blanket with the legs extended straight in front of you. Keep the knees straight with the knee caps facing the sky; do not turn the legs in or out. The back of the knees are in contact with the blanket.
- Bend the left leg and place the sole of the left foot against the inner side of the right thigh, near the pubic bone. Do not let the foot slip underneath the right thigh; it barely

touches it. The left (bent) knee rests on the blanket. The left thigh is at a right angle to the right thigh and the left frontal hip bone is slightly further back than the right one.

- The right leg extends straight out of the right hip joint, with the right foot in line with the right frontal hip bone. The knee is straight and the knee cap faces the sky; the back of the knee is in contact with the blanket. Elongate the heel and big toe bone away from you, and pull the little toe bone towards you, so that the foot is vertical and all the toes are in a line. Perform Pada Bandha with the right foot to support the action in the pelvis.

Second part

- On a Mula Bandha inhalation, lift the pelvis up from the femur heads and bring the weight of the body onto the right buttock bone, so that the left buttock bone is slightly lifted. Turn the pelvis and chest to the right, till the shoulders are perpendicular to the right leg. Root the right buttock bone into the earth, and elongate the spinal column upwards out of the sacro-iliac joints.

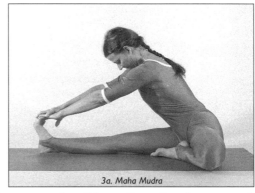
3a. Maha Mudra

- On the exhalation, rotate the pelvis forwards to an angle of about forty-five degrees, and with the left hand hold the outer edge of the right foot, keeping that foot vertical. The right hand rests lightly on the blanket on the right side of the right leg; do not put any weight on that hand. This position is called **Maha Mudra**.

- As the left frontal hip bone is further back than the right one, the spine (trunk) is not perpendicular to the right leg. You have to rotate the trunk towards the right, until the frontal central line (navel-sternum-throat) is in line with the right leg. The left thigh rotates inwards towards the left foot, and the left frontal hip bone rotates towards the navel, while the right one rotates away from the navel towards the right: the left side of waist and rib cage rotate towards the frontal central line, while the right side rotates away from that line towards the right. Beginners often rotate only the shoulders and ribs, but the movement should come from the pelvis.

- Do not pull the knee cap up, but release the tension at the front of the thigh and root the back of the knee into the earth. Extend the back of the leg from the knee to the heel forwards, elongating the heel away from you, and from the knee to the buttock bone backwards. The weight of the body is mainly on the right buttock bone: the left buttock bone is slightly lifted off the blanket, while the left thigh and hip bone rotate inwards.

- The spine, from the sacrum up to the cervical spine, is straight: if there is a deviation to the left it means that the trunk has not been fully rotated. It is very important for the spine to be straight from the beginning, because if there is a curvature to the left, there will be a great strain on the left side of the spine and on the left sacro-iliac joint in the third part of the pose. When the spine is straight and in the center of the back, the width of the rib cage and waist on the left and right side of the spine is equal; if the left side of the back is broader, the spine has curved to the left. Both sides of the back should be evenly long, straight, and parallel to each other.

3b.   *Janu Sirsasana*

Third part

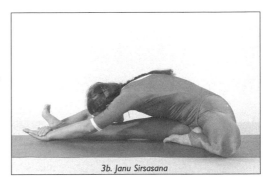

3b. Janu Sirsasana

- When you have reached maximum elongation from the sacrum to the back of the head, and from the pubic bone to the throat, place the head on the shin of the right leg. Keep the right foot vertical. The closer the forehead moves towards the right foot, the better. This position is called *Janu Sirsasana.*

- Turn the palm of the right hand forward, with the thumb and the four fingers form a ring and place the dorsal side of the wrist in the outer arch of the right foot. Turn the palm of the left hand forward as well and insert the fingers of the left hand in the ring formed by the right hand. In this way there is the possibility of future elongation. Many people just clasp the fingers beyond the sole of the foot as in Head Balance, which means that there is no room for future elongation. In the way described above the left hand can keep on sliding forwards within the ring formed by the right hand, till the fingers of the right hand hold the left wrist or even further. It is important to note that, with the right leg extended forward, it is the right hand which forms the ring for the left hand to slide through. This is because, by placing the back side of the right wrist in the small arch, that pressure stabilizes the right foot in its vertical position.

- The lower abdomen arrives first on the right thigh, then the navel; the navel comes to rest exactly on the midline of the right thigh. If this is not the case, but the navel stays on the inner side of the thigh, it means that you have not perfected the first part of this pose.

- After the navel, the sternum has to come to rest on the thigh, close to the knee on the midline of the thigh, not on the inner side. The head is the last to come and rest on the shin. You can either place the forehead on the shin, or, if you are more supple, the chin, so that the eyes look at the right foot. In both cases the neck, shoulders, shoulder blades and arms remain relaxed.

- On each Mula Bandha inhalation, slide the head (and of course the whole trunk) closer to the right foot.

- Hold for one minute; then repeat on the other side.

4. Parivrtta Janu Sirsasana

parivrtta=turned around; janu=knee;
sirsa=head

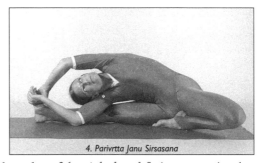

4. Parivrtta Janu Sirsasana

Sit in Maha Mudra (3a) with the right leg extended straight in front of you and proceed:

*   On an exhalation, turn to the left. Rotate the right arm as in Savasana (see page 286) and place the right elbow on the blanket against the inner side of the right knee, with the palm of the right hand facing up to the sky. Turn the whole trunk (pelvis, chest, shoulders and head) to the left.
*   Hold with the right hand the inner arch of the right foot. Extend the left arm up to the sky and elongate it out of the left hip joint; then hold the outer edge of the left foot with the left hand. Insert the head in between the arms and turn completely to the left, till the shoulders are vertically aligned above the right thigh. Look up at the sky.
*   Extend the left thigh out of the left hip joint, keeping the left knee down on the blanket.
*   On each Mula Bandha inhalation, elongate the whole right side of the trunk, from the right groin to the right armpit, forwards towards the right foot. Slide the right elbow closer to the right foot, so that the whole right side of the trunk rests on the thigh.
*   On each exhalation, continue the rotation of the trunk to the left.
*   Hold for one minute; then repeat on the other side.

5. Ardha Baddha Padma Paschimottanasana

ardha=half; baddha=bound; padma=lotus;
paschima=the West, the back of the body;
uttana=intense stretch

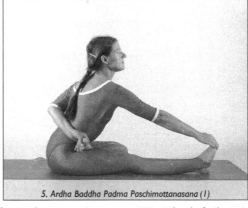

5. Ardha Baddha Padma Paschimottanasana (1)

*   Sit on a blanket with the legs extended straight in front of you. Keep the knees straight with the knee caps facing the sky; do not turn the legs in or out. The back of the knees are in contact with the blanket.
*   Bend the left leg and place the left foot in the groin of the right leg in the same way as for Padmasana (see page 77). The left (bent) knee is close to the right (straight) knee, so that the left thigh makes an angle of forty-five degrees or less with the right one. (Note that in Janu Sirsasana (3b) the left thigh makes an angle of ninety degrees with the right one.) In this way the pelvis is straight and the line between the two frontal hip bones, across the lower abdomen, is at a right angle to the straight leg (which in Janu Sirsasana is not the case).
*   The right leg extends straight out of the right hip joint, with the right foot in line with the right frontal hip bone. The knee is straight, and the knee cap faces the sky; the back of the knee is in contact with the blanket. Elongate the heel and big toe bone away from you, and pull the little toe bone towards you, so that the foot is vertical and all the toes are in a line. Perform Pada Bandha with the right foot to support the action in the pelvis.

- The weight of the body is divided equally between both buttock bones, and the left knee rests on the blanket.
- On an exhalation, rotate the left arm around the back in a large, circular movement and hold the metatarsals of the left foot. As the fingers curl around the metatarsals, the toes should also curl around the fingers, so that the foot holds the hand as much as the hand holds the foot. Keep the left

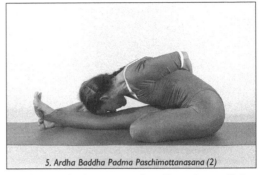

5. Ardha Baddha Padma Paschimottanasana (2)

  shoulder, rib cage, frontal hip bone and groin forward, facing in the direction of the right foot, and keep the left knee close to the right one, and on the blanket.
- On a Mula Bandha inhalation, lift the pelvis up from the femur heads, rooting the buttock bones into the earth and elongating the spinal column upwards out of the sacro-iliac joints.
- On the exhalation, rotate the pelvis forward to about forty-five degrees, and with the right hand hold the outer edge of the right foot, keeping the foot vertical.
- As the pelvis lifts up and moves forwards, the right frontal hip bone moves into the arch of the left foot, so that the heel of the left foot is embedded deep within the flesh of the lower abdomen, between the pubic bone and the navel.
- Do not pull the right knee cap up, but release the tension at the front of the thigh and root the back of the knee into the earth. Extend the back of the leg from the knee to the heel forwards, elongating the heel away from you, and from the knee to the buttock bone backwards.
- After reaching maximum elongation of the spinal column, lower the trunk onto the right leg. This should be done in stages, using the Mula Bandha breathing. On each inhalation, elongate forwards and on each exhalation, lower the trunk further. Lift the lower abdomen up and bring the lower ribs forwards over the foot onto the right thigh.
- The head is the last to come and rest on the shin beyond the knee. You can either place the forehead on the shin or, if you are more supple, the chin, so that the eyes look at the right foot. In both cases the neck, shoulders, shoulder blades and right arm remain relaxed. On each Mula Bandha inhalation, slide the head (and of course the whole trunk) closer to the right foot.
- Hold for one minute; then repeat on the other side.

6. Triangmukhaikapada Paschimottanasana I

tri=three; anga=limb; mukha=face; eka=one; pada=leg,foot; paschima=the West, the back of the body; uttana=intense stretch

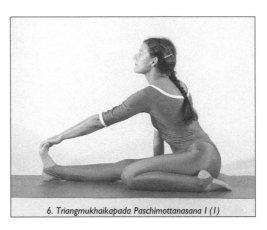

6. Triangmukhaikapada Paschimottanasana I (1)

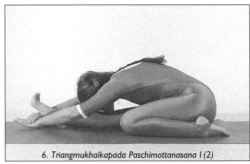

6. Triangmukhaikapada Paschimottanasana I (2)

- Sit on a blanket with the legs extended straight in front of you. Keep the knees straight with the knee caps facing the sky; do not turn the legs in or out. The back of the knees are in contact with the blanket.

- Bend the left leg backwards and place the left foot along the outside of the left hip as in Virasana I (see page 102). The arch of the left foot follows the curve of the left hip, so that the toes point towards the coccyx. The left knee stays next to the right knee, so that the inner knees and thighs remain in contact with each other. The right frontal hip bone has the same height as the left one, and the weight of the body is evenly distributed between both buttock bones. The pelvis is straight and the line between the two frontal hip bones, across the lower abdomen, is at a right angle to the straight leg.

- The right leg extends straight out of the right hip joint, with the right foot in line with the right frontal hip bone. The knee is straight, and the knee cap faces the sky; the back of the knee is in contact with the blanket. Elongate the heel and big toe bone away from you, and pull the little toe bone towards you, so that the foot is vertical and all the toes are in a line. Perform Pada Bandha with the right foot to support the action in the pelvis.

- On a Mula Bandha inhalation, lift the pelvis up from the femur heads, rooting the buttock bones into the earth and elongating the spinal column upwards out of the sacro-iliac joints.

- On the exhalation, rotate the pelvis forward to an angle of about forty-five degrees, and with the left hand hold the outer edge of the right foot, keeping that foot vertical. The right hand rests lightly on the blanket on the right side of the right leg, do not put any weight on that hand.

- Do not pull the right knee cap up, but release the tension at the front of the thigh and root the back of the knee into the earth. Extend the back of the leg from the knee to the heel forwards, elongating the heel away from you, and from the knee to the buttock bone backwards.

- After reaching maximum elongation of the spinal column, lower the trunk onto the right leg. This is done in stages, using the Mula Bandha breathing, so that on each inhalation you elongate forward, and on each exhalation you lower the trunk further, till the rib cage rests evenly on both thighs as in Paschimottanasana (1). Keep the right foot vertical.

- Turn the palm of the right hand forward, with the thumb and the four fingers form a ring and place the dorsal side of the wrist in the outer arch of the right foot. Turn the palm of the left hand forward as well, and insert the fingers of the left hand in the ring formed by the right hand (see the explanation given in Janu Sirsasana (3)). Do not tilt the left shoulder, shoulder blade and the left side of the rib cage up, but keep the whole back parallel to the earth.
- The head is the last to come and rest on the shin beyond the knee. As this pose is more like Paschimottanasana (1) than like Janu Sirsasana (3), the head rests against the inner side of the right shin. You can either place the forehead on the inner side of the shin or, if you are more supple, the chin, so that the eyes look at the right foot. In both cases the neck, shoulders, shoulder blades and arms remain relaxed. On each Mula Bandha inhalation, slide the head (and of course the whole trunk) closer to the right foot.
- Hold for one minute; then repeat on the other side.

7. Triangmukhaikapada Paschimottanasana II

tri=three; anga=limb; mukha=face; eka=one; pada=leg,foot; paschima=the West, the back of the body; uttana=intense stretch

This is basically the same position as the previous one, with the difference that here the left thigh forms an angle of ninety degrees with the right one, and the big toe at the back of the pelvis touches the coccyx as in Upavistha Virasana I (see page 104). One could call this position a reversed Janu Sirsasana (3). In Janu Sirsasana the left thigh is exorotated as in Sukhasana (see page 83), while here the left thigh is endorotated as in Virasana (see page 102). Thus the technique is the same as for Janu Sirsasana (3). Follow the instructions given for that pose.

- Hold for one minute; then repeat on the other side.

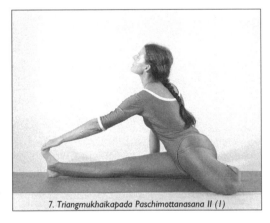

7. Triangmukhaikapada Paschimottanasana II (1)

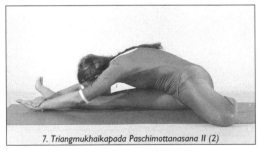

7. Triangmukhaikapada Paschimottanasana II (2)

8. Parivrtta Triangmukhaikapada Paschimottanasana II

parivrtta=turned around; tri=three; anga=limb;
mukha=face; eka=one; pada=leg, foot;
paschima=the West, the back of the body;
uttana=intense stretch

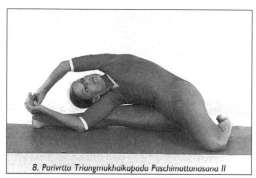

8. Parivrtta Triangmukhaikapada Paschimottanasana II

This position is basically the same as Parivrtta Janu Sirsasana (4). The difference is that here the left leg is endorotated as in Upavistha Virasana I (see page 102), while in Parivrtta Janu Sirsasana (4) the left leg is exorotated as for Sukhasana (see page 83).

* Sit in Triangmukhaikapada Paschimottanasana II (7) with the right leg extended straight in front of you and proceed:
* On an exhalation, turn to the left. Rotate the right arm as in Savasana (see page 286) and place the right elbow on the blanket against the inner side of the right knee, with the palm of right hand facing up to the sky. Turn the whole trunk (pelvis, chest, shoulders and head) to the left.
* Hold with the right hand the inner arch of the right foot. Extend the left arm up to the sky and elongate it out of the left hip joint, then hold the outer edge of the left foot with the left hand. Insert the head in between the arms and turn completely to the left, till the two shoulders are vertically aligned above the right thigh. Look up at the sky.
* Extend the left thigh out of the left hip joint, keeping the left knee down on the blanket.
* On each Mula Bandha inhalation, elongate the whole right side of the trunk, from the right groin to the right armpit, forwards towards the right foot. Slide the right elbow closer to the right foot, so that the whole right side of the trunk rests on the thigh.
* On each exhalation, continue the rotation of the trunk to the left.
* Hold for one minute; then repeat on the other side.

9. Krounchasana

krouncha=heron

This position is basically the same as Triangmukhaikapada Paschimottanasana I (6). The difference is that here the right leg is extended upwards instead of resting on the earth.

* Sit on a blanket with the legs extended straight in front of you. Keep the knees straight with the knee caps facing the sky; do not turn the legs in or out. The back of the knees are in contact with the blanket.
* Bend the left leg and place the left foot along the outer side of the left hip as in Virasana I (see page 102).

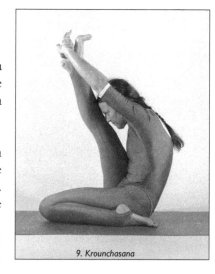

9. Krounchasana

The arch of the left foot follows the curve of the left hip, so that the toes point towards the coccyx. The left knee stays next to the right knee, so that the inner knees and thighs remain in contact with each other. The right frontal hip bone has the same height as the left one, and the weight of the body is evenly distributed between both buttock bones. The pelvis is straight, and the line between the two frontal hip bones, across the lower abdomen, is at a right angle to the straight leg.

- Bend the right leg. Turn the palm of the right hand upward, with the thumb and the four fingers form a ring and place the dorsal side of the wrist in the outer arch of the right foot. Turn the palm of the left hand upward as well, and insert the fingers of the left hand in the ring formed by the right hand (see the explanation given in Janu Sirsasana (3)). Then extend the right leg up towards the sky.
- On each Mula Bandha inhalation, lift the pelvis up from the femur heads, rooting the buttock bones into the earth and elongating the spinal column upwards out of the sacro-iliac joints. On each exhalation, rotate the pelvis further forwards and bring the right leg and the trunk closer to each other.
- The head is the last to come and rest on the shin beyond the knee. You can either place the forehead on the inner side of the shin or, if you are more supple, the chin, so that the eyes look up at the right foot. In both cases the neck, shoulders, shoulder blades and arms remain fairly relaxed. On each Mula Bandha inhalation, slide the head (and of course the whole trunk) up, closer to the right foot.
- Hold for one minute; then repeat on the other side.

10. Akarna Dhanurasana

a=near to; karna=ear; dhanu=bow

This pose is a combination of Paschimottanasana (1) and Krounchasana (9).

- Sit on a blanket with the legs extended straight in front of you.
- Bend forward; with the index and middle finger of the left hand, hold the big toe of the left foot, and with the index and middle finger of the right hand, hold the big toe of the right foot.
- Without turning the trunk or hips, bend the right leg and lift the right foot up next to the right ear. The right knee points backwards and sideways, away from the trunk, at an angle of forty-five degrees. Then extend the right leg up as in Krounchasana (9).
- Hold for one minute; then repeat on the other side.

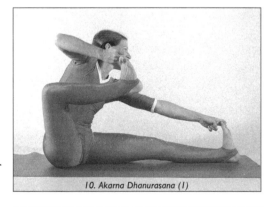

10. Akarna Dhanurasana (1)

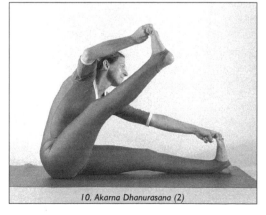

10. Akarna Dhanurasana (2)

11. Marichyasana I

Marichi is the son of Brahman

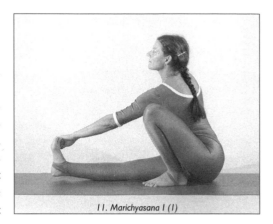

11. Marichyasana I (1)

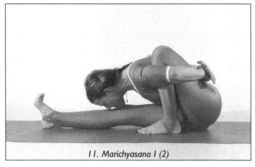

11. Marichyasana I (2)

- Sit on a blanket with the legs extended straight in front of you.
- Bend the left leg, so that the knee points up towards the sky and the left foot rests on the blanket next to the right thigh, with the toes pointing straight forward. In this position, the left buttock bone does not rest on the blanket, but the weight of the body is distributed between the right buttock bone and the left foot.
- The right leg extends straight out of the right hip joint, with the right foot in line with the right frontal hip bone. The knee is straight and the knee cap faces the sky. The back of the knee is in contact with the blanket. Elongate the heel and big toe bone away from you, and pull the little toe bone toward you, so that the foot is vertical and all the toes are in a line. Perform Pada Bandha with both feet to support the action in the pelvis.
- On a Mula Bandha inhalation, lift the pelvis up from the femur heads, rooting the left foot and the right buttock bone into the earth, and elongating the spinal column upwards out of the sacro-iliac joints.
- On the exhalation, rotate the pelvis forward to an angle of about forty-five degrees.
- Rotate the left frontal hip bone, the left side of the rib cage and the left shoulder forward, and place the left shoulder against the inner side of the left knee. Hold with the fingers of the left hand the outer edge of the right foot, keeping that foot vertical. The right hand rests lightly on the blanket on the right side of the right leg, do not put any weight on that hand.
- The inner side of the left knee rests against the backside of the left armpit, and the inner side of the left thigh rests against the left side of the rib cage.
- On each Mula Bandha inhalation, lift the pelvis up from the femur heads, rooting the right buttock bone and the left foot into the earth, and elongating the spinal column upwards out of the sacro-iliac joints.
- On each exhalation, rotate the trunk further towards the right.
- When you have reached the maximum elongation from the sacrum to the back of the head, and from the pubic bone to the throat, rotate the left arm backwards around the left knee in a large, circular movement. Do not elongate and rotate the left arm from the shoulder joint, but rather from the spinal column between the shoulder blades.
- Rotate the right arm backwards as well with a large, circular movement, and clasp the hands on the back. With the left knee bent, it is the left hand which has to hold the right hand. The reason is that in this position the left shoulder is in a slightly dangerous endorotation. By holding the right hand with the left, the muscles of the left shoulder are tensed and are therefore better able to hold the left shoulder in a strong and stable position.

- On each Mula Bandha inhalation, lift the pelvis up from the femur heads, rooting the left foot and the right buttock bone into the earth and elongating the spinal column forwards out of the sacro-iliac joints. On each exhalation, rotate the pelvis further forward and bring the trunk closer to the right leg.
- The head is the last to come and rest on the shin beyond the knee. You can either place the forehead on the shin or, if you are more supple, the chin, so that the eyes look at the right foot.
- Hold for one minute; then repeat on the other side.

12. Marichyasana II
Marichi is the son of Brahman

This is a combination of Padmasana (see page 77) and Marichyasana I (11).

- Sit on a blanket with the legs extended straight in front of you.
- Place the right foot in the left groin as in Padmasana (see page 77).
- Lean the body over on the right hip. Bend the left knee as in Marichyasana I (11) so that the knee points up towards the sky and the left foot rests on the blanket. The left heel touches the back of the left thigh and the toes point straight forward. In this position the left buttock bone does not rest on the blanket, but the weight of the body is distributed between the right hip and thigh, and the left foot.

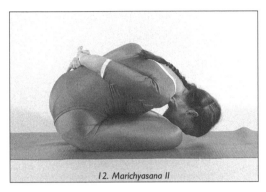
12. Marichyasana II

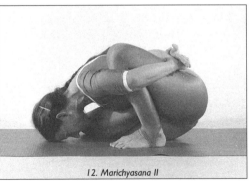
12. Marichyasana II

- On a Mula Bandha inhalation, lift the pelvis up from the femur heads. Root the left foot into the earth, bring the weight of the body forward onto the right thigh and knee, and elongate the spinal column upwards out of the sacro-iliac joints.
- On the exhalation, rotate the pelvis forward to an angle of about forty-five degrees.
- Rotate the left frontal hip bone, the left side of the rib cage and the left shoulder forward, and place the left shoulder against the inner side of the left knee. Elongate the left arm forward out of the left groin.
- The inner side of the left knee rests against the backside of the left armpit, and the inner side of the left thigh rests against the left side of the rib cage.
- On each Mula Bandha inhalation, lift the pelvis up from the femur heads, rooting the right thigh and knee and the left foot into the earth, and elongating the spinal column upwards out of the sacro-iliac joints.
- When you have reached maximum elongation from the sacrum to the back of the head, and from the pubic bone to the throat, rotate the left arm backwards around the left knee in a large, circular movement. Do not elongate and rotate the left arm from the shoulder joint, but rather from the spinal column between the shoulder blades.

- Rotate the right arm backwards as well with a large, circular movement, and clasp the hands on the back. With the left knee bent as in Marichyasana I (11), it is the left hand which has to hold the right. The reason is that in this position the left shoulder is in a slightly dangerous endorotation. By holding with the left hand the right, the muscles of the left shoulder are tensed and therefore are better able to hold the left shoulder in a strong and stable position.
- On each Mula Bandha inhalation, lift the pelvis up from the femur heads, rooting the left foot and the right thigh and knee into the earth, and elongating the spinal column forwards out of the sacro-iliac joints. On each exhalation, rotate the pelvis further forward and bring the trunk closer to the right leg.
- The head is the last to come and rest on the blanket in between the left foot and the right knee.
- Hold for one minute; then repeat on the other side.

13. Ubhaya Padangusthasana

ubhaya=both; padangustha=big toe

13a. Ubhaya Padangusthasana

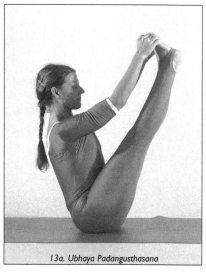

This position is basically the same as the first and second part of Paschimottanasana (1). The difference is that here the legs are extended up towards the sky, and the body balances on the buttock bones.

- Sit on a blanket with the legs extended straight in front of you.
- Bend the knees and hold the big toes with the index and middle fingers of the hands.
- Lean the body slightly backwards and extend the legs up towards the sky, keeping the inner ankles

13a. Ubhaya Padangusthasana

together. Do not bend the lumbar and thoracic spine. This position is an excellent toner for the front and back muscles of the trunk.
- On each Mula Bandha inhalation, lift the pelvis up from the femur heads, rooting the buttock bones into the earth and elongating the spinal column upwards out of the sacro-iliac joints. On each exhalation, rotate the pelvis further forward, so that the weight of the body rolls forwards onto the points of the buttock bones.
- Hold for one minute; then proceed to 13b.

13b. *Urdhvamukha Prasarita Padottanasana I*
urdhva=upwards; mukha=face; prasarita=spread;
pada=leg, foot; uttana=intense stretch

This position is the same as Dvipada Upavistha
Konasana (15a). The difference is that here the
legs are extended up towards the sky and the
body balances on the buttock bones.

- Spread the legs, maintaining the balancing
  position on the buttock bones.
- Follow the same instructions as for the
  previous pose.
- Hold for one minute.

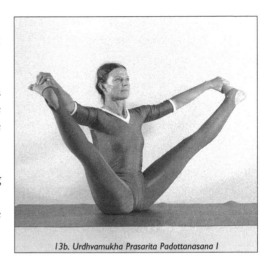
13b. Urdhvamukha Prasarita Padottanasana I

14. Urdhvamukha Paschimottanasana I
urdhva=upwards; mukha=face; paschima=the West,
the back of the body; uttana=intense stretch

This position is the same as the third part of
Paschimottanasana (1). The difference is that here the
legs are extended up towards the sky and the body
balances on the buttock bones.

- Sit in Ubhaya Padangusthasana (13a) and proceed:
- On an exhalation, close the trunk and head with
  the legs as described in Paschimottanasana (1).
  As you are here working upwards against the force
  of gravity, it is harder to keep the back straight
  and elongate the spinal column upwards out of
  the groins and the sacro-iliac joints. Follow the
  instructions given for Paschimottanasana (1).
- Hold for one minute.

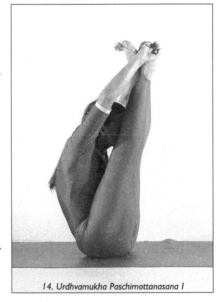
14. Urdhvamukha Paschimottanasana I

15. Upavistha Konasana
upavistha=seated; kona=angle

15a. Dvipada Upavistha Konasana
dvi=two; pada=leg, foot;
upavistha=seated; kona=angle

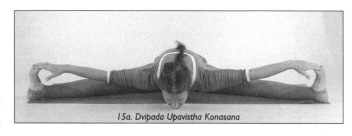
15a. Dvipada Upavistha Konasana

First part
- Sit on a blanket with the legs extended straight in front of you.
- Spread the legs as far apart as possible. Keep the knees straight with the knee caps facing the sky; do not turn the legs in or out. The back of the knees are in contact with the blanket. Elongate the heels and big toe bones away from you, and pull the little toe bones towards you, so that the feet are vertical and the toes point straight up to the sky. Perform Pada Bandha to support the action in the pelvis.
- Do not pull the knee caps up, but release the tension at the front of the thighs and root the back of the knees into the earth. Extend the back of the legs from the knees to the heels forwards, elongating the heels away from you, and from the knees to the buttock bones backwards.
- Root the buttock bones and the coccyx into the earth, together with the back of the thighs, and draw the two frontal hip bones forward and up towards the ribs: rebounce action, extending the pelvis in opposite directions, down and up.

Follow the instructions given in Paschimottanasana (1). The only difference is that in this position, the legs are spread.

Second part
- On an exhalation, rotate the pelvis forward and place the hands on the ankles. The feet remain vertical and the backs of the knees remain in contact with the blanket.
- Follow the instructions given in Paschimottanasana (1). The only difference is that in this position, the legs are spread and thus you can rotate the pelvis more than forty-five degrees forward.
- Do not allow the legs to rotate inward as the body bends forwards: the knee caps continue facing the sky. In this pose, special care must be taken not to tip the coccyx back and up towards the lumbar spine. Keep the coccyx firmly rooted by elongating the buttock bones and coccyx back and *down* as you draw the two frontal hip bones forward and *up*.

Third part
- When you have reached maximum elongation from the sacrum to the back of the head and from the pubic bone to the throat, place the head on the blanket. The further the head moves forward, the better.
- Here too the driving force for the trunk to elongate forwards lies in the pelvis. Rubbing forward on the buttock bones and rooting them, draw the two frontal hip bones forward and elongate the spine horizontally forwards. The chest remains passive; as the spine elongates, the rib cage too moves forwards as a result of the movement of the pelvis and the spine.

- Keep the shoulder blades, shoulders, arms and hands relaxed. Eventually, you can place the chest on the blanket in between the legs. Keep the palms of the hands on the tips of the toes with the fingers straight. Slide the hands further sideways on the toes as the trunk and head slide forwards on the blanket.
- Hold for one to five minutes.

15b. *Ekapada Upavistha Konasana*
eka=one; pada=leg, foot; upavistha=seated; kona=angle

- Start with the first part of Dvipada Upavistha Konasana (15a) and proceed:

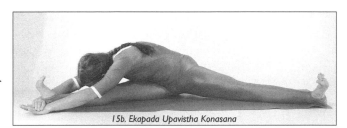

15b. Ekapada Upavistha Konasana

First part
- On a Mula Bandha inhalation, lift the pelvis up from the femur heads, rooting the buttock bones into the earth and elongating the spinal column upwards out of the sacro-iliac joints.
- On the exhalation, rotate the pelvis and trunk towards the right and with the left hand hold the outer edge of the right foot, keeping that foot vertical. The right hand rests lightly on the blanket on the right side of the right leg, do not put any weight on that hand.
- Rotate the trunk toward the right, until the frontal central line (navel-sternum-throat) is in line with the right leg. The left thigh rotates slightly inwards, and the left frontal hip bone rotates toward the navel, while the right frontal hip bone rotates away from the navel to the right: the left side of waist and rib cage rotates towards the right leg, while the right side rotates away from the right leg towards the right. Beginners often rotate only shoulders and ribs, but the movement should come from the pelvis.
- Do not pull the knee caps up; release the tension at the front of the thighs and root the back of the knees into the earth. At the same time, elongate the back of the legs from the buttock bones towards the heels, elongating the heels away from you. The weight of the body is mainly on the right buttock bone. The left buttock bone is slightly lifted off the blanket and the left thigh and frontal hip bone rotate slightly inwards.
- The spine from the sacrum up to the cervical spine is straight; if there is a deviation to the left it means that the trunk has not been fully rotated. It is very important for the spine to be straight from the beginning; if there is a curvature to the left, there will be a great strain on the left side of the spine and on the left sacro-iliac joint in the second part of the pose. When the spine is straight and in the center of the back, the width of rib cage and waist on the left and right side of the spine is equal; if the left side of the back is broader, the spine has curved to the left. Both sides of the back should be evenly long, straight, and parallel to each other.

Second part

- When you have reached maximum elongation from the sacrum to the back of the head, and from the pubic bone to the throat, place the head on the shin of the right leg. The closer the forehead moves towards the right foot, the better. Keep the right foot vertical.
- Turn the palm of the right hand forward, with the thumb and the four fingers form a ring and place the dorsal side of the wrist in the outer arch of the right foot. Turn the palm of the left hand forward as well, and insert the fingers of the left hand in the ring formed by the right hand. In this way there is the possibility of future elongation. It is important to note that on the right side it is the right hand which forms the ring for the left hand to slide through. This is because, by placing the back side of the right wrist in the small arch of the right foot, that pressure stabilizes the right foot in its vertical position (see the description in Janu Sirsasana (3)).
- The lower abdomen arrives first on the right thigh, then the navel; the navel comes to rest exactly on the midline of the right thigh. If this is not the case, but the navel stays on the inner side of the thigh, it means you have not perfected the first part of this pose.
- After the navel, the sternum comes to rest on the thigh, close to the knee on the midline of the thigh, not on the inner side. The head is the last to come and rest on the shin. You can either place the forehead on the shin, or, if you are more supple, the chin, so that the eyes look at the right foot. In both cases the neck, shoulders, shoulder blades and arms remain relaxed. On each Mula Bandha inhalation, slide the head (and of course the whole trunk) closer to the right foot.
- Hold for one minute; then repeat on the other side.

15c. Parivrttaikapada Upavistha Konasana

Parivrtta=turned around;
eka=one; pada=leg,foot;
upavistha=seated; kona=angle

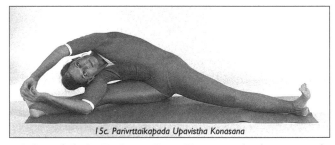

15c. Parivrttaikapada Upavistha Konasana

This position is basically the same as Parivrtta Janu Sirsasana (4). The difference is that here both legs are straight, while in Parivrtta Janu Sirsasana the leg, towards which you are turning, is bent.

- Start with the first part of Ekapada Upavistha Konasana (15b) towards the right leg and proceed:
- On an exhalation, turn to the left. Rotate the right arm as in Savasana (see page 286) and place the right elbow on the blanket against the inner side of the right knee, with the palm of the right hand facing up to the sky. Turn the whole trunk (pelvis, chest, shoulders and head) to the left.
- Hold with the right hand the inner arch of the right foot. Extend the left arm up to the sky and elongate it out of the left hip joint, then hold the outer edge of the left foot with the left hand. Insert the head in between the arms and turn completely to the left, till the two shoulders are vertically aligned above the right thigh. Look up at the sky.
- Extend the left leg out of the left hip joint, keeping the left knee down on the blanket.

- On each Mula Bandha inhalation, elongate the whole right side of the trunk, from the right groin to the right armpit, forwards towards the right foot. Slide the right elbow closer to the right foot, so that the whole right side of the trunk rests on the thigh.
- On each exhalation, continue the rotation of the trunk to the left.
- Hold for one minute; then repeat on the other side.

16. Baddha Konasana II

baddha=bound; kona=angle

(See also page 112.)

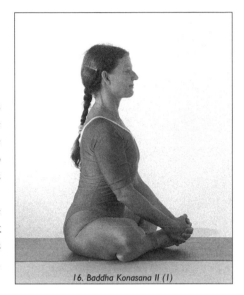

16. Baddha Konasana II (1)

- Sit on a blanket with the knees spread sideways and the soles of the feet united. Hold with the hands the feet and pull the heels as close to the pubic bone as possible. Lower the knees to the blanket by elongating the thighs sideways out of the hip joints.
- Pull the buttock muscles backwards with the hands, so that you are sitting on the buttock bones, not on the flesh. The body weight is divided evenly between both buttock bones. Then hold the feet with the hands again.
- The pelvis is in a vertical position, with the two frontal hip bones in vertical alignment above the groins. The groove of the spine is even from base to top and runs straight upwards.
- On a Mula Bandha inhalation, root the buttock bones, the outer thighs and the outer edges of the feet into the earth, lift the pelvis and trunk up from the femur heads and elongate the spinal column upwards.
- On the exhalation, extend the thighs and knees

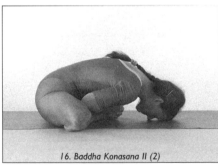

16. Baddha Konasana II (2)

sideways out of the hip joints and bend forward, till the sternum rests on the feet and the head on the blanket. The sternum arrives on the feet before the head arrives on the blanket. Do not lift the buttock bones up, but extend them backwards, spreading them at the same time.
- On each inhalation, extend the buttock bones further backwards and the thighs further sideways. At the same time, elongate the lower abdomen, rib cage, spine and head further forwards.
- On each exhalation, lower the trunk and head with gravity onto the feet and earth.
- Hold for one to five minutes; then come up on an inhalation, raising first the head, then the chest, and then the abdomen.

17. Malasana

mala=garland

- Start with Utkatasana II (see page 100) and proceed:
- Widen the knees, lower the elbows onto the blanket, and then press the inner thighs against the sides of the rib cage.
- On a Mula Bandha inhalation, root the feet into the earth, extend the groins, the buttock bones and the back of the thighs backwards, and elongate the lower abdomen, rib cage, spine, head and hands forwards.
- On the exhalation, rotate both arms backwards with a large, circular movement, and clasp the hands on the back. Or, hold the back of the heels with the hands if you cannot clasp the hands on the back. Then lower the head onto the blanket.
- Hold for one minute; then stand up again in Tadasana on an exhalation.

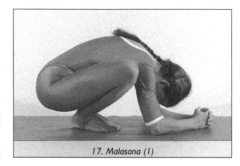

17. Malasana (1)

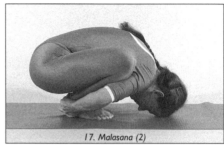

17. Malasana (2)

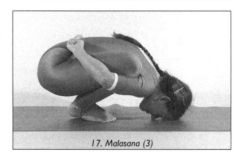

17. Malasana (3)

18. Kurmasana

kurma=tortoise

- Sit on a blanket with the legs extended straight in front of you.
- Widen the legs, until the distance between the feet is slightly more than the width of the shoulders.
- Bend the knees. Turn the legs slightly outwards and insert the shoulders underneath the knees, till the backs of the knees rest on the deltoid muscles. Then extend the arms sideways.

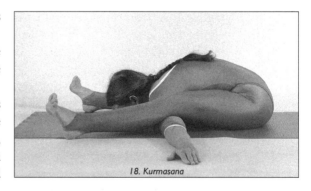

18. Kurmasana

- Roll the legs inwards again, till the knees point straight up towards the sky and the inner thighs press against the side ribs. Extend the legs till they are straight, and elongate the heels forward, keeping the feet vertical.
- Rest the head on the blanket, on either the forehead or the chin. On each Mula Bandha inhalation, elongate the trunk and spine forward from the groins towards the head. On each exhalation, elongate the legs further forwards, so that the knees press down more onto the deltoid muscles, and elongate the arms further sideways.
- Hold for one minute.

19. Ekapada Sirsasana cycle

eka=one; pada=leg, foot; sirsa=head

19a. Ekapada Sirsasana

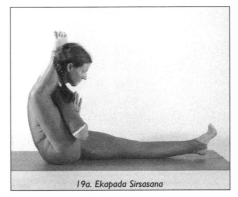
19a. Ekapada Sirsasana

- Sit on a blanket with the legs extended straight in front of you.
- Hold the right foot in both hands and lift it as for Padmasana (see page 77). The right hand supports the right ankle, and the left hand holds the metatarsals of the foot.
- Lift the foot to face level and rotate the knee so that it points sideways, not backwards.
- Place the right hand on the calf muscle of the right leg, and with the thumb push the calf muscle backwards over the shoulder.
- Turn the chest and shoulders towards the left, and insert the right shoulder underneath the knee of the right leg.
- Then lift the right foot over the back of the head, till the outer ankle rests against the back of the neck.
- Lift the face to look forward, not downwards. The back will be bent, but try to keep the bending minimal. Fold the hands in Namasté I in front of the sternum.
- As the tendency in this pose is to roll the pelvis backwards on the buttock bones, you have to counteract that by keeping the left leg firm and performing Pada Bandha with the left foot. In this way you can pull the trunk forward to the vertical line.
- On each Mula Bandha inhalation, elongate the trunk upwards, and on each exhalation maintain that height.
- Hold for a few seconds; then repeat on the other side.

Practice this position for a while till you feel comfortable in it. Then you can try the variations. These variations are done in the Vinyasa mode, that is, proceeding directly from one to the next, using the breathing.

19b. Kala Bhairavasana

Kala Bhairava is Shiva in his aspect as destroyer of the universe

- Start with Ekapada Sirsasana (19a) and proceed:
- Roll onto the left hip and the outer edge of the left foot. Place the left hand behind the body on the blanket, so that the arm forms an angle of ninety degrees with the side of the trunk, and

19b. Kala Bhairavasana

the fingers point away from the left hip. Push the body up on the left hand and the left foot.
- This pose resembles Kasyapasana (see page 190). The left side of the trunk forms one continuous line with the left leg. Extend the right arm up to the sky and look straight forward.
- Root the left hand, performing Hasta Bandha, and the outer edge of the left foot, performing Pada Bandha, to lighten the body.
- Hold for a few seconds; then proceed to 19c.

19c. *Bhairavasana*

bhairava=terrible, formidable

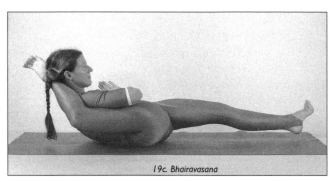

19c. Bhairavasana

- Lower the body again on the left hip and then roll onto the back.
- Press the back of the neck firmly against the outer right ankle, so that the foot does not slip over the head.
- Extend the left leg on the blanket, so that the knee faces straight up towards the sky and the left heel rests on the blanket. Perform Pada Bandha on the left foot to keep the leg straight and firm.
- Hold for a few seconds; then proceed to 19d.

19d. *Skandasana*

Skanda is Kartikeya, the god of war

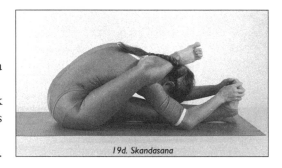

19d. Skandasana

- Come back up again to Ekapada Sirsasana (19a).
- On an exhalation, bend the trunk forward, hold the left foot with the hands and bring the head to the shin.
- Hold for a few seconds; then proceed to 19e.

19e. *Chakorasana I*

chakora is a bird

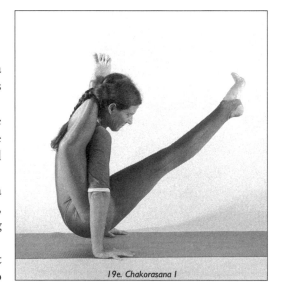

19e. Chakorasana I

- Come back up to Ekapada Sirsasana (19a) and place the hands next to the hips on the blanket.
- Push the whole body up, till you are standing on the two hands only, with the left leg extended straight forward, parallel to the earth. Look straight forward.
- This pose resembles Ekahasta Bhujasana (see page 194). As in Ekahasta Bhujasana, the weight of the straight (suspended) leg is sustained by the abdominal muscles.
- On each Mula Bandha inhalation, root the hands and perform Hasta Bandha to lighten the body.
- Hold for a few seconds; then proceed to 19f.

19f. Ruchikasana
Ruchika is the name of a sage

- Sit down again in Ekapada Sirsasana (19a) and bend the left knee. Place the sole of the foot close to the left buttock bone on the blanket, with the knee pointing up towards the sky.
- Place the hands on the blanket next to you, lift the pelvis up and bring the weight of the body onto the left foot. Then stand up. Keep the right hand on the blanket next to the left foot and hold the left ankle with the left hand. Rest the head on the shin. This pose resembles Ardha Baddha Padmottanasana.
- Hold for a few seconds; then proceed to 19g.

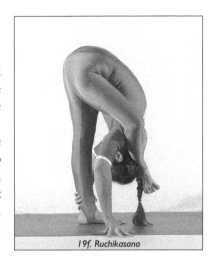
19f. Ruchikasana

19g. Durvasasana
Durvasa is the name of a saint

- On an inhalation, raise the trunk and stand straight up on the left leg.
- In this pose it is very difficult to stand straight. The main issue is to keep the balance and to lift the trunk and head as much as possible.
- Hold for a few seconds; then repeat 19a through 19g on the other side.

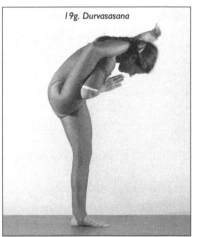
19g. Durvasasana

20. Yoga Nidrasana
nidra=sleep

- Lie on the back on a blanket.
- Bend the legs and spread the knees, so that the backs of the knees rest against the outer sides of the deltoid muscles. Hold the ankles with the hands, with the thumbs pointing inwards towards each other.

20. Yoga Nidrasana

- Raise the head, and insert the shoulders one by one inside the knees. Cross the ankles behind the head or neck.
- Rotate the arms backwards around the thighs, and clasp the hands at the back of the pelvis.
- In this pose the back is bent. Try, however, to straighten it as much as possible, using the Mula Bandha breathing: on each Mula Bandha inhalation, widen the upper chest and shoulders, and extend the feet further backwards, so that the angle in the knees increases. On each exhalation, lower the sacrum further to the earth.

- Hold for a few seconds (you can increase the time to one minute); then change the crossing of the feet.

The following positions are done in the Vinyasa mode, that is, flowing from one into the other, using the breathing:

21. Dvipada Sirsasana

dvi=two; pada=leg, foot; sirsa=head

21a. Dvipada Sirsasana

This is basically the same position as Yoga Nidrasana (20). The difference is that here you are not lying on the back, but are sitting on the buttock bones. Thus the added problem in this pose is that of the balance. This again depends on a finely tuned cooperation between the lower back muscles and the abdominal muscles.

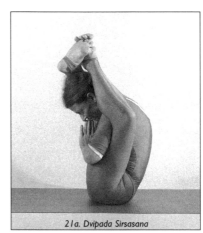

21a. Dvipada Sirsasana

- Start with Ekapada Sirsasana (19a), placing the right foot behind the neck.
- Bend the left leg and bring the left foot back over the head in the same way. Cross the ankles in the neck as in Yoga Nidrasana (20), fold the palms in front of the sternum in Namasté I and look straight forward.
- Hold for a few seconds; then proceed to 21b.

21b. Chakorasana II

chakora is a bird

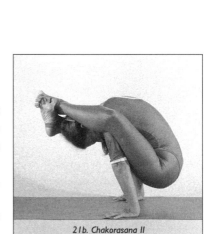

- Place the hands next to the hips on the blanket, slant the body a little forward and push up, till you are standing on the hands. Perform Hasta Bandha in order to lighten the body.
- Keep the grip between the feet and ankles strong, so that the legs will not slip off from the head.
- Hold for a few seconds; thange the crossing of the feet and repeat 21a and b.

21b. Chakorasana II

4.8 Twisting Poses

These positions can be done in <u>three different modes</u>:

a. **Performing each position** separately and holding it for one minute.

b. **Vinyasa**
Connecting two or more positions by flowing from one into the other, using the breathing.

c. **Mala**
Connecting all the positions through Surya Namaskar, using the breathing and holding each of the Twisting Poses for the duration of three breaths.

T w i s t i n g   P o s e s

....

1.	Parivrttaikapada Padmasana I	8. Marichyasana III
2.	Parivrttaikapada Padmasana II	9. Marichyasana IV
3.	Parivrtta Padmasana	10. Marichyasana V
4.	Bharadvajasana I	11. Pasasana
5.	Bharadvajasana II	12. Ardha Matsyendrasana
6.	Vamadevasana	13. Paripurna Matsyendrasana
7.	Yogadandasana	

1. Parivrttaikapada Padmasana I

parivrtta=turned around; eka=one;
pada=leg,foot; padma=lotus

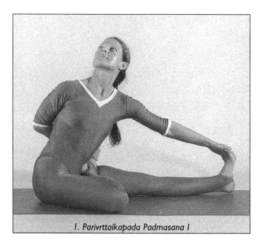

1. Parivrttaikapada Padmasana I

- Sit on a blanket with the legs extended straight in front of you.
- Take the right foot in both hands as for Padmasana (see page 77) and place it in the left groin.
- On a Mula Bandha inhalation root the buttock bones and the right knee into the earth, lift the pelvis up from the femur heads and elongate the whole body upwards. Extend the right arm up to the sky.
- On the exhalation rotate the trunk towards the right, swing the right arm around the back and hold the right foot. Curl the toes of the foot around the fingers, so that the foot holds as much the hand as the hand the foot (Pada Bandha).
- Keep the left leg straight and perform Pada Bandha on both the feet to support the action in the pelvis. With the left hand hold the left foot from the top and turn the head towards the right.
- On each Mula Bandha inhalation elongate the lower abdomen and spinal column further upwards towards the back of the head, rooting the buttock bones and the right knee into the earth.
- On each exhalation rotate the trunk, chest, shoulders and head further towards the right till the chest and shoulders are aligned with the left (straight) leg.
- Hold for one minute. Then repeat on the other side

2. Parivrttaikapada Padmasana II

parivrtta=turned around; eka=one; pada=leg, foot;
padma=lotus

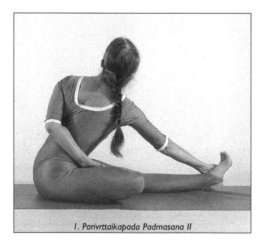

1. Parivrttaikapada Padmasana II

- Sit on a blanket with the legs extended straight in front of you.
- Take the right foot in both hands as for Padmasana (see page 77) and place it in the left groin.
- On a Mula Bandha inhalation root the buttock bones and the right knee into the earth, lift the pelvis up from the femur heads and elongate the whole body upwards. Extend the left arm up to the sky.
- On the exhalation rotate the trunk towards the left, swing the left arm around the back, and hold the right shin.
- Keep the left leg straight and perform Pada Bandha on both feet to support the action in the pelvis. With the right hand hold the left foot from the top and turn the head towards the left.

- On each Mula Bandha inhalation elongate the lower abdomen and spinal column further upwards towards the back of the head, rooting the buttock bones and the right knee into the earth.
- On each exhalation rotate the trunk, chest, shoulders and head further towards the left till the chest and shoulders are aligned with the left (straight) leg.
- Hold for one minute. Then repeat on the other side.

3. Parivrtta Padmasana

parivrtta=turned around; padma=lotus

3a. Parivrtta Siddhasana

For those people who cannot do full Padmasana (see page 77) this Twisting Pose can also be done in Siddhasana (see page 84).

- Sit in Siddhasana with the right foot on the left thigh. The knees should be fairly close together so that both feet stick out on the sides of the thighs. Thus the right knee rests on the left shin and ankle, not on the foot.

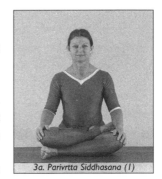
3a. Parivrtta Siddhasana (1)

- On a Mula Bandha inhalation root the buttock bones and the left knee into the earth, lift the pelvis up from the femur heads and elongate the whole body upwards. Extend the right arm up to the sky.
- On the exhalation rotate the trunk towards the right, swing the right arm around the back and hold the right foot. Curl the toes of the foot around the fingers, so that the foot holds as much the hand as the hand the foot (Pada Bandha).
- Cross the left arm over the right thigh, turning the arm as in Savasana (see page 286). Place the back of the wrist against the outer right thigh and hold the left foot. Curl the toes of the foot around the fingers, so that the foot holds as much the hand as the hand the foot (Pada Bandha).
- Turn the head towards the right.

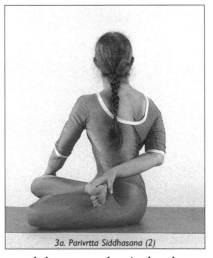
3a. Parivrtta Siddhasana (2)

- On each Mula Bandha inhalation elongate the lower abdomen and spinal column further upwards towards the back of the head, rooting the buttock bones and the left knee into the earth.
- On each exhalation rotate the trunk, chest, shoulders and head further towards the right till the chest and shoulders are perpendicular to the line between the knees.
- Hold for one minute. Then repeat on the other side.

3b. *Parivrtta Padmasana*

This is the same position done in full Padmasana.

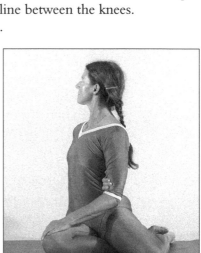

3b. Parivrtta Padmasana

- Sit in Padmasana (see page 77) with the right leg crossing over the left. The knees should be fairly close together so that both feet stick out on the sides of the thighs.
- On a Mula Bandha inhalation root the buttock bones and the knees into the earth, lift the pelvis up from the femur heads and elongate the whole body upwards. Extend the right arm up to the sky.
- On the exhalation rotate the trunk towards the right, swing the right arm around the back and hold the right foot. Curl the toes of the foot around the fingers, so that the foot holds as much the hand as the hand the foot (Pada Bandha).
- Place the left hand on the right knee and turn the head towards the right.
- On each Mula Bandha inhalation elongate the lower abdomen and spinal column further upwards towards the back of the head, rooting the buttock bones and the knees into the earth.
- On each exhalation rotate the trunk, chest, shoulders and head further towards the right till the chest and shoulders are perpendicular to the line between the knees.
- Hold for one minute. Then repeat on the other side.

4. Bharadvajasana I
Bharadvaja is the father of Drona

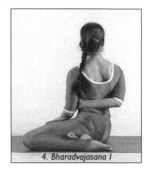

4. Bharadvajasana I

- Sit on a blanket with the legs extended straight in front of you.
- Bend both legs to the left and place them next to the left hip, so that you are sitting on the right hip. The toes of the right foot rest on the Achilles tendon of the left foot. Even though the left buttock bone does not rest on the blanket, it is important to nevertheless bring the weight of the body back onto it, so that the weight is divided evenly on both the buttock bones.
- On a Mula Bandha inhalation root the buttock bones and the knees into the earth, lift the pelvis up from the femur heads and elongate the whole body upwards. Extend the right arm up to the sky.
- On the exhalation rotate the trunk towards the right, swing the right arm around the back, and hold the left upper arm.
- Place the left hand on the right knee and turn the head towards the right.

4. Bharadvajasana I

- On each Mula Bandha inhalation elongate the lower abdomen and spinal column further upwards towards the back of the head, rooting the buttock bones and the knees into the earth.
- On each exhalation rotate the trunk, chest, shoulders and head further towards the right till the chest and shoulders are perpendicular to the line between the knees.
- Hold for one minute. Then repeat on the other side.

5. Bharadvajasana II
Bharadvaja is the father of Drona

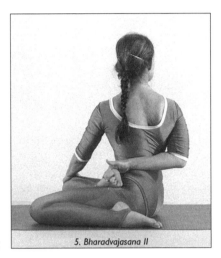

5. Bharadvajasana II

- Sit on a blanket with the legs extended straight in front of you.
- Bend the left leg to the left and place it next to the left hip as in Virasana I (see page 102).
- Take the right foot in both hands as for Padmasana (see page 77) and place it in the left groin. The left knee now points straight forward, and the right knee points at an angle of forty-five degrees to the right.
- In this position both buttock bones and both knees are on the blanket.
- On a Mula Bandha inhalation root the buttock bones and the knees into the earth, lift the pelvis up from the femur heads and elongate the whole body upwards. Extend the right arm up to the sky.
- On the exhalation rotate the trunk towards the right, swing the right arm around the back and hold the right foot. Curl the toes of the foot around the fingers, so that the foot holds as much the hand as the hand the foot (Pada Bandha).
- Place the left hand on the right knee and turn the head towards the right.
- On each Mula Bandha inhalation elongate the lower abdomen and spinal column further upwards towards the back of the head, rooting the buttock bones and the knees into the earth.

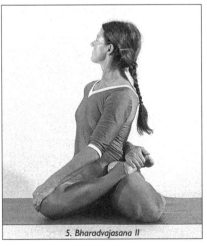

5. Bharadvajasana II

- On each exhalation rotate the trunk, chest, shoulders and head further towards the right till the chest and shoulders are perpendicular to the line between the knees.
- In this pose there is a diagonal action: the left buttock bone and the right knee have to go down simultaneously, so that the rooting is done on a diagonal line: left buttock bone-right knee, and right buttock bone-left knee.
- Hold for one minute. Then repeat on the other side.

6. Vamadevasana

Vamadeva is a name for Shiva

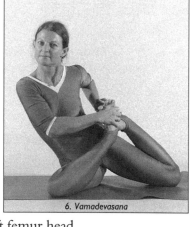

6. Vamadevasana

- Sit on a blanket with the legs extended straight in front of you.
- Bend the left leg backwards as in Upavistha Virasana I (see page 104) till the left thigh makes an angle of ninety degrees with the right one. Bend the right leg as for Sukhasana (see page 83).
- Lift with the left hand the left foot up and rotate the left thigh inwards, turning the arm so that the fingers point forwards and the left elbow points backwards. Hold with the palm of the hand the dorsal side of the left foot. Push the foot till the left heel touches the left femur head.
- Hold with the right hand the dorsal side of the right foot and raise the foot, keeping the knee on the blanket.
- Join the heels and the soles of the two feet together on the outer left hip.
- Hold for a few seconds. Then repeat on the other side.

7. Yogadandasana

danda=staff

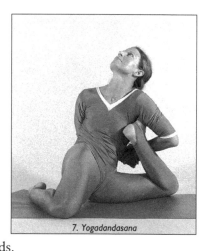

7. Yogadandasana

- Sit on a blanket with the legs extended straight in front of you.
- Bend the right leg as in Virasana I (see page 102).
- Bend the left leg as for Sukhasana (see page 83). Hold the left foot with both hands and raise it, turning the leg as for Padmasana (see page 77).
- Flex the foot at an angle of ninety degrees to the shin. Hold with the right hand the heel and with the left hand the outer edge of the left foot. The left arm crosses over the shin bone. In this way the right hand can push and the left hand can pull the foot backwards.
- Pull the left knee back and down till the outer left thigh rests on the blanket, so that the left thigh rotates even deeper in the left hip joint. The trunk is now resting only on the left hip, while the right hip is raised.
- Release the left hand, lean on the left hip and place the Triceps muscle of the left arm in the arch of the left foot.
- Push with the right hand the left foot still further backwards. At the same time turn the chest and shoulders towards the right, till the sole of the left foot rests in the left armpit.
- Rotate the left arm backwards around the foot. Swing the right arm around the back and clasp the hands on the back. The left hand holds the right one.
- Turn the head and chest to the right.
- Hold for a few seconds. Then repeat on the other side.

8. Marichyasana III

Marichi is a sage

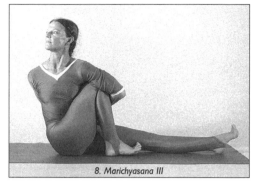

8. Marichyasana III

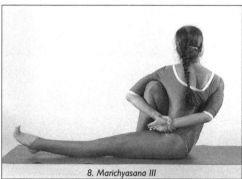

8. Marichyasana III

- Sit on a blanket with the legs extended straight in front of you.
- Bend the right leg so that the knee points up towards the sky and the right foot rests on the blanket next to the left thigh. The toes point straight forward.
- The left leg extends straight out of the left hip joint with the left foot in line with the left frontal hip bone. The knee should be straight with the knee cap facing the sky and the back of the knee in contact with the blanket. Elongate the heel and big toe bone away from you and pull the little toe bone towards you, so that the foot is vertical and all the toes are in a line. Perform Pada Bandha with the left foot in order to support the action in the pelvis.
- On a Mula Bandha inhalation lift the pelvis up from the femur heads, rooting the right foot and the buttock bones into the earth and elongating the spinal column upwards.
- On the exhalation place the right hand back of you on the blanket and rotate the lower abdomen, waist, chest, shoulders and head towards the right.
- Rotate the left arm as in Savasana (see page 286) and place the back side of the left upper arm, close to the arm pit, against the outer side of the right knee or thigh. Keep pointing the right knee straight up to the sky and use the pressure of the left arm against the right outer knee to rotate further towards the right.
- Slide the left arm still further forward on the outer right thigh till the right knee rests in the back side of the left armpit. Do not cross the right knee over the left groin, but keep the right knee, groin, foot and buttock bone all in one line.
- Rotate the left arm backwards around the right shin. Extend the right arm sideways and, with a large, circular movement, swing it backwards around the back. Do not elongate and rotate the right arm from the shoulder joint, but rather from the spinal column between the shoulder blades. Clasp the hands on the back. With the right knee bent it is the left hand which has to hold the right hand. The reason is that in this position the left shoulder is in a slightly dangerous endorotation. By holding the right hand with the left, the muscles of the left shoulder are tensed and are therefore better able to hold the left shoulder in a firm and stable position.
- On each Mula Bandha inhalation elongate the lower abdomen and spinal column further upwards towards the back of the head, bringing the weight of the body forward onto the right foot. Root the buttock bones and the right foot, performing Pada Bandha with both feet to activate the Mula Bandha.
- On each exhalation rotate the trunk, chest, shoulders and head further towards the right till the chest and shoulders are aligned with the left leg. Rotate the right femur head backwards towards the coccyx in order to keep the knee, groin, foot and buttock bone in one line.
- Hold for one minute. Then repeat on the other side.

9. Marichyasana IV

Marichi is a sage

This is basically the same position as Marichyasana III (8). The difference is that here the left leg is bent as in Virasana I (see page 102) instead of being straight as in Marichyasana III (8).

- Sit on a blanket with the legs extended straight in front of you.
- Bend the left leg to the left and place the left foot next to the left hip as in Virasana I (see page 102).
- Bend the right leg so that the knee points up towards the sky and the right foot rests on the blanket next to the left thigh. The toes point straight forward.
- The left thigh extends straight out of the left hip joint, so that the left knee is in line with the left frontal hip bone. The weight of the body is divided evenly on both buttock bones.
- For the rest follow the instructions given in Marichyasana III (8).
- Hold for one minute. Then repeat on the other side.

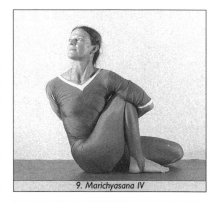

9. Marichyasana IV

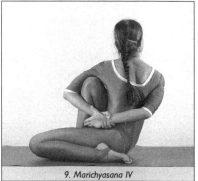

9. Marichyasana IV

10. Marichyasana V

Marichi is a sage

This is basically the same position as Marichyasana III (8). The difference is that here the left leg is bent as in Padmasana (see page 77) instead of being straight as in Marichyasana III (8).

- Sit on a blanket with the legs extended straight in front of you.
- Take the left foot in both hands as for Padmasana (see page 77) and place it in the right groin.
- Bend the right leg so that the knee points up towards the sky and the right foot rests on the blanket. The toes point straight forward.
- In this position the weight of the body is more on the left hip.
- For the rest follow the instructions given in Marichyasana III (8).
- Hold for one minute. Then repeat on the other side.

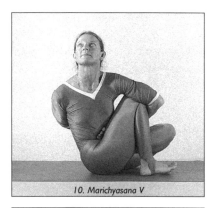

10. Marichyasana V

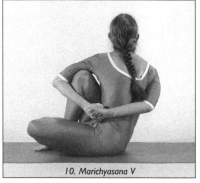

10. Marichyasana V

11. Pasasana

pasa=noose, cord

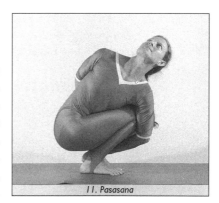

11. Pasasana

- Start with Utkatasana II (see page 100) and proceed:
- On a Mula Bandha inhalation lift the pelvis up from the femur heads, rooting the feet into the earth and performing Pada Bandha. Extend the buttock bones backwards and elongate the spinal column upwards.
- On the exhalation place the right hand back of you on the blanket and rotate the lower abdomen, waist, chest, shoulders and head towards the right. Keep the knees pointing straight forward.
- Rotate the left arm as in Savasana (see page 286) and place the back side of the left upper arm close to the armpit against the outer side of the right knee or thigh. Use the pressure of the left arm against the outside of the right knee to rotate the trunk further towards the right.
- Slide the left arm still further forward on the outer right thigh, till the right knee rests in the back side of the left armpit. Do not move the knees over to the left, but keep the knees, groins, feet and buttock bones all in one line, with the knees pointing straight forward.

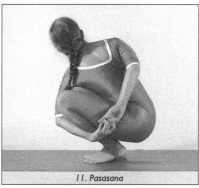

11. Pasasana

- Rotate the left arm backwards around the right shin. Extend the right arm sideways and, with a large, circular movement, swing it around the back. Do not elongate and rotate the right arm from the shoulder joint, but rather from the spinal column between the shoulder blades. Clasp the hands on the back. When turning to the right it is the left hand which has to hold the right hand.
- On each Mula Bandha inhalation elongate the lower abdomen and spinal column further upwards towards the back of the head and bring the weight of the body forward onto the lower spring joints of the feet. Rooting the feet and elongating the buttock bones backwards use the spring joints to rebounce the weight of the body back upwards (Pada Bandha), so that the pose is stable and light at the same time.
- On each exhalation rotate the trunk, chest, shoulders and head further towards the right till the chest and shoulders are aligned with the thighs.
- Hold for one minute. Then repeat on the other side.

12. Ardha Matsyendrasana

*ardha=half; Matsyendra is one of the founders of Hatha Vidya
(matsya=fish; indra=king)*

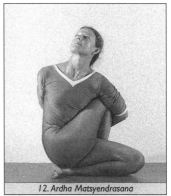

12. Ardha Matsyendrasana

- Sit on a blanket with the legs extended straight in front of you.
- Bend the left leg to the left and place the left foot next to the left hip as in Virasana I (see page 102).
- Place the hands on the blanket next to you, lift the pelvis up and roll the buttock bones onto the left foot. Turn the left foot under in such a way that it makes an angle of ninety degrees with the shin. The foot rests on the outer edge, not on the dorsal side, on the blanket.
- Both the buttock bones rest on the foot, the left one on the inner heel and the right one on the metatarsal of the big toe.
- Swing the right foot over the left thigh and place the right foot next to the outer left thigh, about halfway between the knee and the hip. The toes point straight forward.
- On a Mula Bandha inhalation lift the pelvis up from the femur heads, rooting the right foot into the earth and the buttock bones into the left foot. Elongate the spinal column upwards.

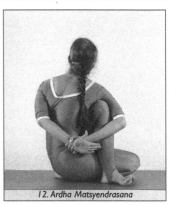

12. Ardha Matsyendrasana

- On the exhalation place the right hand back of you on the blanket and rotate the lower abdomen, waist, chest, shoulders and head towards the right.
- Rotate the left arm as in Savasana (see page 286) and place the back side of the left upper arm close to the armpit against the outer right knee or thigh. Keep pointing the right knee straight up to the sky and use the pressure of the left arm against the outer side of the right knee to rotate further towards the right.
- Slide the left arm still further forward on the outer right thigh till the right knee rests in the back side of the left armpit.
- Rotate the left arm backwards around the right shin. Extend the right arm sideways and, with a large, circular movement, swing it backwards around the back. Do not elongate and rotate the right arm from the shoulder joint, but rather from the spinal column between the shoulder blades. Clasp the hands on the back. When turning towards the right it is the left hand which has to hold the right hand.
- On each Mula Bandha inhalation elongate the lower abdomen and spinal column further upwards towards the back of the head and root the buttock bones and the right foot. Perform Pada Bandha with both feet to activate the Mula Bandha.
- On each exhalation rotate the trunk, chest, shoulders and head further towards the right till the chest and shoulders are aligned with the left thigh. Rotate the right femur head backwards towards the coccyx in order to keep the right buttock bone firmly on the metatarsal of the left foot.
- Hold for one minute. Then repeat on the other side.

The general tendency in this pose is to slide the buttock bones off the foot. This results in a tilting of the pelvis with consequent stress on the downward sacro-iliac joint. Thus special attention has to be given to keeping both buttock bones on the foot.

13. Paripurna Matsyendrasana

paripurna=complete; Matsyendra is one of the founders of Hatha Vidya (matsya=fish; indra=king)

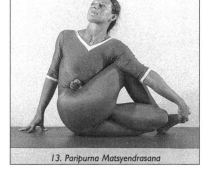

13. Paripurna Matsyendrasana

- Sit on a blanket with the legs extended straight in front of you.
- Bend the left leg and place the left foot in the right groin as for Padmasana (see page 77).
- Bend the right leg and swing the right foot over the left thigh, bringing the weight of the body onto the outer left hip and raising the right hip up. Rest the right foot against the outer side of the left thigh, close to the knee. The toes point straight forward.
- On a Mula Bandha inhalation lift the pelvis up from the femur heads, rooting the left hip into the earth and elongating the spinal column upwards.
- On the exhalation place the right hand back of you on the blanket and rotate the lower abdomen, waist, chest, shoulders and head towards the right.
- Rotate the left arm as in Savasana (see page 286) and place the back side of the left upper arm close to the armpit against the outer side of the right knee. Keep pointing the right knee straight up to the sky and use the pressure of the left arm against the right outer knee to rotate further towards the right.
- Slide the left arm still further forward on the outer right knee till the right knee rests in the back side of the left armpit. Then rotate the arm backwards around the shin and hold the right foot.
- Extend the right arm sideways and, with a large, circular movement, swing it backwards around the back. Hold the left groin.
- On each Mula Bandha inhalation elongate the lower abdomen and spinal column further upwards towards the back of the head, and on each exhalation rotate the trunk, chest, shoulders and head further towards the right.
- Hold for a few seconds. Then repeat on the other side

This Twisting Pose is the most difficult of all. Do not force it, as you can hurt the knee. It may take a long time to master this pose.

4.9 Sirsasana / Head Balance cycle

These positions are done in the *Vinyasa* mode, that is, going from one pose directly into the next one, using the breathing.

Sirsasana cycle
....

1. Salamba Sirsasana I	10. Vajra Sirsasana
2. Urdhva Dandasana	11. Parivrtta Vajra Sirsasana
3. Parivrtta Sirsasana	12. Prasarita Padottana Sirsasana
4. Parivrttaikapada Sirsasana	13. Baddha Kona Sirsasana
5. Parsvaikapada Sirsasana	14. Salamba Sirsasana II
6. Ekapada Sirsasana	15. Salamba Sirsasana III
7. Urdhva Padma Sirsasana	16. Muktahasta Sirsasana
8. Parivrtta Urdhva Padma Sirsasana	17. Baddhahasta Sirsasana
9. Pinda Sirsasana	

Sirsasana or *Head Balance* is one of the best known yoga poses and is often called the king of the postures in traditional texts. It was recommended that this pose be done every day, together with Sarvangasana or Shoulder Balance, for a certain length of time in order to keep the body young, healthy and full of vigor.

Though standing on one's head may look spectacular, it is actually one of the easier positions. The main problem is to find the balance, but once that has been established, the body has exactly the same feeling as in Tadasana. In Tadasana the body is aligned on the force of gravity in spine, pelvis and legs; in Head Balance it is aligned in the same way. Many people stand on their heads with great muscular effort, because they are out of alignment with the force of gravity. As a result they have to use more muscles - and the wrong ones - than necessary to keep the body from falling.

Head Balance is, as the name says, a balance. The legs, pelvis and spine balance on the head and the more they form a straight and continuous line with the neck, the more the body balances on the skeletal structure, not on the upholding force of the muscles.

Practice the straight Head Balance called *Salamba Sirsasana I* first, till that comes naturally, before proceeding to the variations.

1. Salamba Sirsasana I

sa=with; alamba=support; sirsa=head

(See also Part Two: "Comparative Studies of Various Asanas", paragraph 4.13)

- Place a folded blanket on the earth and kneel in front of it.
- Place the elbows and lower arms on the blanket, with the elbows at the same width as the arm pits. Keep them in line; do not keep one elbow further forward than the other. Interlock the fingers and thumbs, and tuck the bottom little finger into the palm of the other hand to make the rim of the hands and wrists equal (photo 1a).

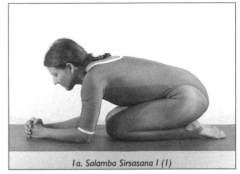
1a. Salamba Sirsasana I (1)

- The wrist has four sides: the inner side (the palm), the back side (the dorsal side), the thumb (radial) side and the little finger (ulnar) side. It was discovered long ago in martial arts that certain points on the wrists induce strength in the arm and the whole body, while other points induce weakness. Both in Karate and in Sword Fighting the point that is of vital importance is the one on the inner wrist, on the side of the little finger, called the *ulnar wrist point*. This is a key point in all martial arts. Anatomically speaking, this point connects three pair of major muscles: the latissimus dorsi, the pectoralis major and the deltoid muscles. It is the combination of these three muscles that lends strength to the arms and trunk, and enables the Karate master to break the bricks, and the Sword master to win a duel. In yoga too this point is of vital importance, especially in a position like Head Balance, as it gives the body stability and endurance.
- Keeping the fingers soft and relaxed and the ulnar wrist points rooted into the earth, place the head on the blanket between the wrists and palms of the hands. The head rests exactly on the top of the skull, halfway between the forehead and the crown, on the fontanel (the thousand-petalled lotus). The face looks straight forward, with the chin and the forehead in vertical alignment.
- Place the knees against the forehead, in between the elbows, with the toes tucked under (photo 1b). Press the elbows against the knees, so that the shoulder blades, the latissimus dorsi and the deltoid muscles widen and the upper back is opened; at the same time, move the shoulder blades towards the waist. If the shoulder blades move towards the spine, the shoulders collapse and the weight of the body will fall into the neck vertebrae.

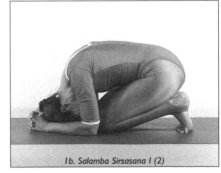
1b. Salamba Sirsasana I (2)

- Root the top of the head into the blanket (Padma Bandha), so that the cervical and thoracic spine elongate up towards the sky. In Head Balance, the rebounce action of the rooting lies in the joint between the first cervical vertebra (the atlas) and the base of the skull. The more the head roots (Padma Bandha), the more this joint opens, giving the thrust for the rest of the spinal column to move up against the force of gravity.

The muscles involved in this elongation of the spine are those vertical ones that run closest to the spinal vertebrae. These muscles should be alerted right from the beginning, so that the body balances in the final pose only on the spinal column and its vertical muscles, not on the shoulders and trapezius muscles, whose fibers run parallel to the earth and are therefore incapable of producing the rebounce force.

In this context it is interesting to note that the big, peripheral muscles of the body, which include the trapezius muscles, are geared for short-term, dynamic action (weight lifting and trapeze work), not for long-term, static action. In Head Balance, where you want to stand for at least five minutes, the body needs to utilize muscles geared for long-term, static action; these are exactly those vertical muscles that run closest to the spinal column.

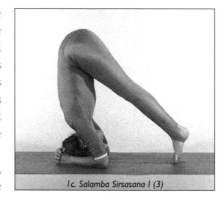

1c. Salamba Sirsasana I (3)

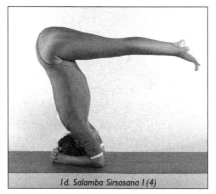

1d. Salamba Sirsasana I (4)

- On an inhalation, raise the knees, keeping the feet on the earth (photo 1c), till the trunk is vertical and the hip joints are in line with the shoulder joints. Do not take the hips back, and do not bend the spine, but keep spine and neck erect.

- On the exhalation, continue the rooting of the head (Padma Bandha) and the elongation of the cervical and thoracic spine, so that the legs are raised to the vertical in one smooth movement, hinging in the femo-iliac joints. The legs are light going up, as it is the vertical spinal muscles that do the work. Keep the knees straight and the feet together (photo 1d and 1e).

- In Salamba Sirsasana I the ears, shoulder joints, hip joints and ankle joints are in vertical alignment, and the entire weight of the body is borne on the head; the elbows, lower arms and hands are used only to maintain the balance.

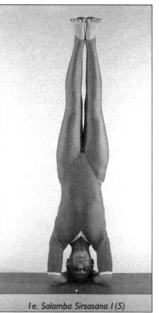

1e. Salamba Sirsasana I (5)

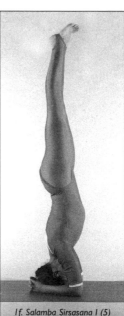

1f. Salamba Sirsasana I (5)

Root the ulnar wrist points into the earth, as it is from here, as well as from the head, that the energy moves up towards the feet to make the connection with the lower spring joints.

- Breathe slowly and easily, using each Mula Bandha inhalation to create the wave upwards that lightens the body, and each exhalation to consolidate that height of the body (photo 1f).

- Elongate the sides of the arm pits, so that the upper arms are almost in line with the sides of the chest; the upper arms and chest should be almost vertical. If the weight of the body is on the front of the trunk (solar plexus) and not on the back (spine and head), the lumbar spine sags, and the chest is not vertical, but slanted, as the lower part is further forward than the upper part. To make the chest vertical, the arm pits and upper ribs have to move forwards, and the lower ribs and lumbar spine backwards.

- This is the same movement as in Tadasana: the straightening of chest and lumbar starts in the pelvis; the only difference is that here the body is upside down. The pelvis is vertical, with the buttock bones pointing straight up towards the sky. If it is tilted forward around the femur heads, the curve in the lumbar spine becomes too pronounced and the weight of the body falls on the front of the trunk. As a result the muscles of the abdomen lose their tone, while the muscles in the lower back become short, narrow and tight. To correct this position make the following movements: keep the ankles and hip joints in line with the shoulder joints, and the knees straight. Then rotate the pelvis backwards, so that the two frontal hip bones move towards the ribs and the coccyx rolls towards the pubic bone. At the same time, bring the lumbar vertebrae back, but not the thoracic vertebrae. In this way the weight of the body is brought onto the back (spine and head) and the head, chest and pelvis are aligned vertically.

- Thus, to create the lightness in the body in Head Balance, the head and the ulnar wrist points have to go down with the force of gravity (rooting), while the spinal column and the legs elongate up against the force of gravity (rebounce, the Normal Force of Newton). To draw the chest out of the shoulder joints, roll the deltoid, triceps and latissimus dorsi muscles forwards towards the face, slightly pressurizing the elbows inwards, and then lift the chest vertically up from the shoulder heads (note that in Tadasana the pelvis is drawn upwards from the femur heads by constricting the tensor fascia lata and the adductors on the inside of the thighs inwards).

- To prevent the pelvis from resting heavily on the lumbar spine, constrict the tensor fascia lata and the adductor muscles of the thighs inwards and elongate the legs up, out of the femo-iliac joints, so that they pull the pelvis up. Keep the legs perpendicular and the knees straight, with the knee caps facing forward, and keep the arches of the feet strong, especially the upper and lower spring joints of the feet, with the toes in line as in Tadasana.

- The neck has the same shape and length as in Tadasana, is soft and natural, and the first cervical and the first thoracic vertebra are in vertical alignment.

- Hold for as long as you can maintain the alignment and lightness. Eventually you should be able to stay up for ten minutes.

- To come down, reverse the process and come back to your original starting point on one smooth exhalation.

When you can stay in this position for five minutes with a certain degree of comfort, you can start to practice the variations:

2. Urdhva Dandasana

urdhva=upwards; danda=staff

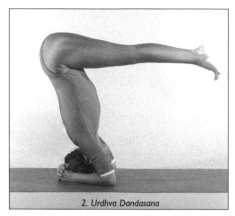

2. Urdhva Dandasana

- Stand in Salamba Sirsasana I (1e) and proceed:
- On an exhalation bring the legs down to an angle of ninety degrees, so that they are parallel to the earth. Keep the back straight and continue rooting the head (Padma Bandha) and the ulnar wrist points. This will help the spinal column to maintain the upward elongation. At the same time, continue rolling the deltoid, triceps and latissimus dorsi muscles forwards, constricting the elbows slightly inwards, so that the shoulder blades remain wide.
- Hold for thirty seconds. On an exhalation, take the legs back up to Salamba Sirsasana I (1e), and proceed to 3.

3. Parivrtta Sirsasana

parivrtta=turned around; sirsa=head

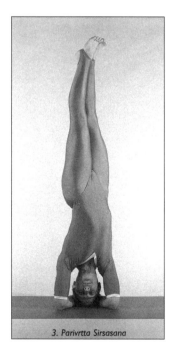

3. Parivrtta Sirsasana

- On an exhalation, rotate the hips towards the right. As they rotate towards the right, the right shoulder and shoulder blade should not yield. Pay special attention to rolling the right deltoid, triceps and latissimus dorsi muscles forward, so that the right elbow stays in line with the right armpit.
- The left and right side of waist and hips should remain parallel to each other; do not lower the left hip as you turn towards the right: the line between the two frontal hip bones remains parallel to the earth.
- Do not curve the lumbar spine forwards by dropping the feet backwards. The line from the bridge of the nose through the sternum, the pubic bone and the middle of the ankles remains vertical.
- Hold for one minute. On an exhalation, come back to the center and repeat on the other side.
- Come back to the center and proceed to 4.

4. Parivrttaikapada Sirsasana

parivrtta=turned around; eka=one; pada=leg, foot; sirsa=head

- Extend the left foot forward and the right foot back.
- On an exhalation, rotate the hips towards the right. As they rotate towards the right, the right shoulder and shoulder blade should not yield. Pay special attention to rolling the right deltoid, triceps and latissimus dorsi muscles forward, so that the right elbow stays in line with the right armpit.

- Spread the legs as much as you can, but keep the feet at the same height from the earth. This means that you have to pay more attention to the right leg, elongating it out of the right sacro-iliac joint. There is a slight curve in the lumbar spine, but do not exaggerate this: the lower abdomen remains in contact with the lower ribs. This is done through the Mula Bandha breathing: the lower abdomen moves back towards the sacrum and then up towards the lower thoracic diaphragm, so that the lower abdomen stays toned and the right leg elongates out of the groin, not out of the waist.
- The left and right side of waist and hips should remain parallel to each other; do not lower the left hip as you turn towards the right: the line between the two frontal hip bones remains parallel to the earth.
- Hold for one minute. On an exhalation, come back to the center and repeat on the other side.
- Come back to the center and proceed to 5.

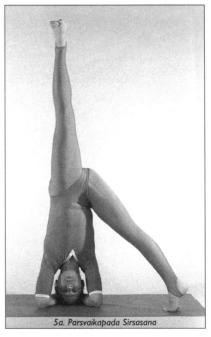

4. Parivrttaikapada Sirsasana

5. Parsvaikapada Sirsasana

parsva=sideways; eka=one; pada=leg, foot; sirsa=head

- On an exhalation, rotate the right leg out and take the foot sideways to the earth. Keep the left side of the trunk and the left leg straight; the knee cap of the left leg and the left groin continue facing straight forward (photo 5a).
- To get a better movement you can hold the right foot with the right hand (photo 5b). Root the head (Padma Bandha) and the left ulnar wrist point and elongate the spine upwards.
- Do not lower the right hip; the line between the two frontal hip bones remains parallel to the earth.
- Hold for thirty seconds. On an exhalation, take the leg up again and repeat on the other side.
- Then proceed to 6.

5a. Parsvaikapada Sirsasana

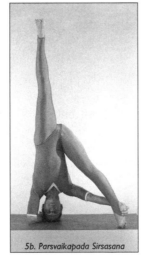

5b. Parsvaikapada Sirsasana

6. Ekapada Sirsasana

eka=one; pada=leg, foot; sirsa=head

- On an exhalation take the right foot straight down, in line with the right armpit. Keep the left side of the trunk and the left leg straight; the knee cap of the left leg and the left groin continue facing straight forward (photo 6a).
- To get a better movement, you can hold the right foot with the right hand (photo 6b). Root the head (Padma Bandha) and the left ulnar wrist point and elongate the spine upwards.
- Do not lower the right hip; the line between the two frontal hip bones remains parallel to the earth.
- Hold for thirty seconds. On an exhalation, take the leg up again and repeat on the other side.
- Then proceed to 7.

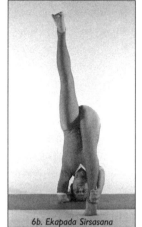

6b. Ekapada Sirsasana

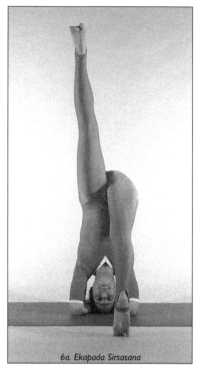

6a. Ekapada Sirsasana

7. Urdhva Padma Sirsasana

urdhva=upwards; padma=lotus; sirsa=head

- Cross the legs in Padmasana (see page 77) and extend the knees up towards the sky. Do not curve the lumbar spine in; performing Pada Bandha to stabilize the hip joints, rotate the pelvis backwards, so that the coccyx rolls towards the pubic bone and the lower abdomen and the two frontal hip bones move towards the lower frontal ribs. Thus the lumbar spine is elongated.
- Extend the thighs out of the hip joints, so that the groins are opened and the knees point straight up towards the sky.
- For the rest, follow the instructions given in Salamba Sirsasana I (1).
- Hold for thirty seconds, and then proceed to 8.

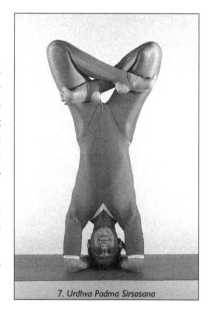

7. Urdhva Padma Sirsasana

8. Parivrtta Urdhva Padma Sirsasana

*parivrtta=turned around; urdhva=upwards; padma=lotus;
sirsa=head*

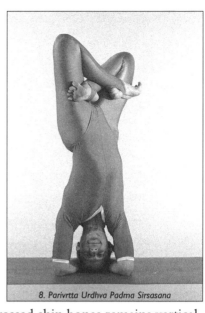

- On an exhalation, rotate the hips towards the right. As they rotate towards the right, the right shoulder and shoulder blade should not yield. Pay special attention to rolling the right deltoid, triceps and latissimus dorsi muscles forward, so that the right elbow stays in line with the right armpit.
- The left and right side of waist and hips should remain parallel to each other; do not lower the left hip as you turn towards the right: the line between the two frontal hip bones remains parallel to the earth.
- Do not curve the lumbar spine forwards by dropping the knees backwards. The line from the bridge of the

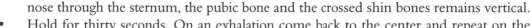
8. Parivrtta Urdhva Padma Sirsasana

nose through the sternum, the pubic bone and the crossed shin bones remains vertical.
- Hold for thirty seconds. On an exhalation come back to the center and repeat on the other side.
- Then proceed to 9.

9. Pinda Sirsasana

pinda=embryo; sirsa=head

- On an exhalation bring the knees down towards the stomach. Even though the back will bend slightly, continue rooting the head (Padma Bandha) and the ulnar wrist points, so that the spinal column maintains a certain elongation.
- Hold for thirty seconds. On an exhalation come back up again. Change the crossing of the legs and repeat 7, 8 and 9.
- Straighten the legs and proceed to 10.

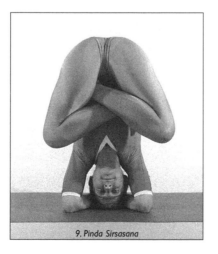
9. Pinda Sirsasana

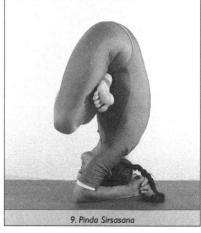
9. Pinda Sirsasana

10. Vajra Sirsasana

vajra=thunderbolt, weapon of indra; sirsa=head

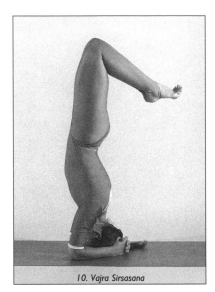

10. Vajra Sirsasana

- Bend the knees backwards without curving the lumbar spine. Performing Pada Bandha to stabilize the hip joints, rotate the pelvis backwards, so that the coccyx rolls towards the pubic bone and the lower abdomen and the two frontal hip bones move towards the lower frontal ribs. Thus the lumbar spine is elongated.
- At the same time extend the thighs out of the hip joints, so that the groins are opened and the knees point straight up towards the sky.
- For the rest follow the instructions given in Salamba Sirsasana I (1).
- Hold for thirty seconds; then proceed to 11.

11. Parivrtta Vajra Sirsasana

parivrtta=turned around; vajra=thunderbolt, weapon of indra; sirsa=head

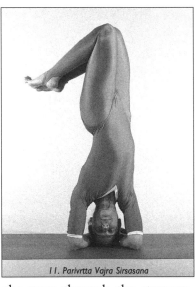

11. Parivrtta Vajra Sirsasana

- On an exhalation rotate the hips towards the right. As they rotate towards the right, the right shoulder and shoulder blade should not yield. Pay special attention to rolling the right deltoid, triceps and latissimus dorsi muscles forward, so that the right elbow stays in line with the right armpit.
- The left and right side of waist and hips should remain parallel to each other; do not lower the left hip as you turn towards the right; the line between the two frontal hip bones remains parallel to the earth.
- Do not curve the lumbar spine forwards by dropping the knees backwards; the line from the bridge of the nose through the sternum, the pubic bone and the inner knees remains vertical.
- Hold for thirty seconds. On an exhalation, come back to the center and repeat on the other side.
- Come back to the center, straighten the legs and proceed to 12.

12. Prasarita Padottana Sirsasana

prasarita=spread, extended;
pada=leg, foot; uttana=intense stretch;
sirsa=head

- Spread the legs to the maximum, keeping the feet at the same height from the earth.
- Hold for thirty seconds; then proceed to 13.

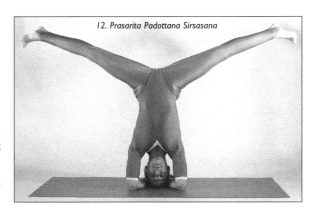

12. Prasarita Padottana Sirsasana

13. Baddha Kona Sirsasana

baddha=bound; kona=angle; sirsa=head

- Join the soles of the feet together as in Baddha Konasana (see page 110) and pull the heels down towards the pubic bone. The toes point straight up towards the sky.
- Hold for thirty second, and then straighten the legs.

When you have reached sufficient balance in these variations, you can try the following ones:

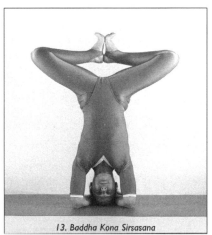

13. Baddha Kona Sirsasana

14. Salamba Sirsasana II

sa=with; alamba=support; sirsa=head

- On an exhalation, release the hands back of the head, bring them forward and place the palms of the hands on the blanket in front of you. The fingers point towards the face, and the wrists and elbows are in line with the armpits, with an angle of ninety degrees in the elbows.
- Root the head (Padma Bandha) and the hands (Hastha Bandha): performing Hasta Bandha activates the arms, shoulders and shoulder blades. Elongate the elbows forward, away from the head, and keep the upper arms and elbows parallel to each other by rolling the deltoid, triceps and latissimus dorsi muscles forwards, and constricting the elbows slightly inwards towards each other.
- Hold for thirty seconds, and then proceed to 15.

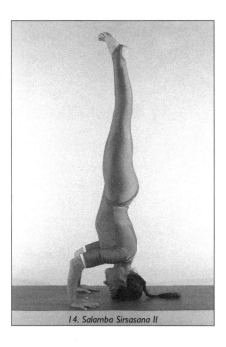

14. Salamba Sirsasana II

15. Salamba Sirsasana III

sa=with; alamba=support; sirsa=head

- Turn the hands the other way round, so that the fingers point away from the face. The wrists and elbows stay in line with the armpits, and the elbows maintain an angle of ninety degrees.
- Root the head (Padma Bandha) and the hands (Hastha Bandha); performing Hasta Bandha activates the arms, shoulders and shoulder blades. Elongate the elbows forward, away from the head, and keep the upper arms and elbows parallel to each other by rolling the deltoid, triceps and latissimus dorsi muscles forwards, and constricting the elbows slightly inwards towards each other.
- Hold for thirty seconds, and then proceed to 16.

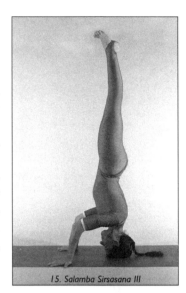

15. Salamba Sirsasana III

16. Muktahasta Sirsasana

mukta=free; hasta=hand; sirsa=head

- Extend the arms in front of you with the back of the hands resting on the blanket and the palms facing upward. The arms and hands can be slightly wider than the armpits to facilitate the balance.
- Hold for thirty seconds, and then proceed to 17.

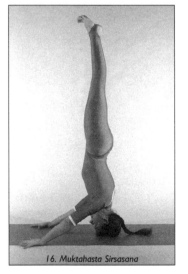

16. Muktahasta Sirsasana

17. Baddhahasta Sirsasana

baddha=bound; hasta=hand; sirsa=head

- Fold the arms in front of the face and clasp the elbows with the hands.
- Hold for thirty seconds. On an exhalation return to Salamba Sirsasana I.

To come down from Salamba Sirsasana I (1), follow the instructions for going up, in the reverse order.

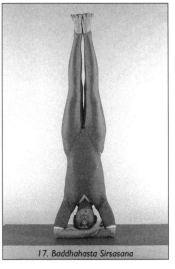

17. Baddhahasta Sirsasana

4.10   Sarvangasana / Shoulder Balance cycle

These positions should be done in the *Vinyasa* mode, that is, going from one pose directly into the next one, using the breathing.

Sarvangasana cycle

1. Halasana
2. Karnapidasana
3. Salamba Sarvangasana I
4. Parsvaikapada Sarvangasana
5. Ekapada Sarvangasana
6. Supta Konasana
7. Parsva Halasana
8. Parsva Karnapidasana
9. Parsva Sarvangasana
10. Parsva Setubandhasana

11. Setubandhasana
12. Ekapada Setubandhasana
13. Urdhva Padma Sarvangasana
14. Parsva Urdhva Padma Sarvangasana
15. Parsva Pinda Sarvangasana
16. Pinda Sarvangasana
17. Salamba Sarvangasana II
18. Niralamba Sarvangasana I
19. Niralamba Sarvangasana II

1. Halasana

hala=plough

(See also Part Two: "Comparative Studies of various Asanas", paragraph 4.13)

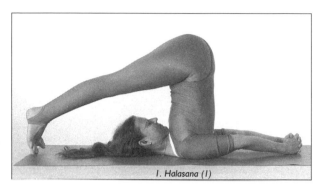

1. Halasana (1)

- Lie on the back on a blanket.
- On an exhalation bring the feet over the head to the blanket. Keep the knees straight and arms extended backwards.
- Clasp the hands as for Salamba Sirsasana I (see page 163) and elongate the wrists away from the shoulders, so that the shoulders are pulled backwards away from the ears. Rotate the upper arms out so that the Deltoid muscles roll underneath the shoulders and the Biceps muscles rotate up towards the sky. Lift the shoulder blades up from the blanket in order to bring the trunk onto the tops of the shoulders.

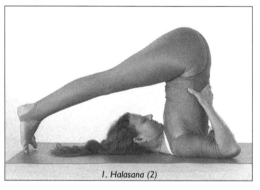

1. Halasana (2)

- Elongate the spine upwards so that all the vertebrae move into the body. The hip joints are in a vertical alignment with the shoulder joints. In order to elongate the spine upwards you have to extend the back of the thighs from the knees towards the buttock bones, spreading the buttock bones and lifting them up towards the sky. Elongate the ulnar wrist points away from you and root them into the earth. This will enable the Latissimus dorsi to lift the chest up and thus to elongate the spine.
- As the spine moves in and the trunk lifts up from the shoulder heads the sternum moves up and forwards towards the chin. Perform Jalandhara Bandha (see page 43) in order to avoid pressing the neck vertebrae onto the earth. Lift the corners of the jaws (not the chin) up by sliding the skull on the first vertebra and then join the chin with the sternum. In this way the first two vertebrae of the neck do not press onto the earth, but are lifted into the neck.
- Rest the feet on the tip of the toes. There should be very little weight on the feet, all the body weight is on the spine and hips. Then place the hands on the back.
- Hold for five minutes. Proceed to 2.

2. Karnapidasana

karna=ear; pida=pressure

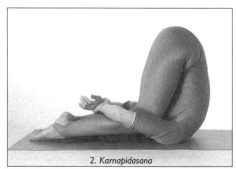

2. Karnapidasana

- On an exhalation extend the arms over the head and bend the knees next to the ears.
- The pelvis has to roll over the head and the back has to bend to bring the knees down.

Keep the feet together with the toes pointing away from the head and clasp the elbows in the knees.
- Hold for one minute.
- If you can do this easily, slide the feet further out to bring the knees down to the blanket over the head. In this way the upper spine between the shoulder blades is elongated even more.
- Extend the arms back again and clasp the hands as for Salamba Sirsasana I (see page 163). Roll the upper arms out and the Deltoid muscles under, and then place the hands back on the back, as close to the shoulder blades as possible.
- Proceed to 3.

3. Salamba Sarvangasana I
sa=with; alamba=support; sarva=whole; anga=body

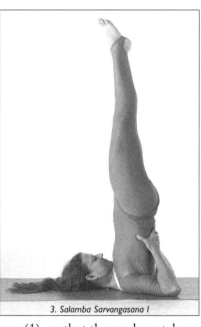

3. Salamba Sarvangasana I

- On an inhalation raise the knees and elongate the spinal column upwards. On the exhalation lift the legs up to Salamba Sarvangasana I, keeping the knees straight and the feet together.
- Seen from the side the ankles, knees, hip joints and shoulder joints are in a vertical alignment.
- Clasp the hands as in Salamba Sirsasana I (see page 163) and extend the arms backwards. Roll the upper arms out so that the Biceps muscles rotate up to the sky and the Deltoid muscles roll underneath the shoulder heads. Root the ulnar wrist points so that the spine in between the shoulder blades elongates upwards.
- Then place the hands back again on the back and lift the chest up from the shoulder heads. Perform Jalandhara Bandha (see page 43) as described in Halasana (1), so that the neck vertebrae do not press on the blanket.
- On each Mula Bandha inhalation lift the chest and trunk up from the shoulder heads and elongate the legs up out of the pelvis. Keep the inner ankles together and the knees facing straight forward.
- On each exhalation maintain the height of the body.
- Hold for five minutes. On an exhalation go back to Halasana (1) and down till you are lying again on the back.

When you can stay for five minutes in this position with a certain degree of comfort you can start to practice the variations:

4. Parsvaikapada Sarvangasana

parsva=sideways; eka=one; pada=leg, foot;
sarva=whole; anga=body

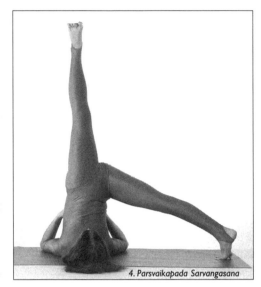

- Stand in Salamba Sarvangasana I (3) and proceed:
- On an exhalation rotate the right leg outwards and take the foot down sideways to the earth.
- Keep the left side of the trunk and the left leg completely straight. The knee cap of the left leg and the left groin should stay facing straight forward.
- Do not drop the right hip. To keep the line between the two frontal hip bones parallel to the earth you have to roll the right femur head back and up towards the left heel.
- Hold for thirty seconds. On an exhalation take the leg up again and repeat on the other side.
- Proceed to 5.

4. Parsvaikapada Sarvangasana

5. Ekapada Sarvangasana

eka=one; pada=leg, foot; sarva=whole; anga=body

- On an exhalation take the right foot straight down to the earth, in line with the right shoulder.
- Keep the left side of the trunk and the left leg completely straight. The knee cap of the left leg and the left groin should stay facing straight forward.
- Do not drop the right hip. To keep the line between the two frontal hip bones parallel to the earth you have to roll the right femur head back and up towards the left heel.
- Hold for thirty seconds. On an exhalation take the leg up again and repeat on the other side.
- Proceed to 6.

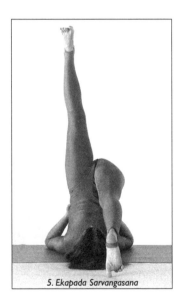

5. Ekapada Sarvangasana

6. Supta Konasana

supta=lying down; kona=angle

- On an exhalation come down to Halasana (1) and spread the legs. Follow the instructions given for Halasana.
- Hold for thirty seconds. Proceed to 7.

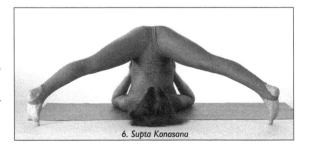

6. Supta Konasana

7. Parsva Halasana

parsva=sideways; hala=plough

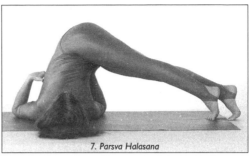
7. Parsva Halasana

- On an exhalation walk the feet towards the right, rotating the hips and spinal column, but not the shoulders. The left foot joins the right foot. Keep the feet vertical and keep only the tips of the big toes on the blanket.
- The shoulders and elbows should remain as in Halasana (1), do not displace the left shoulder and elbow as you walk the feet towards the right.
- Keep the right hip up. Both buttock bones should have the same height from the earth.
- Hold for thirty seconds. Proceed to 8.

8. Parsva Karnapidasana

parsva=sideways; karna=ear; pida=pressure

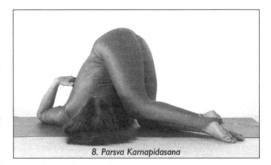
8. Parsva Karnapidasana

- On an exhalation bend the knees next to the right ear.
- The pelvis has to roll over the right shoulder and the back has to bend to bring the knees down. Keep the feet together with the toes pointing away from the head.
- Hold for thirty seconds. Then repeat 7 and 8 on the other side.
- Go up again to Salamba Sarvangasana I (3).
- Proceed to 9.

9. Parsva Sarvangasana

parsva=sideways; sarva=whole; anga=body

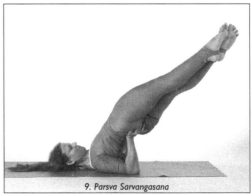
9. Parsva Sarvangasana

- Lower the pelvis and bring the legs halfway down over the head. Turn the hips towards the left and rest the sacrum on the palm of the right hand. The left hip turns backwards, and the right hip turns forwards towards the face.
- Keep the left hand as a support on the left rib cage and lower the legs backwards over the right hand. Keep the knees straight and the upper and lower spring joints of the feet active (Pada Bandha) and in touch with the lower abdomen, so that you do not lose the balance. Eventually the legs will be parallel to the earth.
- Extend the legs out of the groins, not out of the waist. Pull the two frontal hip bones in the direction of the lower frontal ribs, and extend the coccyx towards the heels. In this way the muscles of the lower abdomen stay toned and the lumbar spine stays long.
- Proceed to 10.

10. Parsva Setubandhasana

parsva=sideways; setu=bridge; setu bandha=the construction of a bridge

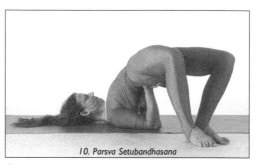

10. Parsva Setubandhasana

- Bend the knees and, keeping the feet together, extend the feet downwards till they reach the blanket. The knees can spread a little as the feet go down, but keep the upper and lower spring joints of the feet active (Pada Bandha) and in touch with the lower abdomen, so that you do not lose the balance.
- Keep rotating the left hip backwards and the right hip forwards towards the face, and keep the support of the left hand on the rib cage.
- If you lose control in this pose and drop onto the blanket, instead of gently landing the feet, it means that you have not used the abdominal muscles correctly. The weight of the legs was supported by the waist and lumbar spine, instead of by the groins and lower abdomen.
- Hold for a few seconds. Then come back up again, keeping the feet together.
- To bring the feet up you have to pull the pubic bone towards the navel, so that the lower abdomen brings the legs up. Join the knees and come back up to Parsva Sarvangasana (9).
- Return to Salamba Sarvangasana I (3) and repeat 9 and 10 on the left side.
- Proceed to 11.

11. Setubandhasana

setu=bridge; setu bandha=the construction of a bridge

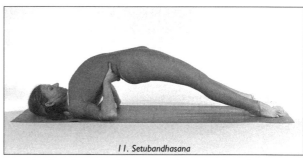

11. Setubandhasana

- To set up the right conditions for going into Setubandhasana it is best to bring the legs first down from Salamba Sarvangasana I (3) into Karnapidasana (2).
- Keep the knees together, reaching over the head to the blanket. Place the hands close to the shoulder blades with the elbows and lower arms parallel to each other.
- Lift the knees and, keeping the knees and feet together and the legs bent, roll the trunk over the hands backwards till the feet reach the blanket back of the trunk. This is a Back Bending position.
- Pull the two frontal hip bones towards the lower ribs and extend the coccyx towards the heels as the feet go down, so that the legs are extended out of the groins, not out of the waist. The muscles of the lower abdomen serve as the 'brakes' for the feet to go down slowly. In all the Back Bendings, the two frontal hip bones and the lower ribs have to maintain their magnetic attraction towards each other in order to keep the length in the lumbar spine. If they lose this contact, the lumbar spine will be compressed in the curve.
- The knees can spread slightly when going down, but keep the feet together and the upper and lower spring joints active (Pada Bandha) and in contact with the lower abdomen, so that you do not lose the balance.

- Extend the legs and place the feet at hip width on the mat. The inner borders of the feet are parallel to each other and the knees are slightly wider than hip width. Keep the feet even, do not keep one foot further forward than the other.
- To create one smooth curve at the front of the body you have to separate the pelvis from the femur heads by rooting the feet (Pada Bandha) and by elongating the legs out of the hip joints. At the same time the coccyx has to extend out of the lumbar spine towards the heels, so that the lumbar vertebrae do not get compressed. The groins should be completely open and should form one continuous line between the upper thighs and the two frontal hip bones.
- Root the back of the head and the back of the upper arms, so that the thoracic spine in between the shoulder blades is elongated and the chest is lifted up from the shoulder heads.
- Resisting the knees slightly backwards towards the shoulders blades and the shoulder blades towards the knees the chest and pelvis have no other choice but to go up. This gives the height and the lightness to the body.
- On each Mula Bandha inhalation lift the trunk by connecting the Pada Bandha, the Mula Bandha, the Uddiyana Bandha and the Jalandhara Bandha, rooting the feet, the head and the arms.
- Hold for one minute. Proceed to 12.

12. Ekapada Setubandhasana

eka=one; pada=leg,foot; setu=bridge;
setu bandha=the construction of a bridge

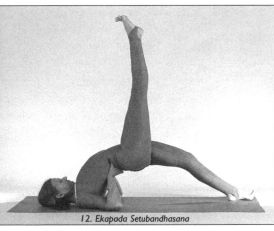

- When you have reached a stable position, bend the right knee and extend the right leg straight up towards the sky. Do not tilt the pelvis. The two frontal hip bones should stay parallel to each other and to the earth.
- The right leg extends upwards in a vertical alignment with the right

12. Ekapada Setubandhasana

  groin, and the left foot and knee extend in alignment with the left groin.
- To get the height and lightness of the pelvis you have to root the left foot (Pada Bandha), elongating the left leg, and elongate the right leg upwards out of the right hip joint. This is in conformity with the principle that the part of the body which is below forms the stable base for the part of the body which is above to elongate upwards against gravity.
- Hold for a few seconds. Then repeat with the other leg.
- On an exhalation walk the feet in towards the head and jump back up to Salamba Sarvangasana I (3), keeping the feet together.
- Proceed to 13.

13. Urdhva Padma Sarvangasana

urdhva=upwards; padma=lotus; sarva=whole; anga=body

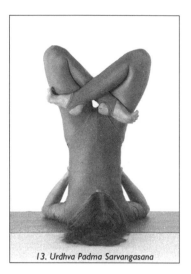

13. Urdhva Padma Sarvangasana

- Cross the legs in Padmasana (see page 77) and extend the knees up towards the sky. In Salamba Sirsasana I you cannot use the hands to cross the legs in Padmasana, but in Salamba Sarvangasana I you can. Therefore you can first learn Urdhva Padmasana in Salamba Sarvangasana I before you try it in Salamba Sirsasana I.
- Performing Pada Bandha in order to stabilize the hip joints rotate the pelvis backwards. The coccyx rolls towards the pubic bone and the lower abdomen and two frontal hip bones move towards the lower frontal ribs. Thus the lumbar spine is elongated.
- Extend the thighs out of the hip joints, so that the groins are opened and the knees point straight up towards the sky.
- For the rest follow the instructions given in Salamba Sarvangasana I (3).
- Hold for thirty seconds. Proceed to 14.

14. Parsva Urdhva Padma Sarvangasana

parsva=sideways; urdhva=upwards; padma=lotus; sarva=whole; anga=body

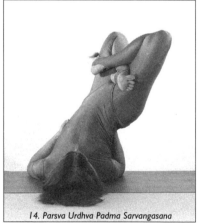

14. Parsva Urdhva Padma Sarvangasana

- Lower the pelvis and bring the crossed legs halfway down over the head. Turn the hips towards the left and rest the sacrum on the palm of the right hand. The left hip turns backwards, and the right hip turns forwards towards the face.
- Keep the left hand as a support on the left rib cage and lower the thighs backwards over the right hand. Keep the upper and lower spring joints of the feet active (Pada Bandha) and in touch with the lower abdomen, so that you do not lose the balance. Eventually the thighs will be parallel to the earth.
- Extend the thighs out of the groins, not out of the waist. Pull the two frontal hip bones in the direction of the lower frontal ribs, and extend the coccyx towards the heels. In this way the muscles of the lower abdomen stay toned and the lumbar spine stays long.
- Hold for thirty seconds. Then repeat on the other side.
- Come back up to Urdhva Padma Sarvangasana (13). Proceed to 15.

15. Parsva Pinda Sarvangasana

parsva=sideways; pinda=embryo; sarva=whole; anga=body

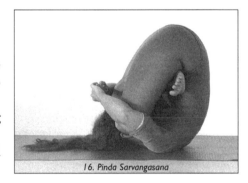

15. Parsva Pinda Sarvangasana

- Lower the pelvis and place the right hip bone on the right hand. Turn the right hip backwards and the left hip forwards towards the face. Then place the right knee next to the right upper arm on the blanket.
- Elongate the left arm sideways, out of the left shoulder joint, as a counterweight for the knees, and root the left ulnar wrist point.
- Continue the rotation of the hips and bring the left knee also down, next to the right ear.
- This whole movement is a diagonal Forward Bending movement, elongating and twisting across the whole spinal column.
- Hold for thirty seconds. Then repeat on the other side.
- Come back to the center. Proceed to 16.

16. Pinda Sarvangasana

pinda=embryo; sarva=whole; anga=body

- On an exhalation bend the back, bring the crossed knees down to the forehead and clasp the arms around the knees.
- Hold for thirty seconds. Change the crossing of the legs and repeat 13, 14, 15 and 16.
- Return to Salamba Sarvangasana I (3). Proceed to 17.

16. Pinda Sarvangasana

17. Salamba Sarvangasana II

sa=with; alamba=support; sarva=whole; anga=body

- Clasp the hands as for Salamba Sirsasana I (see page 163) and extend the arms backwards.
- Extend the wrists away from the shoulders so that the shoulders are pulled backwards away from the ears. At the same time rotate the upper arms out so that the Deltoid muscles roll underneath the shoulders and the Biceps muscles rotate up towards the sky. Root the ulnar wrist points. This enables the Latissimus dorsi to lift the chest up from the shoulder heads and thus to elongate the spine.
- Hold for thirty seconds. Proceed to 18.

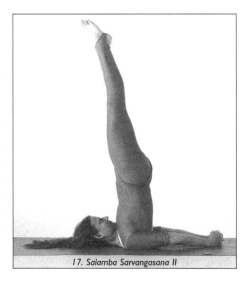

17. Salamba Sarvangasana II

18. Niralamba Sarvangasana I
nir=without; alamba=support; sarva=whole; anga=body

- Raise the arms in an arc of a hundred and eighty degrees over the head to the blanket. Keep the arms parallel to each other and the back of the hands resting on the blanket. Keep the back as straight as possible.
- Hold for thirty seconds. Proceed to 19.

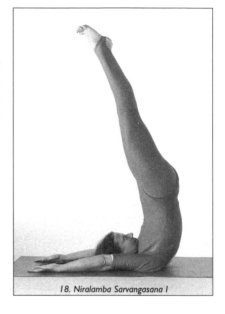

18. Niralamba Sarvangasana I

19. Niralamba Sarvangasana II
nir=without; alamba=support; sarva=whole; anga=body

- Extend the arms up till the palms of the hands rest on the front of the thighs. The fingers point up towards the sky.
- Hold for thirty seconds.

In the last three variations the balance is the main issue, and this depends on the strength and stability of the back and abdominal muscles. Therefore it is important to include them in the daily practice.

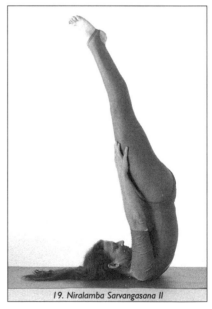

19. Niralamba Sarvangasana II

4.11   Hand Balancings

These positions can be done in <u>four different modes</u>:

a.   Performing each position separately and holding it for thirty seconds.

b.   Vinyasa
Connecting two or more positions by flowing from one into the other, using the breathing.

c.   Mala
Connecting all the positions through Surya Namaskar in the following way, using the breathing:
•   Stand in Tadasana » inhale, extend the arms upwards » exhale, bend down into Uttanasana, inhale, raise the head » exhale, jump back into Chaturanga Dandasana » inhale, go into Urdhvamukha Svanasana » exhale, go into Adhomukha Svanasana, inhale » exhale, go into Vasisthasana I on the right side, stay for three breaths, inhale » exhale, return into Adhomukha Svanasana, inhale » exhale, go into Vasisthasana I on the left side, stay for three breaths, inhale » exhale, return into Adhomukha Svanasana, inhale » exhale, jump forward into Uttanasana » inhale, stand up again in Tadasana, exhale » inhale, extend the arms upwards, etc.

d.   You can also start each one of positions 17 through 26 from Salamba Sirsasana II, finishing by dropping back and pushing up into Urdhva Dhanurasana.

In Tadasana and the Standing Poses, the rebounce force and the resulting elongation upwards with the anti-gravitational lightness and 'bounciness' come through the correct application of the Pada Bandha, that is, the lifting of the talocalcaneonavicular joint and the talocruralis joint, or the lower and upper 'spring' joints.

In Adhomukha Vrksasana and the other Hand Balancings, the same elongation upwards with the anti-gravitational lightness and 'bounciness' come through the correct application of the Hasta Bandha. Hasta Bandha, as described in Chapter 3 on the Bandhas, is the act of rooting the rim of the palm into the earth, that is, the wrist and the fingers, and then 'sucking' the center of the palm upwards. One can compare this to the 'suckers' on the hands and feet of lizards, with which they scale walls and ceilings. This shoots the energy through the arms and shoulders, and thus elongates them.

Hand Balancings

....

1. *Adhomukha Vrksasana*	15. *Padma Mayurasana*
2. *Padma Adhomukha Vrksasana*	16. *Hamsasana*
3. *Pincha Mayurasana*	17. *Bakasana*
4. *Padma Pincha Mayurasana*	18. *Parsva Bakasana*
5. *Vasisthasana I*	19. *Ekapada Bakasana I*
6. *Vasisthasana II*	20. *Ekapada Bakasana II*
7. *Kasyapasana*	21. *Dvipada Koundinyasana*
8. *Visvamitrasana*	22. *Ekapada Koundinyasana*
9. *Dvihasta Bhujasana*	23. *Ekapada Galavasana*
10. *Titthibhasana*	24. *Urdhva Kukkutasana*
11. *Bhujapidasana*	25. *Galavasana*
12. *Ekahasta Bhujasana*	26. *Parsva Kukkutasana*
13. *Astavakrasana*	
14. *Mayurasana*	

1. Adhomukha Vrksasana

adho=downwards; mukha=face; vrksa=tree

1a. Close to the wall

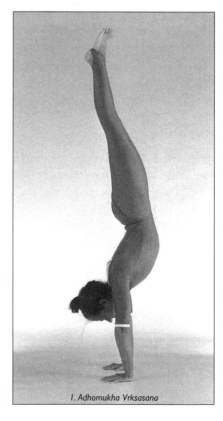

1. Adhomukha Vrksasana

• Kneel down close to a wall, facing it.
• Place the hands on the earth, close to the wall. The arms are parallel to each other, with the hands in alignment with the armpits. Keep the middle fingers parallel to each other and the other fingers and the thumbs spread. Make sure that the hands are even; do not keep one hand further forward than the other. Turn the pits of the elbows forward towards the wall (Savasana rotation of the arms, see page 286).
• On an exhalation, lift the knees, walk the feet closer to the hands and jump up till both the heels are on the wall (change legs each time you jump up on the wall, so as not to create an imbalance in the back muscles by always using the same leg).
• The pelvis is the area in the body which contains the heaviest bone and muscle structure. If the feet jump up fast and the trunk is pulled up by that

speed and the strength of the leg muscles, the pelvis will sag and the result is a 'collision' of the pelvis with the lumbar vertebrae. This will weaken the lumbar vertebrae. The correct way of jumping up into Adhomukha Vrksasana is by pulling the legs and the pelvis up with the back muscles, so that those muscles will get stronger, and the pelvis does not collapse into the lumbar. The pelvis should actually arrive first on the wall, before the heels.

- Keep only the heels on the wall and bring the rest of the body in alignment, with the hip joints straight above the shoulder joints and the middle bones of the hands. Keep the arches of the feet strong (Pada Bandha) and the inner ankles together.
- Keep the top of the head pointing straight downwards, in between the inner arms. Keeping the head flexed backwards gives more curve in the upper thoracic spine, but makes it harder for the shoulders to elongate; on the other hand, keeping the head straight down in between the upper arms gives more freedom in the shoulder blades to slide the chest upwards, out of the shoulder joints.
- Root the hands into the earth and perform Hasta Bandha. This creates the rebounce force in the arms and shoulder joints, so that they elongate automatically. The weight of the body is above the middle bones of the palms, not above the bones of the wrists.
- On each Mula Bandha inhalation, elongate the body vertically upwards from the middle bones of the hands to the middle bones of the feet. Thus the whole body is connected into one unit through the five major Bandhas: lifting the chest up from the shoulder heads, lifting the pelvis up from the lumbar spine, and lifting the legs up from the hip joints.
- On each exhalation maintain that height.
- Hold for one minute.

1b. With two legs

When you have gained confidence jumping up with one leg, you can start to practice jumping with both legs together. Here especially it is obvious that you have to pull the pelvis and legs up with the back muscles, otherwise you will never get up.

- Start as for 1a, but keep the hands slightly further away from the wall and the head flexed backwards.
- On an exhalation jump up, keeping the inner ankles and knees together and pulling the body up with the back muscles. It is very easy to check the strength of those muscles. If the knees and feet spread apart ('frog'-jumping) while jumping up, this is a clear indication of the weakness of the lumbar muscles. Thus the importance of keeping the inner knees and ankles together.
- Root the hands while jumping up, so that the shoulders do not yield: the shoulder joints remain aligned with the palms as the pelvis goes up. Keep the knees bent till the toes are on the wall and the knees, hip joints, shoulder joints and palms are in vertical alignment. Then extend the legs up and proceed as in 1a.

1c. *Away from the wall*

When you have mastered jumping up with both feet, you can take the hands further away from the wall and jump up without allowing the feet to go on the wall. Keep the body just close enough to it to be able to put the feet on it in case you lose balance. Eventually, this pose has to be done in the middle of the room.

- In this free standing version, the head does not point straight down, but is flexed backwards and the eyes look at a point between the two hands. Fix the eyes on that point in order to keep the balance.
- Proceed with the rooting of the hands, the Hasta Bandha and the elongation of the whole body upwards from the middle bones of the hands to the middle bones of the feet, as described above.
- Hold for one minute.

2. Padma Adhomukha Vrksasana
padma=lotus; adho=downwards; mukha=face; vrksa=tree

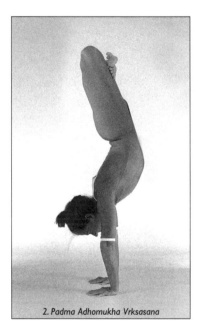

2. Padma Adhomukha Vrksasana

- Start with 1a, close to the wall.
- Cross the legs in Padmasana (see page 77). Keep the knees on the wall, but bring the hips in alignment with the shoulder joints and the palms of the hands.
- For the rest follow the instructions given in Adhomukha Vrksasana (1).

3. Pincha Mayurasana
pincha=chin,feather; mayura=peacock

(See also Part Two: "Comparative Studies of Various Asanas", paragraph 4.13)

3a. *Close to the wall*

- Kneel down on a 'sticky' yoga mat, close to a wall and facing it.
- Turn the arms as for Savasana (see page 286), so that the palms of the hands face upwards. Bend the arms and place the elbows on the mat, in alignment with the armpits. Then turn the palms of the hands down. The middle fingers are parallel to each other and the inner and outer wrists are equally long and parallel to each other. The tips of the middle fingers are on one line with the center of the palms and wrists, the center

of the elbows and the center of the armpits. Make sure that the hands are even; do not keep one hand further forward than the other. Spread the other fingers and extend them on the mat, rooting the knuckles of the fingers together with the ulnar wrist points. Perform Hasta Bandha to activate the shoulder joints and shoulder blades.

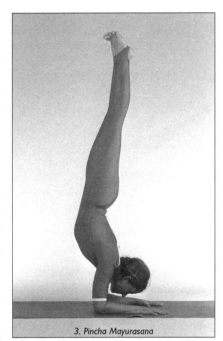
3. Pincha Mayurasana

- On an inhalation, raise the hips and knees and walk the feet in towards the arms, keeping the shoulders in vertical alignment with the elbows: the angle between the upper arms and the lower arms remains ninety degrees. Elongate the groins upwards and raise the pelvis and one leg, till the trunk and the leg are aligned almost vertically with the shoulder and elbow joints. Do not lose the height of the shoulders.
- In this pose it is even more important than in Adhomukha Vriksasana (1) not to jump up with the speed of the foot, dragging the pelvis and back up. The correct way of going into this pose is by using the abdominal and lower back muscles, so that you actually raise the body without jumping. Roll on the lower spring joint of the bottom foot and lift the trunk and bottom leg up into Pincha Mayurasana with the back muscles. Keep both legs straight, till the heels are on the wall (change legs each time you lift up, so as not to create an imbalance in the back muscles by always using the same leg).
- Keeping only the heels on the wall, bring the hip joints in alignment with the shoulder and elbow joints. Keep the arches of the feet strong (Pada Bandha) and the inner ankles together.
- Keep the top of the head first pointing straight downwards in between the inner arms. Keeping the head flexed backwards gives more curve in the upper thoracic spine, but makes it harder for the shoulders to elongate; on the other hand, keeping the head straight down in between the upper arms gives more freedom in the shoulder blades to slide the chest upwards, out of the shoulder joints.
- Root the hands, the ulnar wrist points, the lower arms and the elbows, performing Hasta Bandha. This creates the rebounce force in the upper arms and shoulder joints, so that they elongate automatically. Then flex the head backwards.
- On each Mula Bandha inhalation, elongate the body vertically upwards from the middle bones of the hands to the middle bones of the feet. Thus the whole body is connected into one unit through the five major Bandhas: lifting the chest up from the shoulder heads, lifting the pelvis up from the lumbar spine and lifting the legs up from the hip joints.
- On each exhalation maintain that height.
- Hold for one minute.

3b. *Away from the wall*

- When you have gained confidence on the wall, you can start practicing further away from the wall, without allowing the feet to go to the wall. Keep the body just close enough to it to be able to put the feet on it in case you lose balance. Eventually, this pose has to be done in the middle of the room.
- In this free standing version, the head does not point straight down, but is flexed backwards and the eyes look at a point between the two hands. Fix the eyes on that point in order to keep the balance.
- Proceed with the rooting of the hands, the Hasta Bandha and the elongation of the whole body upwards from the middle bones of the hands to the middle bones of the feet, as described above.
- Hold for one minute.

4. Padma Pincha Mayurasana

padma=lotus; pincha=chin,feather; mayura=peacock

- Start with 3a close to the wall and cross the legs in Padmasana (see page 77). Keep the hips in alignment with the shoulder and elbow joints.
- Hold for one minute; then change the crosslegs.

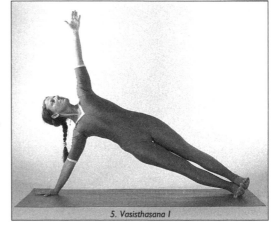

4. Padma Pincha Mayurasana

5. Vasisthasana I

Vasistha is the name of a sage

- Start with Adhomukha Svanasana (see page 216) on a 'sticky' yoga mat and then proceed:
- On an exhalation, roll over on the right hand and the right foot; the outer arch of the right foot is in line with the wrist and middle finger of the right hand.
- The right foot rests on the outer edge, more on the plantar than on the dorsal side of the foot. Place the left foot on the right one, so that the inner ankles touch and all the toes are in line as in Paschimottanasana. Perform Pada Bandha to stabilize the trunk and to lighten the weight of the pelvis on the femur heads.

5. Vasisthasana I

- The distance between the right hand and the right foot is such that the right arm forms an angle of ninety degrees with the chest. Thus the arm is not vertical, but slants forward from the shoulder joint.
- Rotate the right arm as in Savasana (see page 286): the biceps muscle rotates towards the right hand and the triceps muscle towards the ribs.

- Seen from the side, the back of the head is in line with the sacrum and the back of the heels, and the ears, shoulder joints, hip joints, knees and ankles are in one line. Seen from the front, the bridge of the nose is in line with the sternum, the pubic bone and the inner ankles.
- Extend the left arm up towards the sky, in line with the right arm. This means that the arm does not point straight up, but is slanted, so that here too there is an angle of ninety degrees in the left arm pit. Turn the face to look up.
- Do not sink the chest into the right shoulder joint. Create space by rooting the right hand into the earth, performing Hasta Bandha, so that the arm is elongated and the chest is lifted up from the right shoulder head. Do not disturb the alignment of the body, however.
- Do not sink the pelvis into the right hip joint. Create space by rooting the outer edge of the right foot into the earth, performing Pada Bandha, so that the leg is elongated and the pelvis is lifted up from the right femur head.
- On each Mula Bandha inhalation, extend the coccyx towards the heels and elongate the lower abdomen and spine towards the back of the head. On each exhalation, turn the trunk and head further up towards the sky.
- Hold for three breaths. On the fourth exhalation, place the left hand on the mat, at shoulder width from and parallel to the right one, roll over on the right foot, place the left foot at hip width, parallel to the right one, on the mat and return to Adhomukha Svanasana.
- Hold Adhomukha Svanasana for three breaths.
- On the fourth exhalation, turn over on the left foot and repeat on the left side.

6. Vasisthasana II

Vasistha is the name of a sage

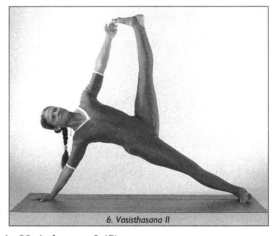

6. Vasisthasana II

- Start with Adhomukha Svanasana (see page 216) on a 'sticky' yoga mat and then proceed:
- On an exhalation, turn over on the right hand and the right foot and go into Vasisthasana I (5).
- Bend the left leg, with the index and middle finger of the left hand hold the big toe (palm facing forward) and extend the leg up towards the sky.
- For the rest follow the instructions given in Vasisthasana I (5).
- Keep the straight lines of the body, especially the line between the back of the head, the sacrum and the right heel. To stay in line, take the head and left leg backwards and the pelvis forwards, without turning it upwards. To avoid sagging the pelvis, you have to root the outer edge of the right foot, and elongate the left leg upwards, out of the left hip joint. That will automatically pull the pelvis upwards.
- Hold for three breaths. On the fourth exhalation, release the left foot, return to Vasisthasana I (5), and then to Adhomukha Svanasana.
- Hold Adhomukha Svanasana for three breaths.
- On the fourth exhalation, turn over on the left foot and repeat on the left side.

7. Kasyapasana

Kasyapa is the son of Marichi and grandson of Brahman

- Start with Adhomukha Svanasana (see page 216) on a 'sticky' yoga mat and then proceed:
- On an exhalation, turn over on the right hand and the right foot and go into Vasisthasana I (5). Cross the left foot as for Padmasana (see page 77), swing the left arm around the back and hold the foot. If you cannot do this, you can start from the mat.
- Sit in Siddhasana (see page 84), with the left foot in the groin of the right leg. Swing the left arm around the back in a circular motion and hold the metatarsal of the left big toe.
- Roll over onto the right hip and extend the right leg, but not fully; keep the knee slightly bent. Place the right hand on the mat in line with the right foot, with the fingers pointing

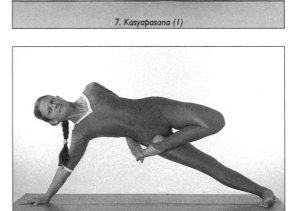

7. Kasyapasana (1)

7. Kasyapasana (2)

in a straight line away from the right hip. The right arm makes an angle of ninety degrees with the chest, and thus is not perpendicular, but slants forward, away from the shoulder joint. The right foot rests on the outer edge, more on the plantar than on the dorsal side.
- On an exhalation, push up on the right hand and foot, till the right leg is straight and in alignment with the trunk. Extend the coccyx towards the right heel, and elongate the left thigh and knee out of the left hip joint. At the same time, elongate the lower abdomen and the two frontal hip bones up towards the ribs. Thus the left groin is opened.
- For the rest follow the instructions given in Vasisthasana I (5).
- Keep the alignment of the body, especially between the back of the head, the sacrum and the right heel. To stay in line, bring the head and left knee back and the pelvis forwards, without turning it upwards. To avoid sagging the pelvis, you have to root the outer edge of the right foot and elongate the left thigh out of the left hip joint. That will automatically pull the pelvis upwards.
- Hold for three breaths. On the fourth exhalation, release the left foot, return to Vasisthasana I (5), and then to Adhomukha Svanasana.
- Hold Adhomukha Svanasana for three breaths.
- On the fourth exhalation, turn over on the left foot and repeat on the left side.

8. Visvamitrasana
Visvamitra is the name of a sage

In the three previous positions the body balances on a unilateral line, that is, either on the right hand and right foot, or on the left hand and left foot. In Visvamitrasana, the body balances on a diagonal line, that is, on the left hand and right foot, or on the right hand and left foot.

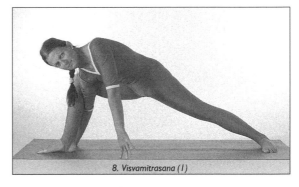
8. Visvamitrasana (1)

- Start with Adhomukha Svanasana (see page 216) on a 'sticky' yoga mat, but keep a shorter distance between the hands and feet. Then proceed:
- As the right hand has to end up in line with the left foot, you have to displace both hands slightly towards the left before swinging the right leg forward. On an exhalation, lean the body weight forward, bend the right arm and, lifting the right hip up, swing the right leg forward in a large, circular movement around the outer side of the right arm, so that the foot

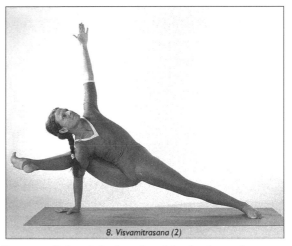
8. Visvamitrasana (2)

lands next to the inner border of the fingers of the right hand, with the knee bent at an angle of ninety degrees and the back of the thigh resting on the deltoid muscle of the right arm.
- Turn the left foot over, so that the sole of the foot rests on the mat, and the inner arch of the left foot is in line with the wrist and middle finger of the right hand.
- Turn over on the right arm and lift the right foot in the direction you are facing, perpendicular to the line between the right hand and the left foot. Then extend the right leg forward in a circular movement, till it is in line with the line between the right hand and the left foot, with the knee straight.
- Extend the left hand up to the sky at an angle of ninety degrees to the chest and look up at the sky.
- For the rest follow the instructions given in Vasisthasana I (5). Keep the alignment of the body, especially the line between the back of the head, the sacrum and the left heel. To stay in line, bring the head back while extending the right leg, and bring the pelvis forwards.
- Hold for three breaths. On the fourth exhalation, place the left hand back on the mat, at shoulder width from and parallel to the right one. Lifting the heel of the left foot and rolling on the ball of the foot, swing the right leg back around the outer side of the right arm in a circular movement, lifting the right hip up, to return to Adhomukha Svanasana. Place the hands back again in their original position, in line with the feet.
- Hold Adhomukha Svanasana for three breaths.
- On the fourth exhalation repeat on the left side.

The next three positions are done in the *Vinyasa* mode, that is, flowing directly from one into the next.

9. Dvihasta Bhujasana

dvi=two; hasta=hand; bhuja=arm

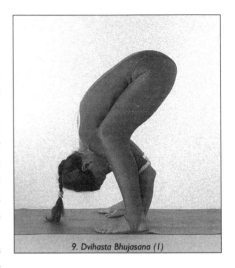

9. Dvihasta Bhujasana (1)

- Start with Adhomukha Svanasana (see page 216) on a 'sticky' yoga mat, but keep a shorter distance between the hands and feet. Then proceed:
- On an exhalation, jump the feet forward around the outer arms in a circular movement, till they land on the mat next to the outer borders of the hands. In this way the distance between the knees is shoulder width. Keep the hips high while jumping, so that you land with the knees just slightly bent.
- Widen the knees a little and, elongating the ribs forward from the groins, place the hands on the back of the calves, with the thumbs on the inner sides of the lower legs, pointing towards each other, and the fingers on the outer sides.
- Insert the shoulders underneath the knees, keeping the hips up and the knees slightly bent. Press the inner thighs against the ribs and the inner knees against the deltoid muscles, and elongate the buttock bones and the back of the thighs up towards the sky. This is Kurmasana (see page 146) standing on the feet.
- Release the hands and place them behind the heels on the mat, with the fingers pointing forwards and the index fingers in line with the back of the heels. Extend the wrists down, lower the pelvis and sit down on the upper arms, near the deltoid muscles.
- Then bring the weight of the body slightly backwards, till the feet lift up from the mat. This is Dvihasta Bhujasana.
- Hold for a few seconds; then proceed to 10.

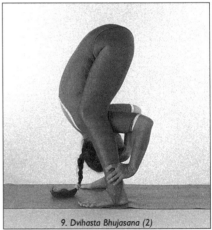

9. Dvihasta Bhujasana (2)

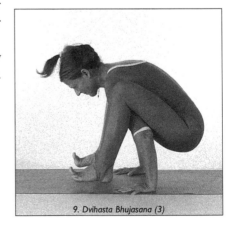

9. Dvihasta Bhujasana (3)

10. Titthibhasana

titthibha=firefly

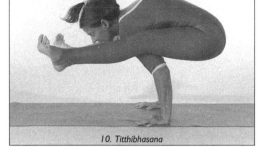

10. Titthibhasana

- Elongate the legs forward, lifting the feet and the pelvis simultaneously: as the lower legs elongate forwards, the buttock bones and the back of the thighs elongate backwards, so that the backs of the legs are extended.
- Press the inner thighs against the ribs, and the inner knees against the deltoid muscles to avoid sliding off the arms. This is Kurmasana (see page 146) standing on the hands: the trunk and the legs, from the buttock bones towards the heels, are parallel to the earth. Perform Pada Bandha to stabilize the legs and pelvis.
- Root the hands, performing Hasta Bandha, so that the arms elongate and the chest is lifted up from the shoulder heads. The back is not straight, but arches upwards: the more you elongate the arms, lifting the chest up from the shoulder heads, the more the back arches upwards (turtle back). Look straight forward.
- Hold for a few seconds; then proceed to 11.

11. Bhujapidasana

bhuja=arm; pida=pressure

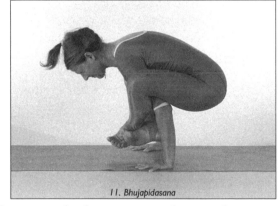

11. Bhujapidasana

- On the exhalation, bend the knees and cross the ankles in front of you. Do not lower the hips as you cross the ankles, but keep extending the buttock bones backwards while pressing the inner thighs against the upper arms.
- Root the hands, performing Hasta Bandha, so that the arms elongate and the chest is lifted up from the shoulder heads. The back is not straight, but arches upwards: the more you elongate the arms, lifting the chest up from the shoulder heads, the more the back arches upwards (turtle back). Look straight forward.
- Hold for a few seconds; then cross the ankles the other way.
- Return to Dvihasta Bhujasana (9). Turn the feet sideways on the upper arms, the right foot towards the right and the left foot towards the left, lift the hips and jump back into Chaturanga Dandasana (see page 57). Keep the head up and bend the arms as you jump, so that the shoulders end up above the hands. Always use the exhalation to jump, and the inhalation to stabilize your position.
- Proceed through Urdhvamukha Svanasana (see page 216) and Adhomukha Svanasana (see page 216).

The next two positions are done in the *Vinyasa* mode, that is, flowing directly from one into the next.

12. Ekahasta Bhujasana

eka=one; hasta=hand; bhuja=arm

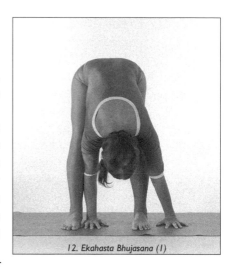

12. Ekahasta Bhujasana (1)

- Start with Adhomukha Svanasana (see page 216), but keep a shorter distance between the hands and feet. Then proceed:
- On an exhalation, jump the feet forward: the left foot ends up in between the two hands, and the right foot swings around the outer right arm in a circular movement to land next to the outer border of the right hand. Thus the hands and feet are on one line. Keep the hips high while jumping, so that you land with the knees just slightly bent.
- Place the right hand on the back of the right calf muscle, with the thumb on the inner side of the lower leg, and the fingers on the outer side, and insert the right shoulder underneath the right knee. Then release the right hand and place both hands behind the feet on the mat, with the fingers pointing forwards.

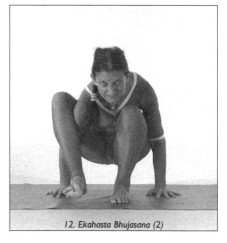

12. Ekahasta Bhujasana (2)

- Extend the wrists down, lower the pelvis and sit down with the right thigh on the right upper arm, near the deltoid muscle. Bring the weight of the body slightly backwards till the right foot lifts up from the mat, keeping the leg bent as in Dvihasta Bhujasana (9).
- Then lift the left foot and extend the leg forward, parallel to the earth.
- Press the inner right thigh against the ribs, and the inner knee against the right deltoid muscle, to prevent the leg from sliding off the arm. Perform Pada Bandha with both feet to stabilize the legs and pelvis.
- Root the hands, performing Hasta Bandha, so that the arms elongate and the chest is lifted up from the shoulder heads. The back is not straight, but arches upwards: the more you elongate the arms, lifting the chest up from the

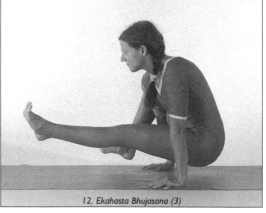

12. Ekahasta Bhujasana (3)

shoulder heads, the more the back arches upwards (turtle back). Look straight forward.
- Hold for a few seconds; then proceed to 13.

13. Astavakrasana

Astavakra is the teacher of King Janaka

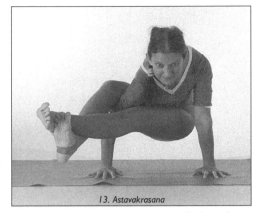

13. Astavakrasana

- Cross the left foot over the right, and extend both legs forwards and slightly sideways; the left foot crosses over the right one, so that the right leg supports the left one.
- Press the inner right thigh against the ribs, and the inner knee against the right deltoid muscle, to prevent the leg from sliding off the arm. Perform Pada Bandha with both feet to stabilize the legs and pelvis.
- Root the hands, performing Hasta Bandha, so that the arms elongate and the chest is lifted up from the shoulder heads. The back is not straight, but arches upwards: the more you elongate the arms, lifting the chest up from the shoulder heads, the more the back arches upwards (turtle back). Look straight forward.
- Hold for a few seconds.
- Release the crossing of the feet and bend the legs again, the left one in between the arms and the right one on the right arm, turning the foot sideways. Then lift the hips, bring the feet back, the left foot through the arms and the right one around the outer side of the right arm, and jump back into Chaturanga Dandasana (see page 57).
- Proceed through Urdhvamukha Svanasana (see page 216) and Adhomukha Svanasana (see page 216), and repeat 12 and 13 on the left side.

14. Mayurasana

mayura=peacock

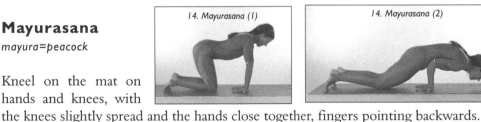

14. Mayurasana (1)

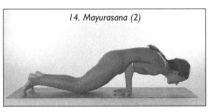

14. Mayurasana (2)

- Kneel on the mat on hands and knees, with the knees slightly spread and the hands close together, fingers pointing backwards.
- Bend the elbows, keeping them close together, lift the knees and pelvis, and place the lower abdomen on the bent elbows: the elbows are in between the two frontal hip bones. Keep the head up.
- Bring the body weight slowly forward, supporting yourself on the toes and hands, till the feet lift off the mat by themselves. The whole body is now supported only on the hands, and makes one line, from the ankles through the knees to the shoulders and ears. The lower arms are not perpendicular to the earth, but slant forwards, with an angle of about a hundred degrees in the elbows.
- Hold for a couple of seconds. On an exhalation, bring the body weight back again, so that the feet go back onto the mat.

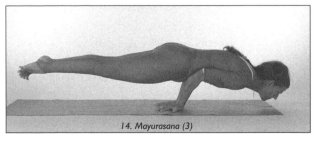

14. Mayurasana (3)

15. Padma Mayurasana

padma=lotus; mayura=peacock

- This is the same position as the previous one, performed with the legs in Padmasana (see page 77).

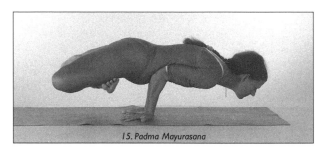

15. Padma Mayurasana

16. Hamsasana

hamsa=swan

- This is the same position as Mayurasana (14), but here the fingers point forward. This produces a tighter angle in the wrist joints.

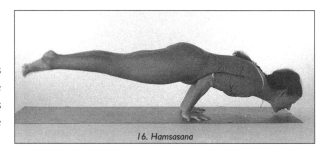

16. Hamsasana

17. Bakasana

baka=crane

- Start with Salamba Sirsasana II (see page 171) and then proceed:
- On an exhalation, lower the legs in between the arms, till the feet are about ten inches from the mat. Keep the knees straight and together.
- Bend the knees between the inner upper arms, keeping the elbows in line with the armpits and an angle of ninety degrees in the elbows.
- Spread the knees, keeping the feet together, and take the shins deep into the armpits. The tibial bones rest on the triceps muscles of the upper arms, and the inner thighs press against the sides of the rib cage. The weight of the body is on the center of the palms.
- Squeeze the knees inwards towards each other, so that the elbows stay in line with the armpits, and keep the inner ankles together, so that all the toes are in line. Perform Pada Bandha with both feet to maintain the compactness of the legs and hips. The upper and lower spring joints of the feet control the hip joints; they are of vital importance

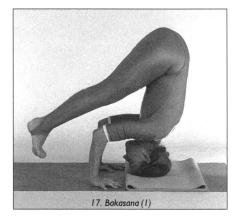

17. Bakasana (1)

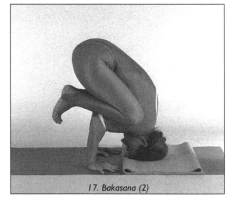

17. Bakasana (2)

in all the Bakasana poses, where you have to maintain the compactness and coherence of the body. Keeping the feet and spring joints inactive would mean that the body would fall apart in the hip joints, and therefore it would be impossible to perform these poses.

- To lift the head up from the mat, bring the weight of the body back onto the wrists. As soon as the head is loose from the mat, however, you have to bring the weight of the body again forward onto the center of the palms. The central point of gravity is in the center of the palms. Thus, to maintain an even and effortless equilibrium, the weight of the body at the front of this central point and at the back of it should be even: the head, shoulders, upper chest and knees at the front of this central point should be in balance with the lower trunk, thighs and feet, which are at the back of it.

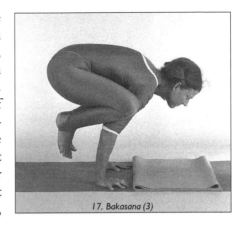

17. Bakasana (3)

- As the head lifts, the feet will go down (see-saw action around the shoulder joints), but do not lower them too much, and do not lose the action in the spring joints (Pada Bandha).

- After reaching the balance, work on the lightness of the pose, the rooting and the elongation. Pressing the tibial bones against the triceps muscles to maintain the compactness of the body, root the hands and perform Hasta Bandha, so that the arms elongate and the chest is lifted up from the shoulder heads. The back is not straight but arches upwards; the more you elongate the arms, lifting the chest up from the shoulder heads, the more the back arches upwards (turtle back). Thus the pose is high and light.

- As Bakasana is the true counterpose for Back Bendings, the back should not be concave but, on the contrary, should make a 'cat-back,' that is, the whole spine, from the base up to the neck, should push up towards the sky. The first thoracic vertebra and the coccyx are at the same height; they form the extreme ends of the bow, while the spine forms the drawn bow itself. This is the reversed bow: whereas in Dhanurasana (see page 215) the bow of the spine is curved into the trunk, here it is curved backwards, out of the trunk. Therefore Bakasanas are the counter poses for Back Bendings, and in both cases the coccyx and first thoracic vertebra form the extreme end points of the bow.

- The neck should be loose; do not try to lift the head up too much: the eyes look at an angle of forty-five degrees forward and downward.

- To come out of the pose, the movement of lowering the head onto the mat and bringing the weight of the body back onto the wrists should be synchronized, so that at all times the weight at the front and back of the central point of gravity is maintained.

- Once the head is on the mat, release the shins from the upper arms by lifting the pelvis and bringing the knees again in between the inner upper arms. Then extend the legs and return to Salamba Sirsasana II.

18. Parsva Bakasana

parsva=sideways; baka=crane

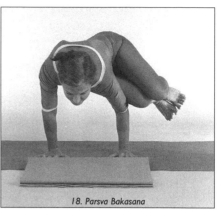

18. Parsva Bakasana

- Start with Salamba Sirsasana II (see page 171) and proceed:
- On an exhalation, lower the legs between the arms, till the feet are about ten inches from the mat. Keep the knees straight and together.
- Bend the knees between the inner upper arms, keeping the elbows in line with the armpits and an angle of ninety degrees in the elbows.
- Then lift the knees slightly above the level of the upper arms and, rotating the back, especially the lumbar spine, swing the legs over the left upper arm, till the outer side of the right thigh rests on the triceps muscle of the left arm. Turn the back enough so that you do not come to rest on the quadriceps muscle of the right thigh, but rather on the fascia lata.
- Keep the inner ankles together, so that all the toes are in line. Perform Pada Bandha with both feet to maintain the compactness of the legs and hips.
- The upper and lower spring joints of the feet control the hip joints; they are of vital importance in all the Bakasana poses, where you have to maintain the compactness and coherence of the body. Keeping the feet and spring joints inactive would mean that the body would fall apart in the hip joints, and therefore it would be impossible to perform these poses.
- Even though the thighs rest only on the left upper arm, the weight of the body is still distributed evenly between both hands, on the center of the palms.
- To lift the head up from the mat, bring the weight of the body back onto the wrists. Keep lifting the feet, though. As soon as the head is loose from the mat, you have to bring the weight of the body again forward, onto the center of the palms. The central point of gravity is in the center of the palms. Thus, to maintain an even and effortless equilibrium, the weight of the body at the front and back of this central point should be even: the head, shoulders, upper chest and knees in front of this central point should be in balance with the lower trunk, thighs and feet, which are behind it.
- As the head lifts, the feet will go down (see-saw action around the shoulder joints), but do not lower them too much, and do not lose the action in the spring joints (Pada Bandha).
- After reaching the balance, work on the lightness of the pose, the rooting and the elongation. Pulling the heels close to the buttocks while keeping the inner ankles together, root the hands and perform Hasta Bandha, so that the arms elongate and the chest is lifted up from the shoulder heads. This rooting, elongation, lightness and lifting will be easier to feel on the right (free) side of the body, but try nevertheless to create some of it on the left side too.
- Here too the spine should push up to the sky, even though in this pose it is much less obvious than in the previous one, due to the turning of the spinal vertebrae. To give an extra accentuation to this turning of the spine, you have to synchronize the lifting of the feet with the lifting of the right shoulder blade, so that the first thoracic vertebra and the coccyx have the same height from the earth. Keep the hips exactly in the middle, in between the two elbows, so that the spine from the coccyx to the back of the head remains perpendicular to the line between the hands.

- The neck should be loose; do not try to lift the head too much; the eyes look at an angle of forty-five degrees forward and downward.
- To come out of the pose, the movement of lowering the head onto the mat and bringing the weight of the body back onto the wrists should be synchronized, so that at all times the weight at the front and back of the central point of gravity is maintained.
- Once the head is on the mat, release the thighs from the left upper arm by lifting the pelvis and bringing the knees again in between the inner upper arms. Then extend the legs and return to Salamba Sirsasana II.
- Repeat on the other side.

19. Ekapada Bakasana I

eka=one; pada=leg,foot; baka=crane

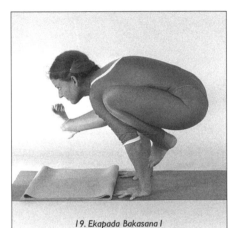

19. Ekapada Bakasana I

This pose is a combination of Bakasana (17) and Titthibhasana (10).

- Start with Salamba Sirsasana II (see page 171) and proceed:
- On an exhalation, lower the legs between the arms, till the feet are about ten inches from the mat. Keep the knees straight and together.
- Bend the knees between the inner upper arms, keeping the elbows in line with the armpits and an angle of ninety degrees in the elbows.
- Lift the left knee and bring the left shin into the left armpit as in Bakasana (17).
- Press the left thigh against the left side of the rib cage, keeping the lower spring joint of the left foot active (Pada Bandha). The weight of the body is on the center of the palms.
- Lift the right knee and turn the right leg out, so that the toes of the right foot point away from the trunk, at an angle of ninety degrees to the right. Then swing the right leg forward in a circular movement, till the inner side of the thigh comes to rest on the deltoid muscle of the right arm. The right knee is still bent, and the right foot is still pointing away from the trunk.
- To lift the head up from the mat, bring the weight of the body back onto the wrists. Keep lifting the feet, though. As soon as the head is loose from the mat, bring the weight of the body again forwards, but not completely onto the center of the palms.
- While lifting the head, extend the right leg forward as in Titthibhasana (10): keeping the toes pointing sideways extend the right foot forward in a circular movement, till the knee is straight and the sole of the right foot faces forward at an angle of forty-five degrees. Thus the left shin bone and the inner right thigh rest on the upper arms.
- After reaching the balance, work on the lightness of the pose, that is, on the rooting and the elongation. Pressing the left shin bone and the inner right thigh against the triceps muscles of the upper arms to maintain the compactness of the body, root the hands and perform Hasta Bandha, so that the arms elongate and the chest is lifted up from the shoulder heads. The back is not straight, but arches upwards; the more you elongate the arms, lifting the chest up from the shoulder heads, the more the back arches upwards (turtle back). Thus the pose is high and light.

- To come out of the pose, the movement of lowering the head onto the mat and bringing the weight of the body back onto the wrists should be synchronized, so that at all times the weight at the front and back of the central point of gravity is maintained.
- Once the head is on the mat, release the left shin and right thigh from the upper arms by lifting the pelvis, and bring the knees again in between the inner upper arms. Then extend the legs and return to Salamba Sirsasana II.

20. Ekapada Bakasana II

eka=one; pada=leg, foot; baka=crane

- Start with Salamba Sirsasana II (see page 171) and proceed:
- On an exhalation, lower the legs between the arms, till the feet are about ten inches from the mat. Keep the knees straight and together.
- On the next exhalation, bend the left knee and bring the left shin into the left armpit as in Bakasana (17). Lift the right

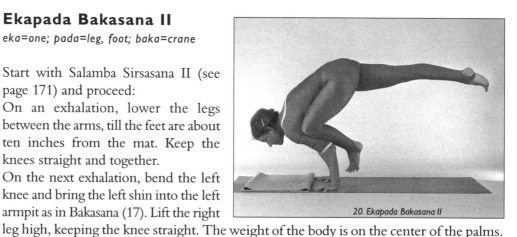

20. Ekapada Bakasana II

leg high, keeping the knee straight. The weight of the body is on the center of the palms.
- To lift the head up from the mat, bring the weight of the body back onto the wrists. As soon as the head is loose from the mat, however, you have to bring the weight of the body again forwards, onto the center of the palms.
- This pose is the hardest of the Bakasana poses, because the weight of the body back of the central point of gravity is greatly increased due to the backward extension of the right leg. Therefore it is imperative to keep the right leg raised high throughout the pose. Press the left shin down on the left arm, performing Pada Bandha to support the action in the pelvis and lower abdomen.
- To come out of the pose, the movement of lowering the head onto the mat and bringing the weight of the body back onto the wrists should be synchronized, so that at all times the weight at the front and back of the central point of gravity is maintained.
- Once the head is on the mat, release the left shin from the left upper arm, lift the pelvis and extend the left leg, joining it with the right one. Then return to Salamba Sirsasana II.

21. Dvipada Koundinyasana

dvi=two; pada=leg, foot; Koundinya is the name of a sage

- Start with Parsva Bakasana (18) on the left arm and proceed:
- After reaching the balance, extend both legs so that they point forward at an angle of forty-five degrees.
- For the rest follow the instructions given in Parsva Bakasana (18).

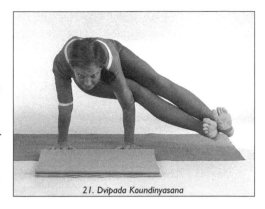

21. Dvipada Koundinyasana

22. Ekapada Koundinyasana

eka=one; pada=leg, foot; Koundinya is the name of a sage

- Start with Parsva Bakasana (18) on the left arm and proceed:
- Cross the left knee behind the right one, and extend the right leg forward. Keep the left knee bent. The right foot points forward in the direction you will be facing, and the left foot points backwards.

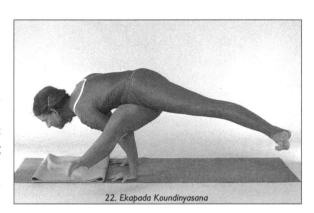

22. Ekapada Koundinyasana

- To lift the head, keep the left leg bent and proceed as usual.
- After reaching the balance, extend the left leg backwards. This means that the weight of the body is increased back of the central point of gravity. If this situation is not corrected, the weight of the left leg will inevitably drag you down. Thus, while extending the left leg backwards, you have to simultaneously bring the chest and shoulders slightly forwards, so that you maintain an even weight at the front and back of the central point of gravity.
- Before lowering the head again, bend the left leg, bringing the chest and shoulders slightly backwards (otherwise there will be too much weight on the front of the central point of gravity and you will fall on your head), and return to Parsva Bakasana.
- To come out of the pose, the movement of lowering the head onto the mat and bringing the weight of the body back onto the wrists should be synchronized, so that at all times the weight at the front and back of the central point of gravity is maintained.
- Once the head is on the mat, release the thighs from the left upper arm by lifting the pelvis and bringing the knees again in between the inner upper arms. Then extend the legs and return to Salamba Sirsasana II.
- Repeat on the other side.

23. Ekapada Galavasana

eka=one; pada=leg, foot; Galava is the name of a sage

This pose is a preparation for Urdhva Kukkutasana (24).

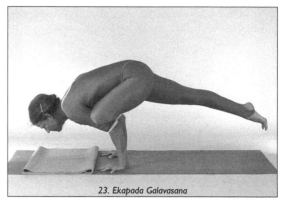

23. Ekapada Galavasana

- Start with Salamba Sirsasana II (see page 171) and proceed:
- Bend the left leg and place the left foot in the right groin as for Padmasana (see page 77).
- Bend the right knee and bring the legs down to the arms. Place the left shin on the triceps muscle of the left arm and the left foot on the triceps muscle of the right arm, hooking the toes around the outer edge of the right upper arm and performing Pada Bandha to stabilize the hips. The right knee is still bent, with the right foot pointing backwards.
- Lower the hips, so that the rib cage rests on the left lower leg, and then extend the right leg backwards.

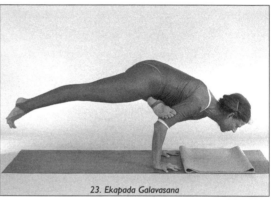

23. Ekapada Galavasana

- To lift the head, proceed as usual. Keep the right leg raised high with the help of the back muscles. The rib cage rests throughout on the lower left leg. Do not lose the grip of the left foot on the outer right arm.
- Before lowering the head onto the mat again, bend the right leg and then proceed as usual.

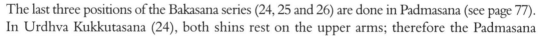

The last three positions of the Bakasana series (24, 25 and 26) are done in Padmasana (see page 77). In Urdhva Kukkutasana (24), both shins rest on the upper arms; therefore the Padmasana should be fairly wide. In Galavasana (25), the crossed shins rest on one arm, and thus the Padmasana has to be tighter. In Parsva Kukkutasana (26) the Padmasana should be very tight.

24. Urdhva Kukkutasana

urdhva=upwards; kukkuta=cock

If you can do Padmasana in Salamba Sirsasana II, this pose is actually the easiest of all the Bakasana poses.

- Start with Salamba Sirsasana II (see page 171), cross the legs in Padmasana (see page 77) and, on an exhalation, lower the legs and place the shins on the triceps muscles of the upper arms, close to the armpits.

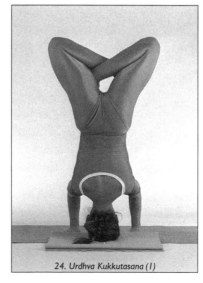

24. Urdhva Kukkutasana (1)

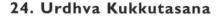

- To lift the head up from the mat, take the pelvis slightly back and down, and proceed as usual.
- Squeeze the thighs inward towards each other, and pull the knees up into the abdomen to maintain the compactness of the pose. Root the hands, performing Hasta Bandha, so that the arms elongate and the chest lifts up from the shoulder heads.
- This position is Yoga Mudrasana I (see page 87) while balancing on the hands, thus the body is parallel to the earth. Like in Bakasana (17), do not make the back concave but, on the contrary, make a 'cat-back', that is, the whole spine, from the base up to the neck,

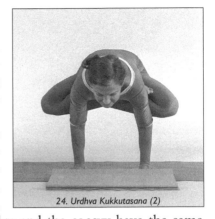

24. Urdhva Kukkutasana (2)

pushes up towards the sky. The first thoracic vertebra and the coccyx have the same height from the earth; they form the extreme ends of the bow, while the spine forms the drawn bow itself.

- The neck should be loose, do not try to lift the head up too much; the eyes look at an angle of forty-five degrees forward and downward.
- To come out of the pose, proceed as usual.

25. Galavasana

Galava is the name of a sage

As mentioned before, the Padmasana here should be tighter than in the previous pose.

- Start with Salamba Sirsasana II (see page 171), cross the legs in Padmasana (see page 77) and proceed:
- On an exhalation, lower the legs to the arms. Turn the hips to the left and place the point where the shins cross each other on the triceps of the left upper arm. The left knee is now on the left side of the left arm, and the right thigh is in between the two arms.
- Pull the right knee up towards the chest, almost as if you want to bite it. This involves strong action of the adductor muscles of the right thigh and of the oblique abdominal muscles.
- To lift the head, proceed as usual.
- This pose is like a twisted Yoga Mudrasana I (see page 87) performed while balancing on the hands. Thus the body is parallel to the earth as in Urdhva Kukkutasana (24).
- Pull the right knee up towards the chest, and keep pointing it straight forward in the direction you

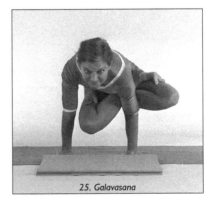

25. Galavasana

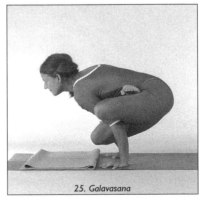

25. Galavasana

are facing, in the middle of the two elbows. Perform Pada Bandha to maintain the compactness of the thighs and hips.
- To come out of the pose, proceed as usual.

26. Parsva Kukkutasana

parsva=sideways; kukkuta=cock

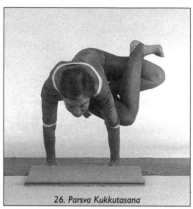

26. Parsva Kukkutasana

As mentioned before, in this position the Padmasana is tightest.

- Start with Salamba Sirsasana II (see page 171), cross the legs in Padmasana (see page 77) and proceed:
- Hook the toes around the outer edges of the thighs, so that the arches and ankles are very strong (Pada Bandha).
- On an exhalation, lower the legs to just above the level of the upper arms. Inhale, and with a strong exhalation swing the legs to the left till the quadriceps muscle of the right thigh comes to rest on the triceps muscle of the left arm. The left knee points upwards.
- To lift the head, proceed as usual.
- To come out of the pose, proceed as usual.

This pose is the most difficult of the Bakasana series, partly because of the extreme twisting of the trunk, and partly because of the balance.

4.12 Back Bendings

Back Bendings

a. Simple Back Bendings
b. Urdhva Dhanurasan
c. Back Bend Variations

4.12a Simple Back Bendings

Simple Back Bendings

1. Urdhvamukha Salabhasana
   a. Arms backwards
   b. Arms sideways
   c. Arms forwards
   d. Makarasana
2. Dvipada Adhomukha Salabhasana
   a. Arms backwards
   b. Arms sideways
   c. Arms forwards
   d. Makarasana
3. Ekapada Adhomukha Salabhasana
   a. Arms backwards
   b. Arms sideways
   c. Arms forwards
   d. Makarasana

4. Dvipada Salabhasana
   a. Arms backwards
   b. Arms sideways
   c. Arms forwards
   d. Makarasana
5. Ekapada Salabhasana
   a. Arms forwards, same side arm and leg up
   b. Arms forwards, opposite arm and leg up
6. Dhanurasana
7. Bhujangasana I
8. Urdhvamukha Svanasana
9. Adhomukha Svanasana
10. Purvottanasana
11. Ustrasana

1. Urdhvamukha Salabhasana

urdhva=upwards; mukha=face;
salabha=locust

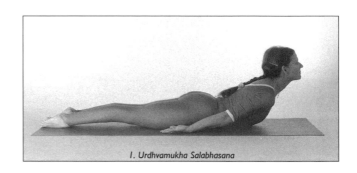

1. Urdhvamukha Salabhasana

1a. Arms backwards

- Lie on the stomach on a blanket with the legs extended straight backwards and the inner ankles together. Extend the arms backwards and clasp the hands on the back.
- On the inhalation, lift the head,

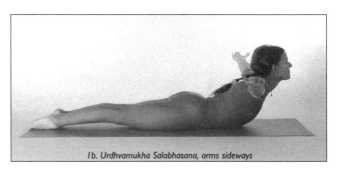

1a. Urdhvamukha Salabhasana, arms backwards

chest and arms up, pulling the body up from the kidney region. Elongate the arms backwards out of the shoulder joints. Do not flex the head too far back, but keep the neck long and fairly relaxed.
- Keep the legs and feet on the blanket and the inner ankles together, rooting the top of the arches into the earth.
- Hold for a few seconds, retaining the breath. On the exhalation, lower the head, chest and arms. Repeat three times.

1b. Arms sideways

- Lie on the stomach on a blanket with the legs extended straight backwards and the inner ankles together. Extend the arms sideways on the blanket, at an angle of ninety degrees to the chest, with the palms of the hands turned down.

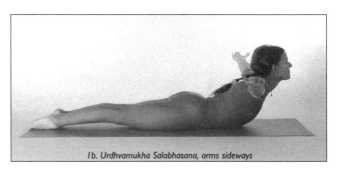

1b. Urdhvamukha Salabhasana, arms sideways

- On the inhalation, lift the head, chest and arms up, pulling the body up from the kidney region. Elongate the arms sideways out of the shoulder joints. To keep the arms at an angle of ninety degrees to the chest, elongate the ulnar side of the wrists more. Do not flex the head too far back, but keep the neck long and fairly relaxed.
- Keep the legs and feet on the blanket and the inner ankles together, rooting the top of the arches into the earth.
- Hold for a few seconds, retaining the breath. On the exhalation, lower the head, chest and arms. Repeat three times.

1c. *Arms forwards*

- Lie on the stomach on a blanket with the legs extended straight backwards and the inner ankles together. Extend the arms forwards on the blanket, keeping them parallel to each other and the palms of the hands turned down.

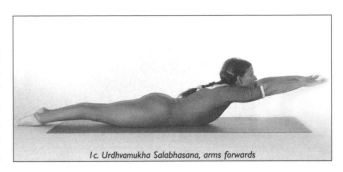

1c. Urdhvamukha Salabhasana, arms forwards

- On the inhalation, lift the head, chest and arms up, pulling the body up from the kidney region. Elongate the arms forwards out of the shoulder joints, keeping them parallel to each other. Do not flex the head too far back, but keep the neck long and fairly relaxed.
- Keep the legs and feet on the blanket and the inner ankles together, rooting the top of the arches into the earth.
- Hold for a few seconds, retaining the breath. On the exhalation, lower the head, chest and arms. Repeat three times.

1d. *Makarasana*
makara=crocodile

- Lie on the stomach on a blanket with the legs extended straight backwards and the inner ankles together. Bend the arms and clasp the hands in the neck.

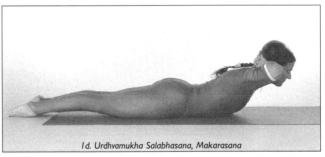

1d. Urdhvamukha Salabhasana, Makarasana

- On the inhalation, lift the head, chest and arms up, pulling the body up from the kidney region. Keep the elbows up. Do not flex the head too far back, but keep the neck long and fairly relaxed.
- Keep the legs and feet on the blanket and the inner ankles together, rooting the top of the arches into the earth.
- Hold for a few seconds, retaining the breath. On the exhalation, lower the head, chest and arms. Repeat three times.

2. Dvipada Adhomukha Salabhasana

dvi=two; pada=leg,foot; adho=downwards; mukha=face; salabha=locust

2a. *Arms backwards*

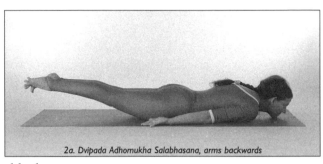

2a. Dvipada Adhomukha Salabhasana, arms backwards

- Lie on the stomach on a blanket with the legs extended straight backwards and the inner ankles together. Extend the arms backwards on the blanket next to the trunk, with the palms of the hands turned down. Rest the forehead or chin on the blanket.
- On the inhalation, lift the legs up, keeping the knees straight and elongating the legs backwards out of the lumbar spine. The inner ankles stay together and the head, trunk and arms stay on the blanket.
- Hold for a few seconds, retaining the breath. On the exhalation, lower the legs. Repeat three times.

2b. *Arms sideways*

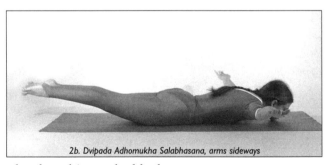

2b. Dvipada Adhomukha Salabhasana, arms sideways

- Lie on the stomach on a blanket with the legs extended straight backwards and the inner ankles together. Extend the arms sideways on the blanket, at an angle of ninety degrees to the chest, with the palms of the hands turned down. Rest the forehead or chin on the blanket.
- On the inhalation, lift the legs up, keeping the knees straight and elongating the legs backwards out of the lumbar spine. The inner knees stay together and the head, trunk and arms stay on the blanket.
- Hold for a few seconds, retaining the breath. On the exhalation, lower the legs. Repeat three times.

2c. *Arms forwards*

- Lie on the stomach on a blanket with the legs extended straight backwards and the inner ankles together. Extend the arms forwards on the blanket, keeping

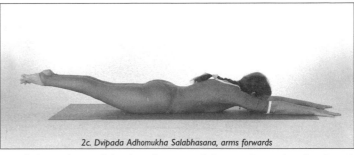

2c. Dvipada Adhomukha Salabhasana, arms forwards

them parallel to each other and the palms of the hands turned down. Rest the forehead or chin on the blanket.
- On the inhalation, lift the legs up, keeping the knees straight and elongating the legs backwards out of the lumbar spine. The inner ankles stay together and the head, trunk and arms stay on the blanket.
- Hold for a few seconds, retaining the breath. On the exhalation, lower the legs. Repeat three times.

2d. *Makarasana*
makara=crocodile

- Lie on the stomach on a blanket with the legs extended straight backwards and the inner ankles together. Bend the arms and clasp the hands in the neck. Rest the forehead or chin on

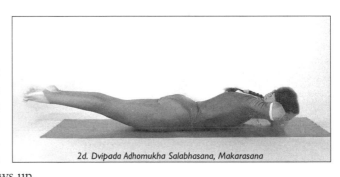

2d. Dvipada Adhomukha Salabhasana, Makarasana

the blanket, but keep the elbows up.
- On the inhalation, lift the legs up, keeping the knees straight and elongating the legs backwards out of the lumbar spine. The inner ankles stay together and the head and trunk stay on the blanket.
- Hold for a few seconds, retaining the breath. On the exhalation, lower the legs. Repeat three times.

3. Ekapada Adhomukha Salabhasana

eka=one; pada=leg, foot; adho=downwards; mukha=face; salabha =locust

3a. *Arms backwards*

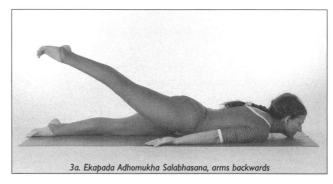

3a. Ekapada Adhomukha Salabhasana, arms backwards

- Lie on the stomach on a blanket with the legs extended straight backwards and the inner ankles together. Extend the arms backwards on the blanket next to the trunk, with the palms of the hands turned down. Rest the forehead or chin on the blanket.
- On the inhalation, lift the right leg up, keeping the knee straight and elongating the leg backwards out of the lumbar spine. Do not tilt the right side of the pelvis up to lift the leg, but use the biceps muscle at the back of the thigh to lift it. Both the frontal hip bones stay on the blanket.
- Hold for a few seconds, retaining the breath. On the exhalation, lower the leg and repeat with the other one. Repeat three times with each leg.

3b. *Arms sideways*

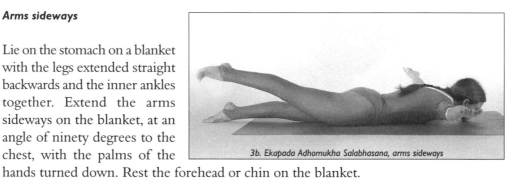

3b. Ekapada Adhomukha Salabhasana, arms sideways

- Lie on the stomach on a blanket with the legs extended straight backwards and the inner ankles together. Extend the arms sideways on the blanket, at an angle of ninety degrees to the chest, with the palms of the hands turned down. Rest the forehead or chin on the blanket.
- On the inhalation, lift the right leg up, keeping the knee straight and elongating the leg backwards out of the lumbar spine. Do not tilt the right side of the pelvis up to lift the leg, but use the biceps muscle at the back of the thigh to lift it. Both the frontal hip bones stay on the blanket.
- Hold for a few seconds, retaining the breath. On the exhalation, lower the leg and repeat with the other one. Repeat three times with each leg.

3c. *Arms forwards*

- Lie on the stomach on a blanket with the legs extended straight backwards and the inner ankles together. Extend the arms forwards on the blanket, keeping them 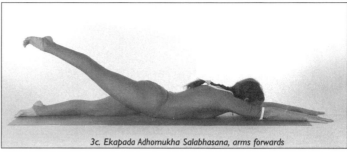 parallel to each other and the palms of the hands turned down. Rest the forehead or chin on the blanket.

3c. Ekapada Adhomukha Salabhasana, arms forwards

- On the inhalation, lift the right leg up, keeping the knee straight and elongating the leg backwards out of the lumbar spine. Do not tilt the right side of the pelvis up to lift the leg, but use the biceps muscle at the back of the thigh to lift it. Both the frontal hip bones stay on the blanket.
- Hold for a few seconds, retaining the breath. On the exhalation, lower the leg and repeat with the other one. Repeat three times with each leg.

3d. *Makarasana*
makara=crocodile

- Lie on the stomach on a blanket with the legs extended straight backwards and the inner ankles together. Bend the arms and clasp the hands in the neck. Rest the forehead or chin on 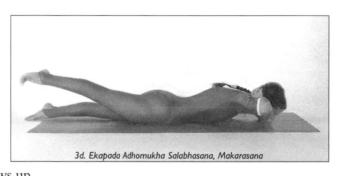 the blanket, but keep the elbows up.

3d. Ekapada Adhomukha Salabhasana, Makarasana

- On the inhalation, lift the right leg up, keeping the knee straight and elongating the leg backwards out of the lumbar spine. Do not tilt the right side of the pelvis up to lift the leg, but use the biceps muscle at the back of the thigh to lift it. Both the frontal hip bones stay on the blanket.
- Hold for a few seconds, retaining the breath. On the exhalation, lower the leg and repeat with the other one. Repeat three times with each leg.

4. Dvipada Salabhasana

dvi=two; pada=leg, foot; salabha=locust

4a. Arms backwards

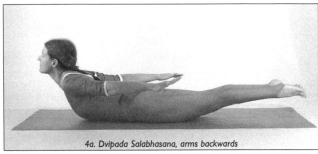

4a. Dvipada Salabhasana, arms backwards

- Lie on the stomach on a blanket with the legs extended straight backwards and the inner ankles together. Extend the arms backwards and clasp the hands on the back.
- On the inhalation, lift the head, chest, arms and legs up, pulling the body up from the kidney region. Elongate the arms backwards out of the shoulder joints, and the legs backwards out of the lumbar spine.
- Keep the knees straight and the inner ankles together, and do not flex the head too far back, but keep the neck long and fairly relaxed.
- Hold for a few seconds, retaining the breath. On the exhalation, lower the head, chest, arms and legs. Repeat three times.

4b. Arms sideways

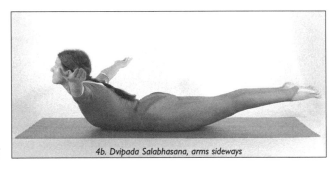

4b. Dvipada Salabhasana, arms sideways

- Lie on the stomach on a blanket with the legs extended straight backwards and the inner ankles together. Extend the arms sideways on the blanket, at an angle of ninety degrees to the chest, with the palms of the hands turned down.
- On the inhalation, lift the head, chest, arms and legs up, pulling the body up from the kidney region. Elongate the arms sideways out of the shoulder joints and the legs backwards out of the lumbar spine. To keep the arms at an angle of ninety degrees to the chest, elongate the ulnar side of the wrists more.
- Keep the knees straight and the inner ankles together, and do not flex the head too far back, but keep the neck long and fairly relaxed.
- Hold for a few seconds, retaining the breath. On the exhalation, lower the head, chest, arms and legs. Repeat three times.

4c. Arms forwards

- Lie on the stomach on a blanket with the legs extended straight backwards and the inner ankles together. Extend the arms forwards on the blanket, keeping them parallel to

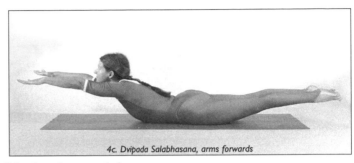

4c. Dvipada Salabhasana, arms forwards

each other and the palms of the hands turned down.
- On the inhalation, lift the head, chest, arms and legs up, pulling the body up from the kidney region. Elongate the arms forwards out of the shoulder joints and the legs backwards out of the lumbar spine. Keep the arms parallel to each other.
- Keep the knees straight and the inner ankles together, and do not flex the head too far back, but keep the neck long and fairly relaxed.
- Hold for a few seconds, retaining the breath. On the exhalation, lower the head, chest, arms and legs. Repeat three times.

4d. Makarasana
makara=crocodile

- Lie on the stomach on a blanket with the legs extended straight backwards and the inner ankles together. Bend the arms and clasp the hands in the neck.

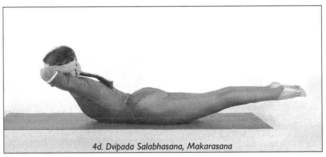

4d. Dvipada Salabhasana, Makarasana

- On the inhalation, lift the head, chest, arms and legs up, pulling the body up from the kidney region. Keep the elbows up and elongate the legs backwards out of the lumbar spine.
- Keep the knees straight and the inner ankles together, and do not flex the head too far back, but keep the neck long and fairly relaxed.
- Hold for a few seconds, retaining the breath. On the exhalation, lower the head, chest, arms and legs. Repeat three times.

5. Ekapada Salabhasana

eka=one; pada=leg, foot; salabha=locust

5a. *Arms forwards, same side arm and leg up*

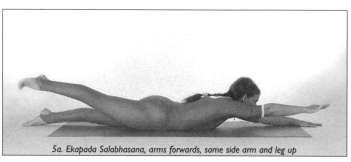
5a. Ekapada Salabhasana, arms forwards, same side arm and leg up

- Lie on the stomach on a blanket with the legs extended straight backwards and the inner ankles together. Extend the arms forwards on the blanket, keeping them parallel to each other and the palms of the hands turned down.
- On the inhalation, lift the head, chest, right arm and right leg up. Do not flex the head too far backward, but keep the neck long and fairly relaxed.
- Do not tilt the right side of the chest and pelvis up to raise the right arm and leg, but use the back muscles and the biceps muscle of the right leg. Both frontal hip bones stay on the blanket and the shoulder blades stay parallel to the earth.
- Keep the knees straight, the right leg in line with the right hip and the right arm in line with the right shoulder. Elongate the right arm forward out of the right shoulder joint, and the right leg backward out of the lumbar spine.
- Hold for a few seconds, retaining the breath. On the exhalation, lower the head, chest, right arm and right leg, and repeat with the other leg and arm. Repeat each side three times.

5b. *Arms forwards, opposite arm and leg up*

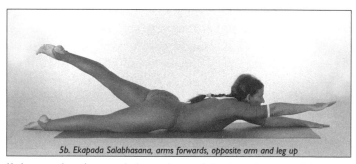
5b. Ekapada Salabhasana, arms forwards, opposite arm and leg up

- Lie on the stomach on a blanket with the legs extended straight backwards and the inner ankles together. Extend the arms forwards on the blanket, keeping them parallel to each other and the palms of the hands turned down.
- On the inhalation, lift the head, chest, right arm and left leg up. Do not flex the head too far backward, but keep the neck long and fairly relaxed.
- Do not tilt the right side of the chest and the left side of the pelvis up to raise the right arm and left leg, but use the back muscles and the biceps muscle of the left leg. Both frontal hip bones stay on the blanket and the shoulder blades stay parallel to the earth.
- Keep the knees straight, the left leg in line with the left hip and the right arm in line with the right shoulder. Elongate the right arm forward out of the right shoulder joint, and the left leg backward out of the lumbar spine.
- Hold for a few seconds, retaining the breath. On the exhalation, lower the head, chest, right arm and left leg, and repeat with the other leg and arm. Repeat each side three times.

6. Dhanurasana

dhanu=bow

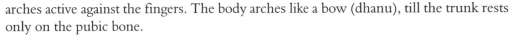

- Lie on the stomach on a blanket with the legs extended straight backwards and the inner ankles together. Bend the knees, and hold the arches of the feet with the hands, curling the toes around the fingers. Keep the feet together and the knees slightly wider than hip width.
- On an inhalation, pull the chest, feet and knees up towards the sky, keeping the

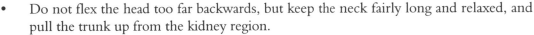

6. Dhanurasana

arches active against the fingers. The body arches like a bow (dhanu), till the trunk rests only on the pubic bone.
- Do not flex the head too far backwards, but keep the neck fairly long and relaxed, and pull the trunk up from the kidney region.
- Hold for a few seconds, rocking the body gently on the Mula Bandha breathing; this gives the lower abdomen an excellent massage.
- On the exhalation, release the feet and lower the body onto the blanket.

7. Bhujangasana I

bhujanga=serpent

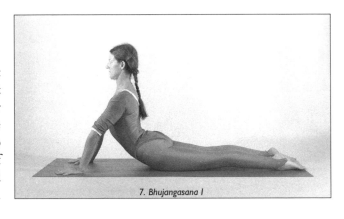

- Lie on the stomach on a blanket with the legs extended straight backwards and the inner ankles together. Place the hands on the blanket next to the head, with the palms of the hands turned down and the fingers pointing forwards. The elbows point backwards.

7. Bhujangasana I

- On a Mula Bandha inhalation, raise the head and chest and straighten the arms. Do not sink the chest into the shoulders, but lift it up against gravity. This is done by performing Hasta Bandha with the hands, so that the arms are elongated. Keep the lower abdomen on the earth and the knees straight.
- On the exhalation, curve the spine and head backwards, and roll the shoulders back by turning the pit of the elbows forwards: this lowers the shoulder blades.
- On each inhalation pull the two frontal hip bones forwards and up to elongate the spine upwards, and on each exhalation curve the spine backwards, creating a round movement which starts in the lower abdomen and ends in the back of the head.
- Hold for a few seconds, breathing normally. On the exhalation, bend the arms and lower the chest and head onto the blanket.

8. Urdhvamukha Svanasana

urdhva=upwards; mukha=face;
svana=dog

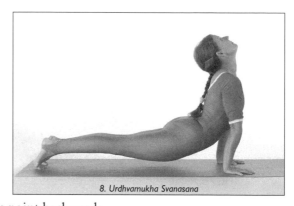

8. Urdhvamukha Svanasana

- Lie on the stomach on a mat with the legs extended straight backwards. Keep the feet at hip width so that the legs are parallel to each other.
- Place the hands on the blanket underneath the shoulders, with the palms of the hands turned down and the fingers pointing forwards. The elbows point backwards.
- Turn the toes under and straighten the knees, lifting them off the blanket.
- On a Mula Bandha inhalation, raise the head, chest and pelvis, straightening the arms till the whole body is supported only on the hands and the balls of the feet. The legs are parallel to the earth, and the knees are straight. Do not sink the chest into the shoulders, but lift it up against gravity. This is done by performing Hasta Bandha with the hands, so that the arms are elongated.
- On the exhalation, curve the spine and head backwards, and roll the shoulders back by turning the pit of the elbows forwards: this lowers the shoulder blades.
- On each inhalation pull the two frontal hip bones forwards and up to elongate the spine upward, and on each exhalation curve the spine backwards, creating a round movement which starts in the lower abdomen and ends in the back of the head.
- Hold for a few seconds, breathing normally. On the exhalation, bend the arms and lower the pelvis, chest and head onto the blanket.

9. Adhomukha Svanasana

adho=downwards; mukha=face;
svana=dog

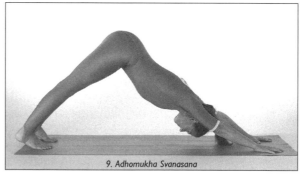

9. Adhomukha Svanasana

- Start with Urdhvamukha Svanasana (8) and proceed:
- On an exhalation, raise the pelvis and extend it backwards, keeping the arms and legs straight, till the body forms a unilateral triangle.
- The hands are at shoulder width, so that the arms are parallel to each other. The fingers point straight forward, with the middle fingers parallel to each other.
- The feet are at hip width, so that the legs are parallel to each other. The inner borders of the feet are also parallel to each other.
- Make sure that your weight is evenly distributed between the two hands and between the two feet.
- Rotate the arms as in Savasana (see page 286), which means that the inner elbows rotate forwards: the biceps muscles rotate outwards, and the triceps muscles rotate towards the ribs.
- Extend the fingers evenly on the earth, almost as if you are going to lift the wrists up.

This is important for the shoulders; elongating the shoulders while carrying weight on the wrists will jam the shoulder joints. Pressing the metatarsals of the fingers down as if you want to lift the wrists up lifts the shoulder blades; then, when you elongate the shoulders, the movement is circular and there is no jamming in the shoulder joints.

- On a Mula Bandha inhalation, lift the heels up and extend the buttock bones upwards, spreading them at the same time. Then extend them backwards and elongate the back of the thighs from the knees to the buttock bones, so that the lumbar vertebrae move in.
- After reaching the maximum elongation, lower the heels onto the mat and lower the head in between the arms to the mat.
- Root the hands and perform Hasta Bandha, so that the arms elongate and the chest and trunk are drawn up from the shoulder heads in the direction of the buttock bones. Thus the shoulders, the arm pits and the spinal column are elongated. At the same time, root the feet and perform Pada Bandha, so that the legs elongate and the pelvis is drawn up from the femur heads. Thus the whole spinal column is elongated harmoniously and the highest point in the body is in the buttock bones.
- On each Mula Bandha inhalation elongate the spine and shoulders further, and on each exhalation lower the head further to the mat. The groove of the spine is even, from the first cervical vertebra to the sacrum.
- Hold for one minute. Then lower the pelvis and return to Urdhvamukha Svanasana (8).

10. Purvottanasana

purva=East; uttana=intense stretch

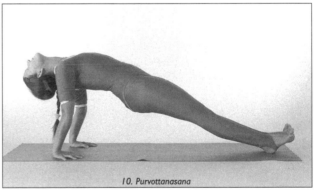

10. Purvottanasana

When the yogi performs the Sun Salutation (Surya Namaskar, see page 56), he faces the East. Therefore, the frontal side of the body is considered the East, the back side of the body the West, the right side of the body the South and the left side of the body the North. In Purvottanasana the East side of the body is extended, while in Paschimottanasana (see page 127) the West side of the body is extended (*paschima=the West*).

- Sit on a mat with the legs extended straight in front of you. Lean the trunk backwards at an angle of forty-five degrees and place the hands on the mat, in line with the shoulders, so that the arms are perpendicular; the fingers point towards the heels.
- On an exhalation lift the pelvis up, till the whole trunk forms one line from the feet to the top of the sternum. The feet are resting on the heels, not on the soles.
- Root the hands and perform Hasta Bandha to elongate the arms and to lighten the chest on the shoulder heads. After elongating the cervical and thoracic spine with Jalandhara Bandha (see page 43), curve the head backwards.
- On an exhalation, lower the pelvis again on the mat and turn the hands around, so that the fingers point away from the trunk, backwards. Then repeat Purvottanasana. This position of the hands gives a more extreme rotation in the shoulder joints.

11. Ustrasana

ustra=camel

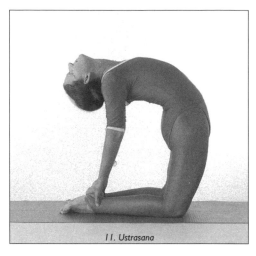

11. Ustrasana

As Ustrasana is an intermediate pose between the Simple Back Bendings and the more advanced ones, it is described here in great detail to lay the foundation for the next series of poses.

- Kneel on a mat with the feet and heels together, and the knees slightly wider than hip width. The stable part of the body is the one which is in contact with the earth; this forms the basis for the mobile part to pull away from, upwards against gravity, or in any other direction.

- In Ustrasana, the basis is formed by the entire lower leg, from the knees to the tips of the toes. On this basis the femur heads have to be fixed in such a way that they, in turn, provide the stable basis for the pelvis and the rest of the body to pull up from. This is done by constricting the outer hips and the inner thighs inwards towards each other while keeping the thighs perpendicular, at an angle of ninety degrees with the lower legs.

- The thighs are like a pillar, and on top of this vertical pillar the spine has to form a crescent moon shape, which has to retain its shape and coherence right from the beginning and throughout the pose.

- Lighten the weight of the body on the femur heads by lifting the pelvis and entire body up from the femur heads (rebounce action). This is done by elongating the inner arches of the feet backwards and rooting them into the earth while performing Pada Bandha, lengthening the thighs, and maintaining the constricting action of the outer hips and inner thighs.

- The act of lengthening the thighs and lifting the pelvis up from the femur heads on the Mula Bandha inhalation pulls the energy upwards along the interior spinal column. Mula Bandha is that lifting of the pelvis, but not only of the physical structure. It is the mula, the root of the body, which has to pressurize upwards, thus shooting the energy upwards. This upward movement of the energy travels along the line of gravity, and thus goes from the base of the pelvis straight up into the kidneys, lifting the kidneys (Uddiyana Bandha) up from the lumbar vertebrae. From the kidneys, still traveling in a straight line upwards, the energy goes up into the top of the sternum, lifting that up to the sky (the lower part of Jalandhara Bandha, see page 43). This is the crescent moon shape: it has to retain its shape and integrity throughout.

- Keeping the thighs perpendicular, extend the arms horizontally sideways. Then elongate them out of the shoulder joints and bring the hands back in a circular movement to hold the heels, curving the spine backwards. Even though the hands hold the heels, there should be no weight on them.

- As the spine curves backwards, the thighs should remain perpendicular. Constrict the outer hips inwards with the support of the Pada Bandha, and pull the two frontal hip bones up towards the ribs, so that on each Mula Bandha inhalation the trunk lifts further up from the femur heads. Keeping the thighs perpendicular helps the body to curve in the kidneys and the thoracic spine, instead of in the lumbar spine.
- The head is the last to curve backwards; this curving backwards of the head has to come out of the action of Jalandhara Bandha, so that the cervical spine retains its length.
- To come out of the pose, return to the original kneeling position: release the hands from the heels and, reversing the process, bring both the shoulder joints and the hip joints simultaneously back to the central line of gravity, keeping the sternum high and the head back: the head is the last to come up again.

4.12b Urdhva Dhanurasana

urdhva=upwards; dhanu=bow

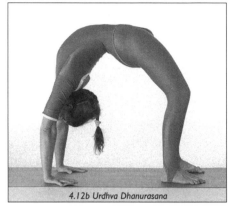

4.12b Urdhva Dhanurasana

Urdhva Dhanurasana is the basis for the more advanced Back Bending positions. We have therefore given quite an extensive description here, so that this will help you to understand the other Back Bendings better.

In no other pose is the interaction between the five Bandhas more obvious than in this pose. Even though in the beginning you can practice pushing up from the earth, you can never attain in that way the full elongation that makes this position one of the most beautiful and elegant of all the asanas. Therefore, once you have gained enough elasticity, start to practice dropping down from Tadasana (see page 49), first onto the wall, and then onto the earth.

Thus, whereas in version **1** the body pushes up from the earth into Urdhva Dhanurasana (for beginners), those who are sufficiently acquainted with the pose and have acquired sufficient suppleness in the spine, hip and shoulder joints, can start practicing this pose going down from Tadasana onto the wall (version **2**).

The final stage is dropping from Tadasana backwards into Urdhva Dhanurasana in the middle of the room (version **3**), after having acquired sufficient understanding and suppleness on the wall.

1. Pushing up from the earth

Lie on the back on a 'sticky' yoga mat and proceed:

- Pull the feet in towards the buttocks till the back of the heels are in contact with the buttocks. The width between the feet is slightly wider than the width of the hips. Keep the feet parallel to each other, do not turn them out, and do not keep one foot further forward than the other, but keep them even, rooting them like in Tadasana. The feet are intimately connected with the spine, especially with the lower part of the spine; if they are weak and do not root, the spine will be weak and out of control, and you will damage the vertebrae by incorrect bending. Keep the knees at the same width as the feet, and rotate the thighs inwards as in Virasana I (see page 102).
- Place the palms of the hands on the mat next to the ears with the fingers pointing towards the shoulders, so that the width between the hands is the same as the width of the shoulders. Keep the hands parallel to each other; do not turn the hands in or out and do not keep one hand further forward than the other, but keep them even. As the feet are rooting into the earth, so too the hands should be rooting. Keep the elbows close to the head, squeezing the ears in between the lower arms, and rotate the upper arms as in Savasana (see page 286), which means that the triceps muscles roll towards the face. The width between the elbows is the same as the width of the shoulders.

- On an exhalation lift the lower part of the pelvis (the coccyx) off the mat, keeping the upper rim of the pelvis and the lumbar area on the mat. The pelvis has to rotate backwards around the femur heads, so that the lumbar spine elongates and the coccyx rolls towards the pubic bone. When you have reached maximum rotation, lift the pelvis and lower part of the trunk off the mat, supporting the body on the feet, shoulders, hands and the back of head. The pubic bone is now the highest point in the body, not the two frontal hip bones. If the two frontal hip bones are higher than the pubis the pelvis has not been rotated enough, and as a result the body bends in the lumbar spine and the groins do not open.

In this context it is important to note that in Forward Bendings the two frontal hip bones move towards the thighs, so that the biceps muscles at the back of the thighs are elongated and the buttock rims (which are at the back of the legs where the legs join the buttocks) are opened. Thus the body bends in the femo-iliac joints, closing with the thighs in the groins like a book. In Back Bendings, the opposite takes place. Here the two frontal hip bones move up in the direction of the ribs, so that the quadriceps muscles at the front of the thighs are elongated and the groins are opened. Thus the body bends in the buttock rims, and the femo-iliac joints are extended.

Do not attempt to go further as long as you cannot do this movement correctly. It is always better to go slowly and imprint the correct movement on the body than to go fast and move incorrectly. Once a wrong habit is created it is very difficult to undo it.

- Raise the body further, until it is only supported on the feet, hands and crown of the head (as in Head Balance). Work again on the backwards rotation of the pelvis: the pubic bone should be higher than the two frontal hip bones. Then push the body completely up till the arms (elbows) are straight.
- As the body goes up, the pubis remains the highest point in the body as long as possible. If the lower ribs are higher, the lumbar spine has lost control, bending is mainly done in the lumbar vertebrae and the shoulder and hip joints do not extend.
- Keep the heels down and the feet parallel to each other. Rotate the knees and thighs inwards, so that the width between the knees remains the same as at the start. Rooting the feet put more weight on the inner edges of the heels and on the big toe bones than on the outer edges of the heels and the little toe bones. If the outer edges of the heels and the little toe bones root more, the adductor muscles on the inside of the thighs become passive and the knees fall apart.
- As the arms are shorter than the legs the knees will not be completely straight. Nevertheless, try to straighten them as much as possible. Rooting the inner edges of the heels and the big toe bones, resist the knees towards the hands, and at the same time elongate the back of the thighs upwards, from the back of the knees towards the buttock bones. The pelvis, rotating backwards around the femur heads, and the back of the thighs, elongating upwards towards the buttock bones, meet in the buttock rims. The result is that the groins at the front of the body open. The lower legs are at right angles to the soles of the feet as in Tadasana.

- Keeping the arms straight and the inner elbows facing each other, bring the shoulder joints in line with the wrist joints. The lower arms are at right angles to the palms of the hands. The shoulder blades are flat and the arms make a continuous line with the sides of the chest. This means that the shoulder joints are fully extended, the arm pits are opened and the sides of the arm pits are elongated; there should be no angle between the upper arms and the chest in the arm pits. The action in the arms is the same as the action in the legs: as the knees rotate towards each other, the inner elbows too rotate towards each other, so that the width between the elbows remains the same as the width of the shoulders. Rooting the palms of the hands, put more weight on the inner edges of the palms and the knuckles of the index fingers than on the outer edges of the palms and the knuckles of the little fingers. If the outer edges of the palms and the little fingers root more, the muscles of the inner arms become passive and the elbows fall apart.
- The pelvis and chest rotate in opposite directions. The pelvis rotates backwards around the femur heads, so that the two frontal hip bones are drawn up towards the lower ribs and the coccyx rolls towards the pubic bone. The pubic bone moves up towards the sky, while the lower legs remain at right angles to the earth. The chest rotates around the shoulder joints in such a way that the lower ribs and the bottom point of the sternum are drawn towards the two frontal hip bones and the upper part of the thoracic spine rolls towards the upper point of the sternum. The upper point of the sternum moves forwards in the direction you are facing, while the arms remain at right angles to the earth.
- The action *from the waist down* is that the legs elongate and the knees resist backwards towards the hands; the backward rotating pelvis and the upward elongating thighs meet in the buttock rims. The result is that the femo-iliac joints are fully extended, the groins are opened and the sides of the hips are elongated. The action *from the waist up* is that the arms elongate and the elbows resist backwards towards the feet; the forward rotating upper chest and the upward elongating arms meet in the shoulder joints. The result is that the shoulder joints are fully extended, the arm pits are opened and the sides of the arm pits are elongated.
- Thus the pelvis and the chest rotate in opposite directions: the coccyx and first thoracic vertebra move away from each other, while the frontal hip bones and the lower ribs (+ bottom end of the sternum) move towards each other. The result is that the whole spinal column is elongated harmoniously and bends evenly in all its vertebrae. *Dhanu* means 'bow': the spine is drawn like a bow between the fulcrum points of the shoulder joints and hip joints.
- This whole movement is based on the rebounce force which comes from the rooting hands and feet: Pada Bandha elongates the legs and lifts the pelvis up from the femur heads, and Hasta Bandha elongates the arms and lifts the chest up from the shoulder heads.
- Keep the head and neck initially straight as in Head Balance; then, when you have reached the maximum height in the shoulder and hip joints, curve the head backwards to look at the heels.

2.   Dropping down from Tadasana onto a wall

- Stand close to a wall with the back towards it and the heels about thirty centimeters distance from it. Keep the feet slightly wider than hip width, with the inner borders of the feet parallel to each other, and keep the feet even. On a Mula Bandha (see page 77) inhalation, raise the arms over the head till they point straight up towards the sky, parallel to each other.
- The most important thing is to create length in the hip joints and the lower abdomen before starting to curve the spine backwards. Thus it is important to start from the 'ski-jumping' stance described in Tadasana (see page 49), in which the body slants slightly forward, so that the lower abdomen is directly above the lower spring joints. Performing Pada Bandha (see page 49), lift the pelvis up on an inhalation, creating space and bounciness in the hip joints. As described in Standing Poses, elongation of the arms over the head starts in the lower spring joints and legs, with the first rebounce 'split' occurring in the ankles, and the second in the hip joints. From here the Mula Bandha inhalation picks up the elongation and carries it on through the whole spinal column, the shoulder blades, the shoulder joints and the arms: keeping the arms parallel to each other and rotating the triceps muscles forward, lift the lower abdomen (Mula Bandha) and kidney region (Uddiyana Bandha, see page 40) on each inhalation.
- Elongate the upper thoracic spine and the cervical spine by performing Jalandhara Bandha (see page 43) at the end of the inhalation, and then curve the head back. Thus the shoulder blades elongate and move into the upper rib cage, and the curve starts in the upper thoracic spine and the cervical spine. Then, vertebra per vertebra, roll the curve down along the thoracic spine. In this way the sternum remains lifted and does not drop into the kidney region.
- As you curve the spine, the weight back of the central line of gravity is increased; therefore you have to simultaneously increase the body weight in front of the central line of gravity in an even measure. This means that the legs, from the slightly forward slanting position of Tadasana, have to start slanting further forward, so that the hip joints are brought in front of the central line of gravity. Keep the legs completely straight, however, and keep the elongation of the legs through the action of the Pada Bandha.
- Up till now the groins are still in, and the trunk forms a crescent moon on top of the femur heads, with the spinal column drawn like a bow from the coccyx up to the first cervical vertebra. Do not pull the coccyx into the lumbar spine, but elongate it out of the lumbar spine as you lower the curve from the thoracic into the lumbar spine.
- Then drawing the frontal hip bones up in the direction of the lower ribs, continue curving the spine, till the groins are completely opened and the whole front of the body, from the front of the ankles to the pit of the throat, forms one even, round line.
- Finally place the hands on the wall with the fingers pointing downwards, but do not put any weight on them.
- To come up again you have to bring the whole body back to the central line of gravity. Thus you have to reverse the process, taking first the femur heads and groins back to the wall while pulling at the same time the frontal hip bones up, so as to maintain the integrity of the curve in the kidney region and in the upper chest.

When you feel comfortable doing this pose close to the wall, you can start walking the feet further away, till the heels are about fifty centimeters away from the wall. Then repeat all the steps described above. Again place the hands on the wall at the end, keeping the legs completely straight. Press the hands lightly against the wall, and on each Mula Bandha inhalation, which starts with the Pada Bandha and the elongation of the legs, lift the chest further up, out of the lumbar spine. Then slide the hands further down, without bending the knees and without collapsing the chest.

• To come back up follow the same steps as described above.

When you feel comfortable doing this pose at this distance from the wall and have gained enough control in the feet, the legs and the hip joints, you can move the feet still further away from the wall (one meter) and again follow the above described steps. Curve the body backwards with the legs straight, till the hands are on the wall.

• When you have reached the deepest point in the curve where you can still keep the knees straight, start walking the hands down on the wall. As the hands go down, the knees start to bend gradually, but only as much as necessary to facilitate going down. Keep the heels on the mat and keep the action in the lower spring joints (Pada Bandha) so as to maintain the rebounce effect in the ankles, knees and hip joints.

• Finally place the hands on the mat with the arms straight and the pits of the elbows facing each other. Keep the palms of the hands flat on the earth with the middle fingers pointing straight towards the heels, and keep the head straight in between the arms with the forehead touching the wall.

• By rooting the hands, performing Hasta Bandha, and applying a slight pressure with the forehead against the wall the arms elongate as in Adhomukha Vrksasana (see page 184). Thus the chest is lifted up from the shoulder heads by the rebounce action in the shoulder joints.

• By rooting the feet and performing Pada Bandha, the legs elongate as in Tadasana. Thus the pelvis is lifted up from the femur heads by the rebounce action in the femur joints. The knees are bent just enough to accommodate for the difference in length between the legs and the arms.

• The name of this position is *Urdhva Dhanurasana*, which means the 'upward bow'. In this pose we can discern two bows, a short one and a long one. The short one is the bow or curve between the coccyx and the first cervical vertebra, in which the whole spine elongates and curves harmoniously. The long bow is the curve which starts on the front of the ankles and runs across the front of the knees, the frontal hip bones, the lower ribs and the elbows towards the wrists. Even though the knees are bent, this bow should also be as harmonious as possible, which means that the frontal hip bones are at the same height from the earth as the lower ribs. Therefore the knees should bend minimally, because it is the angle in the knees which determines the height of the frontal hip bones: the more the knees are bent, the lower the hip bones are.

3. Dropping down from Tadasana onto the earth

When you have reached sufficient control in this pose on the wall, you can learn to do it in the middle of the room. Follow the steps given under **2**.

- To take the hands down to the earth you have to keep lifting the pelvis up from the femur heads with the Mula Bandha breathing, while bending the knees. This means that the frontal hip bones keep contact with the lower ribs. Then drop the hands to the earth.
- Before curving the head backwards, lift the chest up from the shoulder heads by rooting the hands and performing Hasta Bandha, so that the arms elongate and the shoulder blades are lifted. Keep the head initially in between the upper arms. Once you have created the rebounce effect in the shoulder joints curve the head back and bring the shoulder joints vertically above the hands.
- Rooting the feet and performing Pada Bandha elongate the legs, keeping the chest stable. Thus the lumbar spine is elongated as the pelvis is lifted up from the femur heads.
- To come back up to Tadasana, you have to reverse the process.

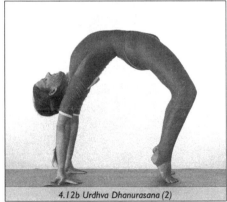

4.12b Urdhva Dhanurasana (1)

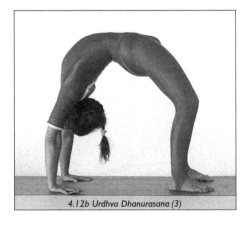

4.12b Urdhva Dhanurasana (2)

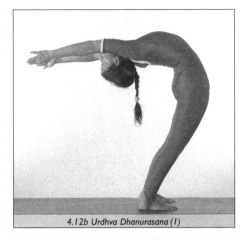

4.12b Urdhva Dhanurasana (3)

4.12c   Back Bend Variations

These positions can be done in <u>three different modes</u>:

a.   Performing each position separately and holding it for a few seconds.

b.   Vinyasa
Connecting two or more positions by flowing from one into the other, using the breathing.

c.   Mala
Connecting all the positions through Surya Namaskar, using the breathing and holding each of the Back Bend Variations for the duration of three breaths.

Back Bendings Variations

1. *Ekapada Urdhva Dhanurasana*
2. *Dvipada Viparita Dandasana*
3. *Ekapada Viparita Dandasana I*
4. *Mandalasana*
5. *Ekapada Viparita Dandasana II*
6. *Chakra Bandhasana*
7. *Vrschikasana I*
8. *Vrschikasana II*
9. *Kapotasana*
10. *Laghu Vajrasana*
11. *Padangustha Dhanurasana*
    a. *Padangustha Dhanurasana I*
    b. *Padangustha Dhanurasana II*
12. *Rajakapotasana*
    a. *Rajakapotasana I*
    b. *Rajakapotasana II*
    c. *Bhujangasana II*
13. *Gherandasana*
14. *Kapinjalasana*
15. *Ganda Bherundasana*
16. *Ekapada Rajakapotasana I*
17. *Ekapada Rajakapotasana II*
18. *Ekapada Rajakapotasana III*
19. *Ekapada Rajakapotasana IV*
20. *Natarajasana*
    a. *Natarajasana I*
    b. *Natarajasana II*

1. Ekapada Urdhva Dhanurasana

eka=one; pada=leg, foot; urdhva=upwards;
dhanu=bow

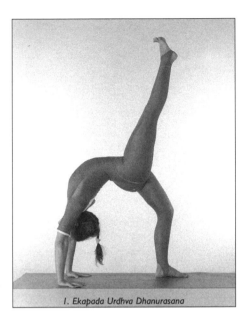

1. Ekapada Urdhva Dhanurasana

- Start with Urdhva Dhanurasana (see page 220) and then proceed:
- Root the left foot further into the earth, performing Pada Bandha, and raise the right leg with bent knee. Keep the weight even on both hands, and continue rooting them, performing Hasta Bandha to maintain the lightness and curve in the chest.
- Keep the two frontal hip bones parallel to each other, as well as parallel to the earth. Then elongate the right leg up towards the sky.
- For the rest follow the instructions given for Urdhva Dhanurasana.

2. Dvipada Viparita Dandasana

dvi=two; pada=leg, foot; viparita=reverse;
danda=staff

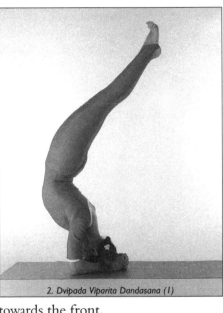

2. Dvipada Viparita Dandasana (I)

- Start with Salamba Sirsasana I (see page 163) on a 'sticky' yoga mat and then proceed:
- Bend the knees backwards, keeping the groins in: as in Urdhva Dhanurasana (see page 220), you have to bring the curve first into the upper back.
- Before curving a joint, however, you have to elongate it, creating the feeling of an 'airbag' inside it. In this pose, you have to pay special attention to rooting the head (Padma Bandha), together with the ulnar wrist points. Collect the upper arms inwards towards the center, so that the shoulder joints form the stable basis; then lift the chest up from the shoulder heads, rotating the triceps and latissimus dorsi muscles towards the front.
- Elongate the thoracic spine, and move the shoulder blades deep into the rib cage; then curve the upper thoracic spine. To bring the curve into the lumbar spine, you have to bring the chest forwards, retaining, however, the attraction between the frontal hip bones and the lower ribs.
- In all the Back Bendings, the two frontal hip bones and the lower ribs have to retain their magnetic attraction towards each other to keep the length in the lumbar spine. If they lose this attraction, the lumbar spine will be compressed in the curve. Thus, there is again a crescent moon shape, this time with the shoulder joints as the lower point (the base) and the hip joints as the top points.

- To drop backwards, constrict the outer hips inwards and elongate the upper thighs upwards out of the hip joints: then bend the knees, till the trunk forms one curve from the top of the knees to the arm pits. Thus the groins are completely open and form one continuous line between the upper thighs and the frontal hip bones. Then drop the feet onto the mat.
- Place the feet slightly wider than hip width, with the inner borders parallel to each other, and keep them in alignment; do not keep one foot further forward than the other.
- To create one smooth curve at the front of the body, from the frontal hip bones to the arm pits, separate the pelvis from the femur heads by rooting the feet (Pada Bandha) and elongating the legs; at the same time, extend the coccyx out of the lumbar spine towards the heels, so that the lumbar vertebrae do not become compressed.
- To lighten the chest up from the shoulder heads, root the top of the head (Padma Bandha) and the ulnar wrist points as in Salamba Sirsasana I (see page 163), so that the thoracic spine in between the shoulder blades elongates. Do not push the lower ribs forwards, but lift the chest up vertically.

2. Dvipada Viparita Dandasana (2)

2. Dvipada Viparita Dandasana (3)

- To get the even curve of the bow, the first thoracic vertebra has to move towards the sternum, while at the same time the coccyx moves out of the lumbar spine towards the heels; in this way the attraction between the frontal hip bones and the lower ribs, on the front of the body, is maintained.
- By resisting the knees slightly backwards towards the shoulders, and the shoulder blades towards the knees, the chest and pelvis have no other choice but to go up: this gives height and lightness to the body.
- Use the Mula Bandha breathing to attain further height: on each inhalation the body becomes lighter by connecting the Pada Bandha, the Mula Bandha, the Uddiyana Bandha and the Jalandhara Bandha, rooting the feet, the head and the ulnar wrist points.
- On an exhalation, walk the feet further out on the mat and extend the legs, till the knees are straight. Keep the feet at hip width, evenly forward with the inner borders of the feet parallel to each other. This pose is called Dvipada Viparita Dandasana, which means the Reversed Walking Stick.
- Hold for a few seconds, and then proceed to 3.

3. Ekapada Viparita Dandasana I

eka=one; pada=leg, foot; viparita=reversed;
danda=staff

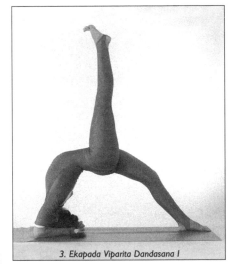

3. Ekapada Viparita Dandasana I

- When you have reached a stable position, lift the right leg up with bent knee and then extend it straight up towards the sky. Do not tilt the pelvis; the two frontal hip bones stay parallel to each other and to the earth.
- The right leg extends upwards in vertical alignment with the right groin, while the left foot and knee are extended in alignment with the left groin.
- To get height and lightness in the pelvis, root the left foot (Pada Bandha), elongating the left leg, and at the same time elongate the right leg upwards out of the right hip joint. This is in conformity with the principle that the part of the body which is below, forms the stable base for the part of the body, which is above, to elongate upwards against gravity.
- Hold for a few seconds. Place the foot back on the mat and repeat with the other leg. Return to Dvipada Viparita Dandasana (2) and then proceed:
- Walk the feet in towards the head. On an exhalation, jump back up to Salamba Sirsasana I, keeping the head on the mat and the feet together. From Salamba Sirsasana I, come down in the usual way.

4. Mandalasana

mandala=circle

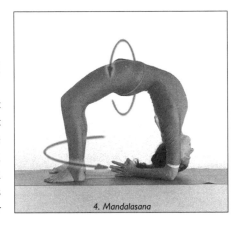

4. Mandalasana

- Start with Dvipada Viparita Dandasana (2) and then proceed:
- Walk the feet towards the left. Turn the left foot ninety degrees outwards and place the right foot on the left ankle. Shift the body weight onto the left foot and, lifting the right hip up vertically, roll it over the left hip, till the right foot is again down on the mat, next to the left foot. Both legs are now straight again and at an angle of ninety degrees to the left side of the trunk.
- Walk the feet to the front, till they are in front of your face.
- Keeping the legs straight, walk the feet around to the right, till the legs are at a ninety degree angle to the right side of the trunk.
- Place the left foot on the right ankle. Shift the body weight onto the right foot, lift the left hip up vertically and roll it over the right one, till the left foot is down on the mat again, next to the right foot.
- Continue walking, till you are back again in Dvipada Viparita Dandasana (2).
- Repeat the same procedure, walking the other way around.

- The front of the body is considered the East side of the body (purva), as it faces the rising sun in Hindu worship. Thus, when the feet are in front of the face, they are on the East side of the body. When the feet are behind the head (in Dvipada Viparita Dandasana) they are at the West side of the body (paschima). When the feet are on the left side of the body they are in the South and when they are on the right side of the body they are in the North. *Mandala* means 'circle'. Thus the feet describe a complete circle around the head (the North Pole).

5. Chakra Bandhasana
chakra=wheel; bandha=bound

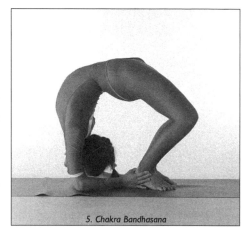

5. Chakra Bandhasana

- Start with Dvipada Viparita Dandasana (2) and then proceed:
- Lift the head and hands up, bring the body weight forward onto the elbows, and walk the feet in towards the head. Keep the head between the arms initially, rooting the elbows to create the rebounce in the shoulder joints.
- On an inhalation, lift the chest up vertically from the shoulder heads, and on the exhalation, bring the upper chest, the arm pits and the shoulder blades forwards over the elbows. Resist the kidney region slightly backwards towards the heels to prevent the lower ribs from collapsing forwards, in which case they would lose the magnetic attraction to the frontal hip bones: the upper ribs and the upper part of the sternum should go faster and further forward than the lower ribs and the lower point of the sternum.
- Keeping the chest stable and the head lifted between the upper arms, raise the heels and walk the feet further in towards the hands, hold the ankles and then lower the heels again.
- To maintain the height and lightness of the body, especially of the pelvis, root the feet. By performing Pada Bandha, the legs elongate up towards the pelvis on the rebounce force. At the same time, the coccyx has to extend out of the lumbar spine towards the knees. Thus the pelvis rotates backwards around the femur heads, and the two frontal hip bones are drawn towards the lower ribs. The upwards elongating legs, and the backwards rotating pelvis, meet in the buttock rims (at the back of the upper thighs where the thighs and gluteus muscles meet). The result is that the groins are opened and the pelvis is lifted.
- To complete the pose, curve the head backwards and look at the heels.
- On an exhalation release the ankles, place the head back on the mat and return to Dvipada Viparita Dandasana (2), and then proceed to 6.

6. Ekapada Viparita Dandasana II

eka=one; pada=leg, foot; viparita=reversed;
danda=staff

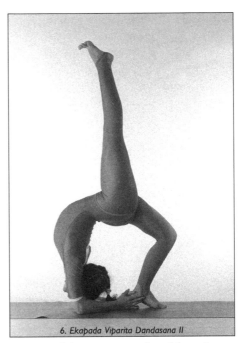

6. Ekapada Viparita Dandasana II

- Start with Dvipada Viparita Dandasana (2) and then proceed:
- Lift the head and hands up, bring the body weight forward onto the elbows and walk the feet in towards the head. Keep the head between the arms initially, rooting the elbows to create the rebounce in the shoulder joints.
- On an inhalation, lift the chest up vertically from the shoulder heads, and on the exhalation, bring the upper chest, the arm pits and the shoulder blades forwards over the elbows. Resist the kidney region slightly backwards towards the heels to prevent the lower ribs from collapsing forwards, in which case they would lose the magnetic attraction to the frontal hip bones: the upper ribs and the upper part of the sternum should go faster and further forward than the lower ribs and the lower point of the sternum.
- Keeping the chest stable and the head lifted between the upper arms, raise the heels and walk the feet further in towards the hands. Hold the left ankle and lower the heel again.
- Lift the right leg up with bent knee and then extend it straight up towards the sky. Do not tilt the pelvis; the two frontal hip bones stay parallel to each other and to the earth.
- The right leg extends upwards in vertical alignment with the right groin, while the left foot and knee remain in alignment with the left groin.
- To get height and lightness in the pelvis, root the left foot (Pada Bandha), elongating the left leg, and at the same time elongate the right leg upwards out of the right hip joint. This is in conformity with the principle that the part of the body, which is below, forms the stable base for the part of the body, which is above, to elongate upwards against gravity.
- Hold for a few seconds. Place the foot back on the mat and repeat with the other leg. Return to Dvipada Viparita Dandasana (2), and then proceed:
- Walk the feet in towards the head. On an exhalation, jump back up to Salamba Sirsasana I, keeping the head on the mat and the feet together. From Salamba Sirsasana I, come down in the usual way.

7. Vrschikasana I
vrschika=scorpion

7a. Close to a wall

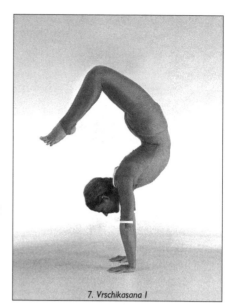

7. Vrschikasana I

*   Start with Adhomukha Vrksasana (see page 184) close to a wall (between thirty and fifty centimeters distance from the wall) and then proceed:
*   Bend the knees, place the toes on the wall and lift the head, curving the spine. Push the wall lightly with the toes as you lift the head, at the same time rooting the hands and performing Hasta Bandha, so that the chest is lifted up from the shoulder heads.
*   Walk the feet down on the wall and raise the head further up towards the feet.
*   Return to Adhomukha Vrksasana and come down again.

When you have gained enough confidence on the wall, and have mastered Adhomukha Vrksasana in the middle of the room, you can try this pose in the middle of the room.

7b. In the middle of the room

*   Start with Adhomukha Vrksasana (see page 184) in the middle of the room and then proceed:
*   Bend the knees and curve the spine. Raising the head further up, bring the feet down to the head. Root the hands and perform Hasta Bandha, so that the chest is lifted up from the shoulder heads.

This position resembles the scorpion as it stings its own head.

8. Vrschikasana II
vrschika=scorpion

8a. Close to a wall

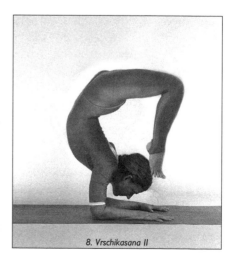

8. Vrschikasana II

*   Start with Pincha Mayurasana (see page 186) close to a wall (about thirty centimeters distance from the wall) and then proceed:
*   Bend the knees, place the toes on the wall and lift the head, curving the spine. Push the wall lightly with the toes as you lift the head, at the same time rooting the ulnar wrist points and the hands, performing Hasta Bandha, so that the chest is lifted up from the shoulder heads.

- Walk the feet down on the wall and raise the head further up towards the feet.
- Return to Pincha Mayurasana and come down again.

When you have gained enough confidence on the wall, and have mastered Pincha Mayurasana in the middle of the room, you can try this pose in the middle of the room.

8b.   *In the middle of the room*

- Start with Pincha Mayurasana (see page 186) in the middle of the room and then proceed:
- Bend the knees and curve the spine. Raising the head further bring the feet down to the head. Root the ulnar wrist points and the hands, performing Hasta Bandha, so that the chest is lifted up from the shoulder heads.

This position resembles the scorpion as it stings its own head.

9. Kapotasana
kapota=pigeon

(For an additional, detailed description, see Part Two: "Comparative Studies of Various Asanas", paragraph 4.13)

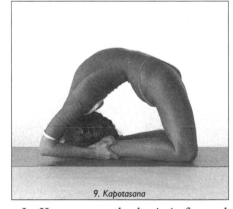

9. Kapotasana

- Kneel on a blanket with the feet and heels together and the knees slightly wider than hip width. The stable part of the body is the one which is in contact with the earth; this forms the basis for the mobile part to pull away from, upwards against gravity, or in any other direction. In Kapotasana, the basis is formed by the entire lower leg, from the knees to the tips of the toes.
- On this base, the femur heads have to be fixed in such a way that they, in turn, form a stable basis for the pelvis and the rest of the body to lift up from. This is done by constricting the outer hips and the inner thighs slightly inwards towards each other, while keeping the thighs perpendicular, at an angle of ninety degrees to the lower legs.
- Thus the thighs are like a pillar, and on top of this vertical pillar the trunk has to create a crescent moon shape which has to retain its shape and coherence right from the beginning and throughout the pose.
- Lighten the weight of the body on the femur heads by lifting the pelvis and trunk up from the femur heads (rebounce action). To do this, you have to elongate the inner arches of the feet backwards and root them into the earth while performing Pada Bandha; at the same time elongate the thighs, maintaining the squeezing action at the outer hips and inner thighs.
- The act of elongating the thighs and lifting the pelvis up from the femur heads with the Mula Bandha inhalation, pulls the energy upwards along the interior spinal column. Mula Bandha is that lifting of the pelvis, but not only of the physical structure. It is the mula, the root of the body, which has to pressurize upwards, thus shooting the energy upwards.

This upward movement of the energy travels along the line of gravity, and thus goes from the base of the pelvis straight up into the kidneys, lifting the kidneys (Uddiyana Bandha) up from the lumbar vertebrae. From the kidneys, still traveling in a straight line upwards, it goes into the top of the sternum (Jalandhara Bandha), lifting that up to the sky. This is the crescent moon shape: this crescent moon has to retain its shape and integrity throughout. On a Mula Bandha inhalation, raise the arms over the head.

- To go down into Kapotasana, the body has to balance around the central line of gravity: as the trunk and arms curve back and down, the upper thighs have to move forwards (maintaining the squeezing action of the outer thighs inwards) to balance the weight of the body, until the moment when the pelvis forms one continuous curve with the thighs through the groins. Whereas in the initial crescent moon shape the trunk formed one curve from the two frontal hip bones to the collar bones, and the groins were dipped inwards, this curve now starts at the knees, and continues through the groins up to the collar bones, forming one smooth and even line.

- Then, 'hanging' from the upper thighs, the groins and the iliopsoas muscles, bring the hands to the feet and hold the heels. Keep the upper arms parallel to each other, the elbows on the blanket and the top of the head in the arches of the feet. Do not put any weight either on the hands or on the elbows; the entire body weight should be suspended from the thighs, groins and iliopsoas muscles.

- On each Mula Bandha inhalation, root the top of the feet into the earth, thus elongating the thighs upwards, so that the angle in the back of the knees increases. This lifts the pelvis up from the femur heads, allowing the wave of the Mula Bandha breathing to create a deeper curve in the kidney region and the upper chest. The head too can, in its turn, move deeper into the arches, thus closing the circle from the Pada Bandha to the Padma Bandha.

- To come out of the pose, release the hands from the heels and, reversing the process, bring both the shoulder joints and the hip joints simultaneously back to the central line of gravity, by bringing the thighs back to the vertical line. Keep the head back and the sternum raised high to come back to the original kneeling position. In this way, the length in the lumbar spine and the curve in the kidney region and upper chest are maintained, and the trunk ends up in the same crescent moon shape as from where it started. The head and arms are the last to come back up again.

10. Laghu Vajrasana

laghu=small, beautiful; vajra=thunderbolt, the weapon of Indra

- Kneel on a blanket with the feet and heels together and the knees slightly wider than hip width. Place the hands on the front of the thighs, close to the knees.
- Follow the instructions given in Kapotasana (9) to create the curve in the spine. Then take the head down into the arches of the feet, crawling the fingers down on the front of the

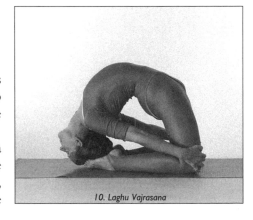

10. Laghu Vajrasana

thighs towards the knees to maintain the curve. When the head rests in the arches, the fingers are holding the top front portion of the knees.

In this position one can clearly recognize the bow: the wooden part of the bow is the curving trunk, which starts between the knees and runs over the pubic bone, the lower point of the sternum, the upper point of the sternum and the forehead, and the string of the bow is formed by the extended arms, which pull the shoulder joints and knees towards each other: the closer these are pulled towards each other, the higher the curve of the wooden part of the bow.

11. Padangustha Dhanurasana
padangustha=big toe; dhanu=bow

11a. Padangustha Dhanurasana I

* Start with Bhujangasana I (see page 215) and then proceed:
* Bend the right knee and turn the right foot out so that it is at an angle of ninety degrees to the ankle, with the toes pointing sideways, away from the trunk.
* Support yourself on the left hand, turn the right arm as for Savasana (see page 286), and with the right hand hold the right foot: the palm of the hand covers the top of the foot, and the fingers curve around the inner arch.

11a. Padangustha Dhanurasana I

* Rotate the arm in the shoulder joint, till the elbow points up towards the sky. In order to help this movement, and to take the load off the shoulder joint, pull the right leg up to the sky, so that the right foot pulls the right arm up, not vice versa. Both the right hand and the right foot now point up towards the sky.
* Keeping the upwards extension of the right leg, lift the left hand off the earth, bend the left leg and hold the left foot in the same way as described above; the trunk rolls from the Bhujangasana I (see page 215) position forwards onto the stomach.
* Repeating the same procedure as above, rotate the left arm in the shoulder joint, till both hands and feet point up towards the sky: this is the bow when it is slack. To draw the bow (for shooting the arrow), both the hands and the feet have to elongate up towards the sky.
* The wooden part of the bow is formed by the entire spinal column, from the coccyx to the first cervical vertebra, while the arms and legs form the string of the bow. The juncture where the hands hold the arches of the feet forms the point where the arrow would be notched.
* On each Mula Bandha inhalation, draw the lower abdomen up into the kidney region (Uddiyana Bandha), and still further upwards into the upper thoracic spine and the cervical spine (Jalandhara Bandha): this allows the spine to curve deeper backwards. Then look up. In this final pose the trunk rests on the stomach, in between the two frontal hip bones and the lower ribs.

- Curl the toes around the fingers (Pada Bandha), so that the feet hold the hands as much as the hands hold the feet, and elongate the arches up towards the sky. As in Kapotasana (9) and Laghu Vajrasana (10), the knees should be kept slightly wider than hip width.
- Hold for a few seconds, and then proceed to 11b.

11b. Padangustha Dhanurasana II

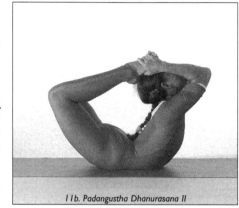

11b. Padangustha Dhanurasana II

- Bend the elbows and knees and pull the feet to the head, thus closing the circle from the Pada Bandha to the Padma Bandha.
- Keep the upward extension of the thighs out of the hip joints, and of the upper arms out of the shoulder joints, so that the wooden part of the bow (the spinal column) stays tightly bent.
- Hold for a few seconds. Return to Padangustha Dhanurasana I.
- As the bow is tightly strung, do not release both hands at the same time to come out of this pose, but release first one hand and place that hand and foot back on the earth to support the trunk. Then release the other hand and foot and return to Bhujangasana I (see page 215).

12. Rajakapotasana
rajakapota=king of the pigeons

12a. Rajakapotasana I

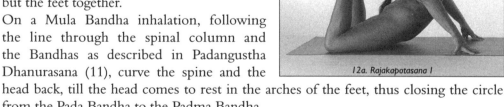

12a. Rajakapotasana I

- Start with Bhujangasana I (see page 215) and then proceed:
- Bend the knees to an angle of about eighty degrees, supporting yourself on the hands. Keep the knees slightly wider than hip width, but the feet together.
- On a Mula Bandha inhalation, following the line through the spinal column and the Bandhas as described in Padangustha Dhanurasana (11), curve the spine and the head back, till the head comes to rest in the arches of the feet, thus closing the circle from the Pada Bandha to the Padma Bandha.
- Here too, the Pada Bandha stabilizes the femur heads, so that you can draw the pelvis forwards and upwards on the inhalation, thus elongating and curving the spinal column into an even and harmonious bow.

Hold for a few seconds, and then proceed to 12b.

12b. *Rajakapotasana II*

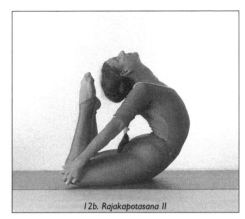

12b. Rajakapotasana II

- Lift the right hand, supporting yourself on the left hand, and bring the right hand back in a circular movement to hold the right shin bone, close to the right knee (on the tuberositas of the knee).
- Resist the right shin bone against the hand to stabilize the right side of the body, lift the left hand and bring it back in a circular movement to hold the left shin, close to the left knee (on the tuberositas). At this point the body rests only on the lower abdomen, the groins and the upper thighs.
- To prevent the body from rolling forwards onto the stomach, the shins have to continue resisting backwards against the hands, so that they pull the hands, the arms and the shoulders backwards: thus the body stays in balance. Keep the head in the arches of the feet.
- Hold for a few seconds, and then proceed to 12c.

12c. *Bhujangasana II*
bhujanga=serpent

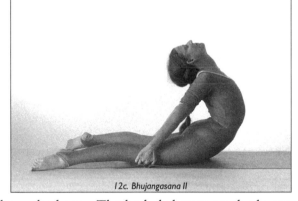

12c. Bhujangasana II

- Increase the resistance of the shins backwards against the hands and extend the legs, till the knees are straight and the feet are on the earth, with the toes pointing straight backwards.
- While extending the knees, you have to crawl the fingers from the tuberositas of the shins over the knee caps, till you are holding the thighs just above the knees. The body balances on the lower abdomen, the pubic bone and the groins, and the head and chest remain curved backwards.
- Hold for a few seconds.
- To come out of this pose, release the knees one hand at a time to prevent the trunk from falling forwards (see Padangustha Dhanurasana (11)).

13. Gherandasana

Gheranda is the name of a sage, author of the Gheranda Samhita.

This pose is a combination of Bhekasana (see page 108) and Padangustha Dhanurasana I (11a).

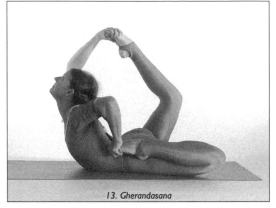
13. Gherandasana

- Start with Padangustha Dhanurasana I (11a) and then proceed:
- Keep the right hand and the right foot raised high to maintain the balance on the abdomen. Release the left hand, bend the left knee and bring the left arm down and backwards in a circular movement to hold the left foot again. The palm of the hand now covers the top portion of the foot and pushes it down to the earth, next to the left hip. The left elbow points upwards and slightly sideways, but keep the shoulders in line, the sternum central and the collar bones even; the left arm is now in the same position as in Bhekasana (see page 108).
- At this point the right side of the body performs Padangustha Dhanurasana I (11a), and the left side Bhekasana (see page 108).
- Release the left hand, and return to Padangustha Dhanurasana I (11a) with the left hand and foot.
- Release the right hand and foot, and repeat Gherandasana on the other side.

14. Kapinjalasana

Kapinjala is a kind of partridge

This pose is a combination of Vasisthasana I (see page 188) and Padangustha Dhanurasana I (11a). In this position one leg is taken behind the central line of gravity; therefore you have to pay special attention to compensating the body weight at the front of the central line of gravity.

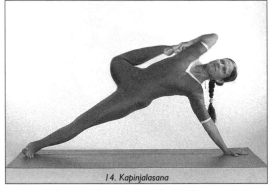
14. Kapinjalasana

- Start with Vasisthasana I (see page 188) on the right hand and the right foot and then proceed:
- Bend the left knee, and with the left hand hold the left foot as described in Padangustha Dhanurasana I (11a) . Then rotate the upper arm in the shoulder joint, till it is next to the left ear, and the left hand holds the left foot behind the left shoulder.
- Rotate the left thigh inwards, so that the two frontal hip bones stay forward in an even line. This is Padangustha Dhanurasana I (11a). At this point the right side of the body performs Vasisthasana I (see page 188) ,and the left side Padangustha Dhanurasana I (11a).
- In addition to the curve, the problem in this pose is the balance. If you do not bring the pelvis and chest forwards, while taking the left leg back into the Padangustha Dhanurasana I curve, the body weight behind the central line of gravity is not compensated and you will therefore lose your balance backwards.

15. Ganda Bherundasana

ganda=cheek; bherunda=terrible, formidable

15a. Close to the wall

- Kneel on a 'sticky' yoga mat close to the wall, facing it.
- Place the hands about thirty centimeters from the wall on the mat, keeping them at shoulder width, with the fingers pointing straight forward towards the wall.
- Bend forward like an animal drinking water, place the chin on the mat, and bend the elbows, till the shoulders are ten centimeters above the hands.
- Supporting the whole body weight on the chin and hands, jump the feet up on the wall. Then extend the knees so that the body forms one smooth curve from the shoulder blades to the back of the heels; the rib cage is wedged in between the inner upper arms.
- To get a deeper curve in the upper spine, bring the sternum gradually down towards the mat in between the hands, rooting the hands and performing Hasta Bandha to lighten the chest.
- The weight of the body has to be balanced evenly at the front and the back of the central line of gravity; thus, as the sternum sinks down, the pelvis has to lift up from the lumbar spine and move closer to the wall.

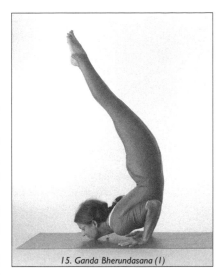

15. Ganda Bherundasana (1)

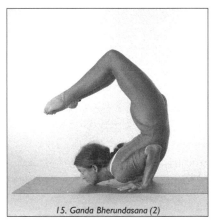

15. Ganda Bherundasana (2)

15b. Away from the wall

- Perform Ganda Bherundasana further away from the wall and then proceed:
- Bend the knees and walk the feet down on the wall.
- When you have reached your deepest curve, take the feet one by one away from the wall, balancing only on the chin and hands.
- Pull the feet in towards the head and place the soles of the feet on the head, thus closing the circle from the Pada Bandha to the Padma Bandha.
- To come out of the pose, place the feet back on the wall again and come down, one foot at a time.

The next three positions are basically the same; the main difference is that in the first one (Ekapada Rajakapotasana I) the bent leg is bent as in Janu Sirsasana (see page 129), in the second (Ekapada Rajakapotasana II) it is bent as in Marichyasana I (see page 138), and in the third (Ekapada Rajakapotasana III) it is bent as in Triangmukhaikapada Paschimottanasana I (see page 134). One could therefore consider these three positions the 'back-face' positions of those three Forward Bending positions.

16. Ekapada Rajakapotasana I

eka=one; pada=leg, foot; rajakapota=the king of pigeons

In this pose the frontal leg is bent as in Janu Sirsasana (see page 129).

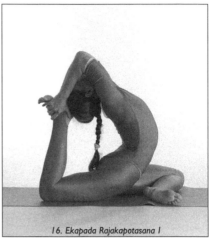

16. Ekapada Rajakapotasana I

First part

- Sit on a mat and extend the right leg straight behind you, keeping the foot and knee in line with the back of the right groin (the buttock rim). The foot points straight backwards, the big and small toes rest evenly on the mat, and the back of the knee faces straight up to the sky.
- Bend the left leg at an angle of forty-five degrees to the trunk, and place the left foot in front of the right groin. Shift the weight of the trunk onto the right hip, and pull the left hip slightly backwards: thus the right hip joint and groin are elongated.
- At the same time, move the two frontal hip bones over towards the right, till the right frontal hip bone is in line with the outer edge of the right groin; both hip bones point forward evenly and have the same height from the earth.
- Extend the left thigh sideways out of the left hip joint and rotate it slightly inward. Thus the left knee is not only extended sideways, but is also rolled forwards on the tuberositas of the left tibia.
- The trunk, from the navel upwards, faces straight forward. Keep the weight of the trunk on the right hip, and rotate the right frontal hip bone, waist and rib cage forwards; thus the two sacro-iliac joints at the back of the pelvis are aligned.
- The pelvis should be almost vertical; if the right hip joint does not elongate sufficiently, the tendency is for the pelvis to fall forward, so that the two frontal hip bones collapse into the groins. To bring the pelvis close to a vertical position, pull the two frontal hip bones *back* and *up* in the direction of the ribs (the typical Back Bending movement). Be careful, however, not to twist the right side of the pelvis backwards.
- On a Mula Bandha inhalation, elongate the spinal column upwards out of the sacro-iliac joints. Root the buttock bones and the thighs into the earth, performing Pada Bandha with both feet, to get the rebounce action in the pelvis; thus the pelvis is lifted up from the femur heads, giving the thrust for the spinal column to elongate.
- On the exhalation, rotate the trunk and spinal column towards the left, until the right shoulder, the right side of the rib cage and the right waist are in alignment with the outer edge of the right groin, and the right frontal hip bone is above the right groin, one thirds distance from the right hip joint, and two thirds distance from the pubic bone.
- The spinal column forms a straight and even groove from the sacro-iliac joints to the cervical spine; it should not deviate to the left. To draw the groove up into the upper thoracic spine, elongate the ears out of the cervical spine. Elongate also the cervical vertebrae upwards and keep the head straight, in alignment with the chest. Keep the shoulders and shoulder blades down and relaxed.

Second part

- Place the right hand on the mat, next to the right thigh, to stabilize your position, and bend the right leg. On a Mula Bandha inhalation, raise the left arm over the head and elongate it out of the left sacro-iliac joint. Never make short movements in yoga: always first create length and lightness in the joints before bending them; this is especially important in the Back Bending Positions.

- On the exhalation, bend the left arm and hold the right foot with the left hand. Even though the left hand holds the right foot, this is only meant to give you a frame within which to elongate and rotate; do not use the hand, the arm and the shoulder muscles to pull the spine and trunk upwards and to rotate them towards the left. That is only done on the breathing.

- On the next Mula Bandha inhalation, elongate the right arm upwards out of the right sacro-iliac joint and hold the right foot also with the right hand.

- When you have reached maximum elongation of the spinal column, start to curve the neck and chest backwards to take the head into the arch of the right foot. As usual, go in stages, using the Mula Bandha breathing: on each inhalation, elongate upwards, and on each exhalation, curve the head and chest further back and down. Curving the neck to take the head back into a back arch starts always with Jalandhara Bandha, so that the cervical and upper thoracic vertebrae are elongated before curving.

- In this whole process the movement is circular: on the inhalation, the lower abdomen moves forwards and up, and the chest moves up and curves back; on the exhalation, the head curves back and down. Thus, seen from the side, there is one smooth curve from the groins to the collar bones. In Back Bendings, one should always look at the front of the body: the line at the front of the body should be round and even. This is only the case if you use the wave of the Mula Bandha breathing correctly.

- Keep the neck, shoulders, shoulder blades and arms relaxed, and place the forehead in the arch of the right foot.

- Hold for a few seconds, and then repeat on the other side.

17. Ekapada Rajakapotasana II

eka=one; pada=leg, foot; rajakapota=the king of pigeons

In this pose the frontal leg is bent as in Marichyasana I (see page 138).

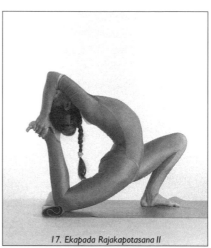

17. Ekapada Rajakapotasana II

- Kneel on a mat and bring the left foot forward, till there is an angle of ninety degrees in the left knee.
- Bend the left knee further, till the back of the left thigh is almost in touch with the calf muscle. As the pelvis is lowered, the right groin is completely opened.
- Keep the two frontal hip bones facing straight forward, and the pelvis and chest as vertical as possible. In all Back Bending positions, the two frontal hip bones move towards the lower ribs; this is to make sure that the extension is in the groins, not in the waist. Thus the lumbar spine is protected as the curve is brought into the hip joints.
- Place the hands next to you on the mat and, supporting yourself for balance on the fingers, curve the head and spine backwards as described in Ekapada Rajakapotasana I (16).
- Bend the right knee, so that the foot points up towards the sky. On a Mula Bandha inhalation, elongate the left arm up over the head, out of the left sacro-iliac joint. On the exhalation, hold the right foot with the left hand, curling the toes around the fingers, so that the foot holds the hand as much as the hand holds the foot. Perform Pada Bandha with both feet for the stability and rebounce of the body, and to lighten the pelvis on the femur heads.
- On an inhalation, elongate the right arm up, resisting the right leg backwards, and hold the right foot also with the right hand. The body now balances on the left foot and the right knee. Keep the left heel down, and the right frontal hip bone parallel to the left one. For the rotation of the right thigh and hip, follow the instructions given in Ekapada Rajakapotasana I (16).
- Using the Mula Bandha breathing and the action of the Pada Bandha in both feet, lift the pelvis up from the femur heads on each inhalation, rotating it backwards, so that the pubic bone moves forwards, and the two frontal hip bones move up towards the ribs: this brings the curve automatically into the upper back, and allows the head to curve deeper backwards. Rest the forehead into the arch of the right foot.
- Hold for a few seconds, and then repeat on the other side

18. Ekapada Rajakapotasana III

eka=one; pada=leg, foot; rajakapota=the king of pigeons

In this pose the frontal leg is bent as in Triangmukhai-kapada Paschimottanasana I (see page 134).

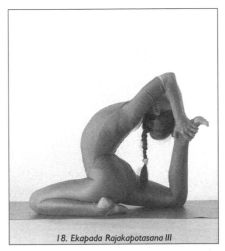

18. Ekapada Rajakapotasana III

- Sit in Virasana (see page 102) and then proceed:
- Extend the right leg straight backwards. Due to the Virasana position of the left leg, the tendency to drop the upper part of the pelvis and the waist forward onto the left thigh is greater in this pose than in the two previous ones. Therefore you have to pay extra attention to the backward rotation of the pelvis, in which the pubic bone moves *forwards* and *up* towards the navel, and the two frontal hip bones move *up* towards the lower ribs: this brings the extension in the right groin, not in the waist.
- For the rotation in the right thigh and hip, follow the instructions given in Ekapada Rajakapotasana I (16).
- As all the Back Bending positions are bow positions, the accent is always on the extreme endpoints of the bow: these are the coccyx and the first cervical vertebra. To curve the whole spine evenly, the parts of the spine closest to those extreme points should be curved in the same measure as the middle part. This is done by drawing the two frontal hip bones *up* towards the ribs, at the same time drawing the ribs *down* towards the two frontal hip bones: thus the central parts of the bow (the lumbar spine and the lower thoracic spine) are lengthened, and the curve is brought into the sacro-iliac joints and into the upper thoracic spine.
- As said before, the tendency in this pose is to collapse the waist forward. By lengthening the spine as described above, the trunk retains its vertical position and its height.
- For the rest follow the instructions given in Ekapada Rajakapotasana I (16).
- Hold for a few seconds, and then repeat on the other side.

19. Ekapada Rajakapotasana IV

eka=one; pada=leg, foot; rajakapota=the king of pigeons

- Start with Hanumanasana (see page 123) with the left leg extended forward and the right leg back and then proceed:
- Supporting yourself on the fingers, bend the right leg.
- For the rest follow the instructions given in Ekapada Rajakapotasana I (16).

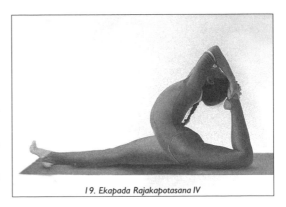

19. Ekapada Rajakapotasana IV

20. Natarajasana

nata=dance; raja=king; Nataraja is a name of Shiva, lord of dance and destruction (the Tandava is the dance of destruction)

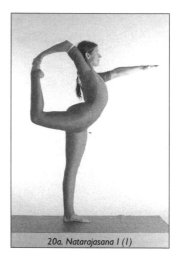

20a. Natarajasana I (1)

Natarajasana is the last pose described in this book, and is also one of the most beautiful, elegant and symbolic poses in yoga: when performed correctly, the body takes on the shape of a tall wine glass. Yoga has always been considered a tool for reaching out to the Universal Force, in which the body becomes the recipient for that Force. In many traditions, including the Christian and Sufi traditions, the Universal Force is compared to wine, which fills the human glass to produce Divine ecstasy. Thus the ritual of drinking wine in the Catholic Church and in the famous Sufi poem, the Rubayat of Omar Khayyam.

Natarajasana, as the last pose in this book, symbolizes the wine glass formed by the human body to be filled with the Universal Force. As the wine glass is completely transparent, the human body and mind too should be as transparent and empty as the crystal wine glass to receive the Divine ecstasy. This has been the aim of this book, to bring the attention of the student from the physical body to the transparent side of us, the one that we have called the *Body of Light*.

20a. Natarajasana I

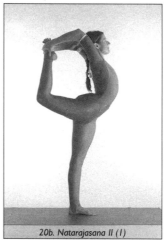

20b. Natarajasana II (1)

*   Stand in Tadasana (which is the first asana described in this book) and proceed:
*   Bend the right knee backwards and, holding with the right hand the right foot as described in Padangustha Dhanurasana I (11a), lift the foot up behind the trunk.
*   For the rest follow the instructions given in Ekapada Rajakapotasana I (16).
*   In this human wine glass, the foot of the glass is formed by the left, vertical leg. The glass itself is formed by the trunk and arms on the one side, and the right thigh and lower leg on the other side. To make this glass vertical and even, the upward elongation of the spinal column, from the coccyx to the back of the head, has to be equal to the upward elongation of the right leg, from the buttock rim to the arch of the right foot. Thus the top of the head, the hands and the right foot are equally high, and reach up to the sky in an even and harmonious way.

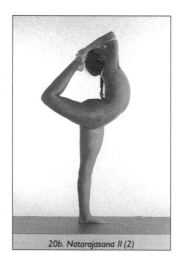

20b. Natarajasana II (2)

20b. Natarajasana II

*   To close the wine glass at the top, curve the head backwards and place the arch of the foot on the top of the head. Thus the circle is closed.

4.13   Comparitive studies of various asanas

Let us now discuss a few asanas and compare them to each other in order to show that, in reality, the body knows only very few movements. These movements are: bending forward, bending backward, bending sideways and twisting around the vertical axis of the spine. One can add the movements of turning the body upside down, like in Head balance, Shoulder balance, Full arm balance, Elbow balance, etc.

Within these major groups of movements we can play around with an enormous amount of positions or asanas, using the *Seven Vital Principles of Practice*, in particular the force of gravity (rooting), to achieve slightly different effects on the body, even though the positions themselves are intrinsically the same or similar.

Comparitive studies of various asanas

1. Playing with gravity
    a. Salamba Sirsasana and
       Pincha Mayurasana
    b. Halasana, Uttanasana,
       Urdhvamukha Paschimottanasana II
       and Paschimottanasana
    c. Paschimottanasana and
       Upavistha Konasana
    d. Kapotasana and
       Urdhva Dhanurasana

2. Front face - Back Face
    a. Janu Sirsana and
       Ekapada Rajakapotasana
    b. Uttanasana and
       Urdhva Dhanurasana

3. Beauty and freedom in yoga

I. Playing with gravity

1a. Salamba Sirsasana and Pincha Mayurasana

Salamba Sirsasana is sometimes called the king of the asanas, as Salamba Sarvangasana is called the queen. One can also say that Salamba Sirsasana is a solar position (the *ha* part of Hatha Yoga) as it heats the body, while Salamba Sarvangasana is a lunar position (the *tha* part of Hatha Yoga) as it tends to cool the body. Salamba Sirsasana in itself is not a complex pose, neither is it a very tiring one if one uses the external and internal forces intelligently. After all, it is Tadasana upside down, and thus subject to the same forces as Tadasana.

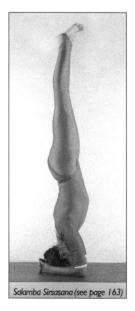

Salamba Sirsasana (see page 163)

The external force is the force of gravity. This force acts not only vertically downwards on the body but contains also a rebouncing aspect, as we have seen. Both the force of gravity and its rebouncing aspect can only function through those parts of the body which are exactly vertical, and this is where, in Salamba Sirsasana, many people get themselves into trouble. This is because they have the impression that, to stand on your head, you need to use the arm and shoulder muscles, which are exactly those muscles that you should *not* use.

Let us have a look at the arm and shoulder muscles. In Salamba Sirsasana I the arms are bent at the elbows at an angle less than ninety degrees, with the shoulders not vertically above the elbows, but a little backwards of them. This is very different from a pose like Pincha Mayurasana where the shoulders are *directly* above the elbows and the arms are bent at an angle of ninety degrees in the elbows. This means, on the one hand, that the head is lifted off the earth. On the other hand it means that the arms can use the gravity/rebounce action, as the upper arms, Deltoid muscles and shoulder joints are in exact vertical alignment.

In Salamba Sirsasana this is not the case. As the shoulder joints are slightly backwards of the elbow joints the force of gravity exerts a tremendous pressure on those joints, a pressure that for most people is expressed in a sagging of the shoulders onto the neck. The reason for this is that muscles in general, and the big, peripheral muscles in particular, are not geared for static action, but only for dynamic action. In weight lifting the muscles of the arms and other parts of the body are used in a dynamic way, thus increasing their capacity of load carrying. Most asanas, on the other hand, are static poses, and thus need a different action.

In Salamba Sirsasana the Deltoid muscles, which cover the shoulder joints, have no vertical rooting support like in Pincha Mayurasana, where the vertical rooting support is formed by the bones of the upper arms. The other muscle used by most people to hold the body up is the Trapezius muscle. This muscle forms a kind of diamond shape at the back of the chest, running from the cervical and thoracic spinal column sideways towards the shoulders. This big, peripheral muscle is vital for many movements.

In Salamba Sirsasana, as it runs for the most part parallel to the earth, it forms however a kind of 'hanging bridge' between the spinal column and the shoulders. On this 'hanging bridge' the force of gravity exerts its pressure at an angle of ninety degrees to the fibers of the muscle. As these fibers are not geared for long term action, after a short while the Trapezius will sag and the weight of the body will 'leak' into the cervical vertebrae.

Because the body has been counting on these big muscles to hold its weight up against gravity, it has not provided a 'back up' in case of failure. Thus, in order to be able to stay for some time in Salamba Sirsasana (ten minutes or more) without damaging the neck vertebrae, we have to approach it differently.

We have to go back to rooting, or the use of the gravity/rebounce force, and let that force do the work for us. Thus we have to find those muscles that *are* able to co-operate with that force, and not sag underneath it. Those muscles are the long muscles (the Erector spinae) that run alongside the entire spinal column. In Salamba Sirsasana those muscles are aligned with the gravity/rebounce force and therefore can utilize that force through the action of rooting. These muscles, however, can only be reached if we move the outer, big muscles out of the way. Those outer, big muscles are the Trapezius and the Latissimus dorsi muscles that form the outer layer of the back. These muscles have to move sideways, away from the spinal column. This is done mainly by rolling the Triceps muscles of the upper arms inwards towards the face (without displacing the elbows), and rolling the Latissimus dorsi muscles forwards, which is experienced as a widening of the entire back. Once those muscles are out of the way, the interior muscle, the Erector spinae, can go into action, elongating its fibers along the line of gravity.

Elongation can only take place, however, if you move a muscle in two opposite directions. Thus, in order to move the entire spinal column upwards along the line of gravity, something else has to move downwards along the line of gravity. That something is the head. Here we come to the crux of the matter. The more you root the head down into the earth, the more you save the neck in Salamba Sirsasana. The act of rooting the head enables the neck and upper thoracic spine to pick up the rebounce force so that they can elongate upwards, away from the earth towards the sky. Before doing this rooting movement into the earth, you can experiment standing in Tadasana and placing a book on the top of your head. The book should be exactly on the middle of the head. You can feel with your fingers a kind of dip on the top of the head halfway between the forehead and the crown of the head. This is the fontanel, or the exact spot where the three joints of the skull meet at the top of the skull. Once you have placed the book on that spot, push it gently upwards towards the sky with the head without raising the shoulders, using only the spinal muscles. This movement starts with the rooting of the feet into the earth and the activating of the Pada Bandha. From there the rebounce force travels upwards through the legs, the lower abdomen and the chest towards the head (and the book).

To make sure that you do not tilt the head forwards or backwards, imagine that you have to elongate your ears upwards into the book. In this way both the back and the front of the neck extend upwards evenly. One can also feel the elongation in the upper back, on the spinal column in between the shoulder blades, as well as a lateral stretch between the shoulder blades themselves. Thus, not only are the ears, shoulder joints, hip joints and ankle joints all in a vertical alignment in Salamba Sirsasana, but the body is very light due to the fact that it is not holding itself up with the gross peripheral muscles, but only with the gravity/rebounce force. It is precisely the spinal column which, elongating upwards away from the downward rooting head, pulls the peripheral muscles, like the Trapezius and Deltoid muscles, with it upwards. Thus the shoulders are lifted and the angle in the elbows is increased, but not by the action of those same muscles, but by the action of the Erector spinae.

The next step is to make sure that the back plate and the front plate of the body are parallel to each other. The back of the pelvis should not collapse into the lumbar spine, thus pushing the lumbar vertebrae into the body. Curving the lumbar spine too much forward results in an over-extension at the front of the body, especially in the region between the lower ribs and the navel. This eventually weakens the abdominal muscles as well as the lumbar spine itself. The neck and thoracic vertebrae pick up the rebounce force of the rooting head in the first joint, the one between the skull and the atlas (the first cervical vertebra). This rebounce force, as it travels upwards, tends to slow down somewhere in the lower thoracic/upper lumbar region. Thus the internal spinal muscles in that region have to be on the alert to pick up the thread from there and continue up towards the sky, not letting that rebounce force collapse in the lumbar, thus dragging the lumbar vertebrae forward into the abdomen. In other words, the pelvis should sit lightly on the lumbar vertebrae, and the bowl of the pelvis, as in Tadasana, should be vertical, not slanted.

At the lower end of the spinal column we have the coccyx. One of the main issues in yoga is that the coccyx should never collapse into the fifth lumbar vertebra. Many people interpret this as meaning that you have to 'tuck the coccyx under'. This, however, drags the lumbar vertebrae too far back, eventually resulting in a loss of the lumbar curve. The curves of the spinal column have to be respected at all cost. Though they should not be too deep, they should not be eliminated either. Thus the correct interpretation is that the coccyx should move away from the lumbar vertebrae through internal (ex)tension, not through flexion. This is facilitated by the action of the legs. If the legs are passive in Salamba Sirsasana their weight will sink heavily into the femur-iliac joints, thus compressing those joints and collapsing the pelvis into the lumbar vertebrae.

The legs, with the ankles in a vertical alignment with the hip joints, should be elongated upwards, out of the femur-iliac joints, so that space is created in those joints and the heads of the femurs sit lightly in the femur-iliac joints, not sink into them. To get the feeling in the legs and consequently in the lower back, you have to constrict the upper thighs slightly inwards so that, at the back, the Gluteus muscles are widened across the sacro-iliac joints, thus pulling the big diamond-shaped ligamental plate that crosses over the lumbar spine (the lumbar aponeurosis) backwards. This action, in its turn, pulls the lumbar spine backwards and thus saves it from collapsing forward into the front of the body. By then elongating the inner thighs upwards you can feel the extension on the hip joints and the lumbar spine.

The *breathing* is vital in all the asanas. In general, the rule is that you use the inhalation to open the body, while you close the body on the exhalation. But when there is more force needed for a certain action, it is better to exhale, using the exhalation as a kind of jet to propel you through the movement. In using the Mula Bandha breathing in Salamba Sirsasana the wave action of the inhalation facilitates the elongation upwards of the spinal column towards the sky, while the exhalation consolidates your position.

Pincha Mayurasana is also a vertically upside down position, but with a different action from Salamba Sirsasana. In the first place, due to the fact that in this position one stands on the lower arms and not on the head, it is not possible to hold this pose for as long as Salamba Sirsasana. Usually one holds it for about one minute. Where in Salamba Sirsasana I the hands are clasped, here the lower arms run parallel to each other and the hands rest straight on the earth with the palms facing downwards and the middle fingers parallel to each other. This means that the outer and the inner edges of the wrists are even.

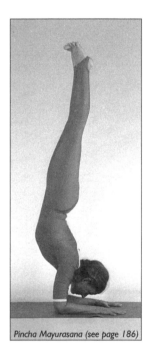

Pincha Mayurasana (see page 186)

Here we run into the first problem. If the shoulders are stiff it is hard to maintain this once the body is raised to a vertical position. The hands tend to move towards each other, so that the lower arms are no longer parallel to each other. For the hands to remain in their original position the shoulders need to be able to form a straight line through the upper arms and rib cage, with the shoulder joints vertically above the elbow joints and an angle of ninety degrees in those joints. Thus it is advisable to work first on loosening and lengthening the shoulder joints before attempting Pincha Mayurasana.

To go up into Pincha Mayurasana you have to keep the hands extended firmly on the earth and the head lifted. The rooting action of the ulnar wrist points and of the hands (Hasta Bandha) here is vital, as it will support the shoulders (rebounce) and will prevent the hands from slipping towards each other. Then raise the body up into Pincha Mayurasana.

Here we run into the second problem. Most people jump up. This means that the speed of the leg which jumps pulls the trunk up into the vertical position. The pelvis, being the heaviest part to pull up, though, tends to sag in the process and thus collides with the lumbar spine and the sacro-iliac joints. Moreover, because most people do not change legs each time they jump up, one side of the lumbar spine becomes stronger over time while the other side becomes weaker and compressed. You can easily verify this for yourself by jumping up next time with the leg that you never use. Thus, unwittingly, one can even create conditions of scoliosis through thoughtless practice.

Instead of jumping up with speed, there is a different way. Keeping the arms firmly planted on the earth with the ulnar wrist points and hands rooted and the shoulders in a vertical alignment with the elbows, raise the trunk and one leg as high as you can. You have to aim at being as close to the vertical as possible. Then, using the flexibility of the lower spring joint of the bottom foot rather than the force of the leg muscles, lift yourself up into Pincha Mayurasana.

With a little bit of practice you can raise the body up without jumping, by just continuing the lengthening upwards of the spinal column and the lower abdomen. Change leg every time you go up. In this way it is the spinal column and the pelvis which pull the bottom leg up, not the bottom leg jumping up which pulls the trunk and pelvis. Thus the pelvis does not collide with the lumbar, and the lumbar vertebrae and sacro-iliac joint are safe.

Once you are in the vertical position, you have to find again, like in Salamba Sirsasana, the central line of gravity, so that you can lift the chest up from the shoulder heads (the upper arms now being the base from which to pick up the rebounce action) and continue that action through the spinal column and legs. The part of the body which now has to cooperate with gravity is, of course, the lower arms.

It is advisable, if the shoulders are really stiff, to practice this pose by keeping the head forward in between the arms, in the direction you are facing. In this way you free the shoulder blades so that you can pull the chest up from the shoulder heads. Keeping the head flexed backwards blocks the shoulder blades and shoulders and thus makes it harder to pull the chest up. While going up, the shoulders should remain vertically above the elbow joints. Many people collapse in the shoulders while going up and thus end up on their foreheads or face as the ninety degree angle in the elbows collapses.

1b.   *Halasana, Uttanasana, Urdhvamukha Paschimottanasana II and Paschimottanasana*

Looking at these poses superficially one would consider them four different poses. Looking at them in a more holistic way, however, one can easily see that they are one and the same pose, subjected to the force of gravity in different ways.

In *Halasana* gravity pushes the pelvis and spine down into the neck and shoulders, in *Uttanasana* it pulls the spine out of the pelvis, liberating the lumbar and shoulders, in *Urdhvamukha Paschimottanasana II* it pushes the legs into the pelvic joints and in *Paschimottanasana* it pulls the body down onto the legs. Even though the shape of the body in all these poses is more or less the same, the effect of gravity is different.

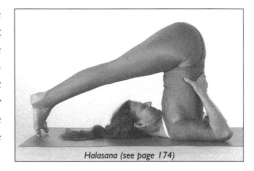
Halasana (see page 174)

To liberate the energy body we have to elongate the physical body always in *opposite* directions, not just in one direction. This involves a stable part and a mobile part which elongates out of the stable part. The stable part of the body is always that one which is in contact with the earth, from which it derives its stability, so that the mobile part can move away from it.

Thus, in *Halasana*, the stable part is formed by the neck, shoulders, upper arms and feet, which rest on the earth, while the mobile part is formed by the spine and pelvis. As gravity pulls down in a straight line through the pelvis and the spine, which are vertically above the shoulders, they have to move upwards in a straight line, away from the shoulders. This is only possible if those stable parts co-operate fully with gravity, that is, if they root into the earth. The more those stable parts root into the earth, the more the mobile parts can elongate upwards along the line of gravity towards the sky.

In *Uttanasana* the stable part is formed by the soles of the feet. Thus, like in Tadasana, we have to root the soles of the feet into the earth, so that the ankles can lift. This lift is carried upwards through the legs and femur heads towards the lower abdomen. By then lifting the pelvis up from the femur heads on a Mula Bandha inhalation a wave is created for the spine to elongate forwards and downwards.

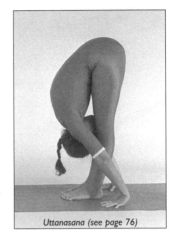

Uttanasana (see page 76)

In *Urdhvamukha Paschimottanasana II* the stable part is formed by the back and the head, which rest on the earth. The mobile part is formed by the legs. In this pose one is tempted to pull the feet straight down to the earth along the line of gravity. In this way, however, we do not create any space in the lumbar vertebrae. So here too the spinal column and the legs should meet exactly in the femur-iliac joints. This happens by elongating the lumbar spine, or more

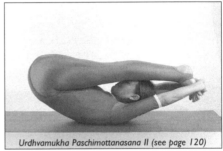

Urdhvamukha Paschimottanasana II (see page 120)

precisely the groins and the pubic bone, backwards as you pull the legs down. In other words, the lumbar vertebrae should not press onto the earth in this pose, but there should still be the slight natural curve of the lumbar spine, just above the pelvic rim at the back.

In *Paschimottanasana* the stable part is, of course, the back of the legs and the buttock bones. So here too, the more those buttock bones and the back of the legs root into the earth, the more the rest of the pelvis and the trunk can lift, as it were, up from the femur heads and buttock bones, creating again a wave action which carries the whole spinal column forward before gravity drops the trunk onto the legs.

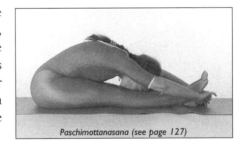

Paschimottanasana (see page 127)

These are simple physical adjustments in these poses, in which you have applied the principle of rooting. This rooting has to be guided by the breathing. Doing the asanas without the breath is like doing wind surfing without wind: you go nowhere.

Inhalation is that part of the breathing which helps the spine to elongate, to lift up from the stable underground. It is that part of the breathing which elongates the body in the opposite direction of the rooting action, so all the elongating and upward movements are done on the inhalation. Thus, in Halasana you elongate the spine upwards on the inhalation, in Uttanasana you elongate it forward, in Urdhvamukha Paschimottanasana II you elongate the lumbar and thoracic spine on the earth and in Paschimottanasana you elongate it forward.

Exhalation is that part of the breathing which by nature follows gravity, in which the ribs drop with gravity, thus emptying the lungs. In Halasana this means moving the spine forwards from the back to the front to bring the sternum closer to the chin, without pushing the chin down, however, which is a common mistake. The chin should always lift up on the sternum towards the sky in the Jalandhara Bandha movement (see page 43), so that here too you maintain the slight natural curve of the neck vertebrae just underneath the skull. In Uttanasana the exhalation helps to drop the whole trunk down to the earth, after you have elongated it forward on the inhalation. In Urdhvamukha Paschimottanasana II the legs come down, and in Paschimottanasana the trunk drops onto the legs.

Thus, on each inhalation and exhalation you create a wave, which ripples throughout the whole trunk. This wave-like action of the inhalation starts always in the lower abdomen, and is carried upwards along the interior length of the spinal column to the top of the head, after which it is attenuated during the exhalation along the line of gravity.

Using rooting and breathing in this way is the first step on the road to an awareness and usage of the *Energy Body* or *Body of Light*.

1c.   *Paschimottanasana and Upavistha Konasana*

The word *paschima* means 'the back of the body' or 'the west'. The back of the body is considered in India the west side as one faces the east for sun worship and thus the front of the body represents the east.

Paschimottanasana is the basic pose from which is derived a whole series of variations. Most of these variations are one-legged variations, in which the hip joint of the bent leg is either rotated inward or outward. In Paschimottanasana both legs are extended straight forward with the inner ankles touching each other and the feet placed in such a way that all the toes are in one line, as in Tadasana. And as in Tadasana, the heels and balls of the feet are in line, in this case in a vertical alignment. You can pull the Gluteus muscles backwards and sideways with your hands, so that you feel that you are sitting on the bones rather than on the flesh. In this way you can understand better whether the body weight is divided equally over the two buttock bones. Due to certain habitual patterns you may feel that you have more weight on one buttock bone than on the other. You can correct this by shifting the weight of the trunk over the legs to the bone which has less weight. The center line of the Quadriceps muscles, the central eye of the knee caps, and the central line of the tibia bones have to face straight upwards towards the ceiling.

Paschimottanasana is a Forward Bending movement. This means that the trunk has to hinge forward in the hip joints. Due to either shortness at the back of the hamstrings or to a certain configuration of the pelvis, this is sometimes not possible. Thus the trunk is bent forward from the lumbar vertebrae, leaving the pelvis in a rigid, upright position. This is the classical humpback position that especially beginner students show.

Therefore, as the root of Forward Bending is in the back of the legs, the most direct approach is to start by softening and lengthening the back of the legs. The Biceps muscles at the back of the thighs are attached to the upper rim of the pelvis and so pull the rim of the pelvis backward if they are tight. This tightness of the Biceps muscles is for the largest part caused by civilized living, which means the use of chairs as well as by certain sports, like bicycling, jogging, canoeing, etc.

There are several positions that can help to lengthen those muscles, like Adho Mukha Svanasana, Uttanasana, and Prasarita Padottanasana. In these positions the gravity helps to pull the weight of the trunk forward and thus the back of the legs can elongate more easily, whereas in Paschimottanasana one has to work against gravity to do this.

As the body has to hinge forward in the hip joints and not in the waist area, you have to bring the movement first down into the lower abdomen. Holding the feet firmly without pulling them perform the Mula Bandha breathing. In this breathing the inhalation starts in the lower abdomen with the pulling up of the pelvic floor in general and for women the uterus in particular. This means that the pressure in the lower abdomen is brought slightly backwards towards the sacro-iliac joints. Thus these joints are widened slightly and do not collapse. From there the air moves upwards along the inner lumber spine into the kidney region, widening the lumbar region and the kidneys.

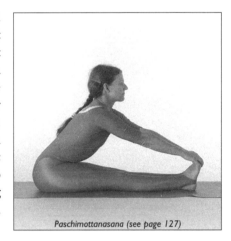

Paschimottanasana (see page 127)

The air then moves upwards along the inner thoracic spine into the upper chest, thus widening and lifting the upper chest. It finally moves up into the back of the head. In this way the body is elongated on each inhalation from the base of the pelvis to the head in a forty-five degree angle, like a jet plane taking off. In this movement the two frontal hip bones are brought forward and lifted towards the rib cage. Note that the pubic bone too is brought slightly forward and *up*. If the pubic bone is brought forward and *down* the sacro-iliac joints collapse and the lower abdomen loses its power.

With the exhalation the body goes down towards the legs with gravity, while maintaining the length on the front from pubic bone to throat. In other words, the trunk should not curl back into itself while going down into the final pose. When finally the face comes to rest on the shin bones this has to be well beyond the knees. The more the length at the front is maintained the closer the face will come to the feet.

Even in the final pose you should maintain the soft, even breathing. Each inhalation creates a gently rippling movement from the base of the pelvis along the inner line of the spine towards the head, while on each exhalation the weight of the trunk is abandoned to gravity. Using the breathing in this way you will find that the body can elongate further and further forward without using the arm muscles or the shoulders to pull. The arms should not pull, but you can include the shoulders and arms in the rippling motion of the breathing, elongating the hands further and further forward beyond the feet. When you do eventually clasp the hands beyond the feet you should turn the palm of one hand facing forward and with the thumb and fingers form a ring in which you insert the fingers of the opposite hand. In this way there is no limit to the elongation as the hand can slide further and further forward through the ring of the other hand. Keep the palm of the sliding hand straight, facing the earth, with the fingers pointing straight forward. Here too, however, you should not create one-sided habits. Change hands at regular intervals so as to get an even movement on both sides of the trunk.

The body is a finely tuned network of information. The minute you put your hands on something the body automatically transfers part of its weight to the hands and through the hands to the support on which the hands are resting.

There are three places where you can clasp the hands around the feet. You can rest them on top of the balls of the feet, clasp them in the arches or rest them on the earth. Many people prefer the first. This is because, by resting the hands on the balls of the feet, part of the weight of the trunk is transferred through the hands to the feet. This softens the lower back, which makes it easier to elongate it, and can be helpful for those students who need to soften the lower back in order to make it move forward. It is counter-productive, however, for those students who are already very flexible in Paschimottanasana, in which case keeping the hands on top of the feet weakens the lower back even further and therefore creates an even more unstable situation in the lumbar spine and sacro-iliac joints. For those people it is advisable to clasp the hands in the arches so that, as there is no support for the hands, the weight of the trunk, arms and hands is sustained by the lower back. Thus the lower back is strengthened.

Even though there are many similarities between Upavistha Konasana and Paschimottanasana, the difference is great.

In *Upavistha Konasana* there is an angle of ninety degrees or more between the legs so that the femur heads fit differently into the hip joints and the sacro-iliac joints have a greater tendency to collapse, due to the fact that the lower abdomen can go down to the earth in between the legs, unlike in Paschimottanasana. Therefore it is easier to let the pubic bone roll too far forward and down. Thus it is even more necessary to keep elongating the coccyx backwards away from the lumbar spine in order to maintain the length at the front of the lower abdomen.

Many people experience discomfort in this position along the inner thighs as the Adductor muscles and the Gracilis muscles are greatly stretched. So here the softening and lengthening has to take place mainly along the inner line of the thighs and knees. One has to pay extra attention to elongating the inner ankles and the metatarsals of the big toes away from the groins, keeping the feet in a vertical position and the toes well spread. The elongation of the metatarsals of the big toes is connected to the inner groins, while the spreading of the other toes and especially of the little toes brings a greater awareness to the muscles around the outer hip joints.

This pose is slightly dangerous for the inner knees and the back of the thighs. To make it safer you have to pull the knee caps strongly up so that you maintain the control over the muscles of the legs. In this way you may go less forward but there is also less chance of hurting a leg muscle. For those students who are flexible and go easily forward it is advisable to keep the legs very strong and the arms spread sideways, resting the palms or wrists just lightly on the tips of the toes so that all the body weight is supported by the lower back.

Using the Mula Bandha breathing and at the same time slightly elongating the legs out of the hip joints elongate the whole trunk upwards and forward before going down on an exhalation to the earth in between the legs. Like in Paschimottanasana the trunk should not curl into itself while going down but should maintain the length at the front so that eventually with a bit of practice you can rest the chest on the earth.

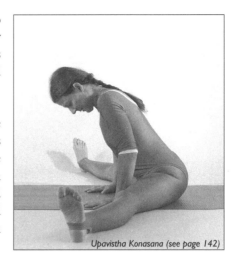
Upavistha Konasana (see page 142)

1d. Kapotasana and Urdhva Dhanurasana

As the technique for Urdhva Dhanurasana is basically the same as for Kapotasana, which is a complex position, it is useful to have a look at Kapotasana first. The main difference between the two is that *Kapotasana* starts from a kneeling position, while *Urdhva Dhanurasana* starts from Tadasana.

The art of the asanas is to liberate the energy trapped within the body by elongating all the joints of the physical body. To do this, we have to differentiate between the stable part(s) of the body and the mobile part(s). The stable part of the body is the one which is in contact with the earth. This forms the basis for the mobile part to pull away from, upwards against gravity, or in any other direction.

In *Kapotasana* (as well as in Ustrasana, which is the same position, but with the arms down), the basis is formed by the entire lower leg, from the knees to the tips of the toes, with the knees slightly wider than the hip joints. This is very important. Many people suffer in Kapotasana and Urdhva Dhanurasana from a sharp pain at the outside of the knees. This is because, when the hips are stiff, the ligaments at the outside of the knees are overstretched. Moreover, keeping the knees in line with the hips or even more narrow than the hips eventually will put a

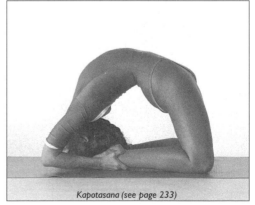
Kapotasana (see page 233)

load on the femur-iliac joints, producing stress there. Keeping the knees slightly wider than the hip joints gives a better, more natural, angle to the femur heads, and thus takes the stress off from those joints and from the knees. The feet and heels are kept together, however, with the toes pointing backwards.

This forms the basis. From here on we have to fix the femur heads in such a way that they, in their turn, form the stable basis for the pelvis and the rest of the body to pull up from. This is done by constricting the outer hips and the inner thighs slightly inwards, from the inner knees up to the inner groins, keeping the thighs perpendicular at an angle of ninety degrees with the lower legs.

To understand this movement better, imagine that you have a block in between the knees and squeeze it, at the same time lifting the arms up over the head. Hold the wrist of one arm and pull it upwards out of that same side femur head, so that you feel the elongation from the outer knee throughout the whole side of the body up to the wrist. Then do the same thing with the other arm and repeat this several times until you feel that you have reached maximum elongation.

This is very important. Many people make the mistake of straight away pushing the groins forward by putting their hands on the hips or at the back of the thighs, thus increasing the angle at the back of the knees. The thighs are like a pillar, and on top of this vertical pillar we have to create a crescent moon shape. This crescent moon shape has to retain its shape and coherence right from the beginning and throughout the pose. Lighten the weight of the body on the femur heads by lifting the pelvis and entire body up from the femur heads (rebounce action). This is done by elongating the inner arches of the feet backwards and rooting them into the earth while performing Pada Bandha, lengthening the thighs and maintaining the squeezing action at the outer hips and inner thighs.

The act of lengthening the thighs by lifting the pelvis up from the femur heads with the Mula Bandha inhalation pulls the energy upwards along the interior spinal column. Mula Bandha is that lifting of the pelvis, but not only of the physical structure. It is the *mula*, the root of the body, which has to pressurize upwards, thus shooting the energy upwards. This upward movement of the energy travels along the line of gravity, and thus goes from the base of the pelvis straight up into the kidneys, lifting the kidneys up from the lumbar vertebrae.

From the kidneys, still traveling in a straight line upwards, it goes up into the top of the sternum, lifting that up to the sky. This is the crescent moon shape. This crescent moon has to retain its shape and integrity throughout.

To go into Kapotasana from here we have to balance the body around the central line of gravity. As the trunk goes back and down, the upper thighs have to move forward (maintaining the squeezing action at the inner sides of the thighs) to balance the weight of the body, until the moment when the pelvis 'clicks' with the femur heads.

Where in the initial crescent moon shape the trunk showed one round line from the pubic bone to the top of the sternum, and the groins were dipped inwards, this round line now starts at the knees and continues through the groins up to the top of the sternum, making one smooth and even curve.

This is in strong opposition to the way many people start, putting the hands on the hips or the back of the thighs and then pushing the trunk/groins forward. The result of this pushing forward is the immediate collapse of the crescent moon shape as the chest sinks down onto the kidney and lumbar area, while the head comes up to balance the uneven distribution of the body weight around the central line of the gravity. In this way the lumbar vertebrae and sacro-iliac joints are completely compressed and there is no smooth curve at the front of the body, but a jarred line of angles and bones (iliac crests and lower frontal ribs). With a little bit of practice (relaxed and with the breathing) one can take the hands all the way down to the earth.

In *Urdhva Dhanurasana* the start is the same. Stand with the feet at hip width or even slightly wider (again to protect the fitting of the femur heads in the femur-iliac joints). Fix the femur heads so that they in their turn can function as a stable underground for the pelvis to lift up from. Using a Mula Bandha inhalation lift the arms straight up over the head, hold the wrist of one arm with the hand of the other, and pull that arm out of the same side femur-iliac joint. Repeat this action several times, until you feel that you have reached maximum elongation. Keeping the legs straight, vertical,

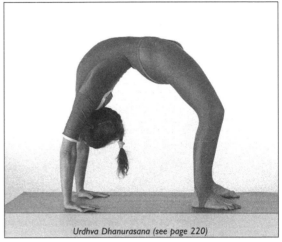

Urdhva Dhanurasana (see page 220)

create that crescent moon shape by lifting the pelvis up from the femur heads. There should be one smooth curve from the pubic bone up to the top of the sternum. (There is again a dip in the groins). Then go back and down in the same way as for Kapotasana till the hands reach the earth. At this point the smooth and even curve starts at the feet and continues through the knees, groins, and lower ribs up to the throat. For a more detailed description of this pose see Urdhva Dhanurasana (page 220).

2. Front face - Back face

2a. *Janu Sirsasana and Ekapada Rajakapotasana*

It is interesting to note that many asanas have a 'front face' and a 'back face'. That is, that the same pose has a forward form and a backward form.

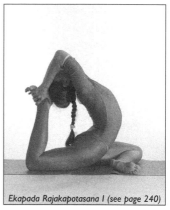

Ekapada Rajakapotasana I (see page 240)

Let us start with two positions which are fairly complicated, but at the same time very interesting. These positions, when performed wrongly, can easily harm the body,

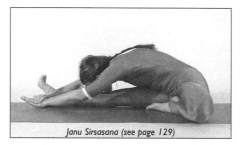

Janu Sirsasana (see page 129)

but, when performed correctly, can be of immense help in cases of scoliosis. Both in Janu Sirsasana and Ekapada Rajakapotasana I, two positions which at first sight seem very different, the emphasis is on correct alignment of the hip joints, the sacro-iliac joints and the lumbar vertebrae. If there is no proper alignment of these joints, these positions can lead to problems, especially in the sacro-iliac joints, but also in minor degree in the lumbar vertebrae.

Let us look at *Janu Sirsasana* first. Sit on a blanket and extend the right leg straight in front of you with the foot and knee in line with the right groin. The right foot should be vertical and the big and small toes (the inner and outer borders of the foot) should be at equal distance from the trunk. The right knee should face straight up to the sky so that the inner and outer knee at the back rest evenly on the blanket. Bend the left leg and place the left foot against the inner side of the right thigh. There should be an angle of ninety degrees between the left and right thigh, and the sole of the left foot also makes an angle of ninety degrees with the left shin. Do not let the left foot slip underneath the right thigh.

In this position we have already a distortion of the pelvis, as the left hip joint is further back than the right. Proceeding with Janu Sirsasana without to a certain degree correcting this situation is precisely what would put a great strain on the left sacro-iliac joint and on the left side of the lumbar vertebrae, over-stretching them disproportionately to the right side. Thus, we cannot maintain the weight of the body equal on both buttock bones, but have to shift it onto the right one, even to the point of slightly lifting the left buttock bone off from the blanket. The left knee, however, has to stay on the blanket. In this way we get an opening or an elongation in the left groin and hip joint. As the weight of the body is shifted onto the right buttock bone, the left frontal hip bone also moves closer to the right thigh, while the right frontal hip bone moves over to the right, to come into alignment with the outer edge of the right thigh. Thus both the frontal hip bones will point evenly forward and have the same height from the earth.

Simultaneously with moving the left frontal hip bone over to the right, the left femur has to be elongated out of the left hip socket. This includes a forward rotation of the left thigh, which means that the left knee is not only extended sideways, but is also rolled forwards on the tuberositas of the left tibia. As the trunk, from the navel upwards, has to face straight forwards in the direction of the right foot, the left frontal hip bone, waist and rib cage should be rotated forwards at the same time as the weight of the body is shifted onto the right buttock bone. Only in this way does the left sacro-iliac joint come into a better alignment with the right one, and is thus less hyper-extended, as this extension is shifted to the left hip joint instead.

In this respect it is interesting to note that, if there is a problem in performing this preliminary movement, that is, elongating and rotating in the left hip joint, experience has shown that this is almost a sure indication of an already existing arthritis of the left hip joint, or a tendency to such.

Once the left sacro-iliac joint is eased, the whole spinal column has to elongate upwards. This movement has to start precisely from those sacro-iliac joints, thus the urgent necessity to first bring those into alignment. Not only does the whole spinal column have to elongate upwards out of the pelvis but, as mentioned previously, it also has to rotate towards the right. To get a better feeling of this hold the outer edge of the right foot with the fingers of the left hand, and keep the right hand loosely on the earth next to the right thigh.

Then, using the Mula Bandha breathing, start elongating the spinal column and turning. On the inhalation, which starts always in the lower abdomen, the pelvis is, as it were, lifted up from the femur heads, while at the same time the buttock bones are slightly extended backwards and downwards (with only the right one in touch with the blanket). On the exhalation the whole spinal column (and consequently the whole trunk), from the sacro-iliac joints upwards, is turned towards the right, until the right arm pit, the right side of the rib cage, and the right waist are in alignment with the outer edge of the right thigh. Thus the right frontal hip bone is above the right groin close to the right hip joints, one third distance from that joint and two thirds distance from the pubic bone.

At this point, seen from the back, the spinal column should form an even groove from the sacro-iliac joints to the cervical spine, and should run straight without any sign of deviation to the left. In order to create the groove also in the upper thoracic spine, the ears have to be elongated out of the cervical spine, leaving, of course, the shoulders and shoulder blades down and relaxed. Needless to say that the drive for this elongation and rotation comes entirely from the breathing, which creates the wave of the movement from the base upwards. Even though the left hand holds the outer edge of the right foot, this is only meant to give you a frame within which to elongate and rotate. Do not use the hand, the arm and the shoulder muscles to pull the spine and trunk upwards and to rotate them.

In this initial upward elongation the head has to stay in alignment with the chest, and the cervical spine has to stay natural. Do not push the cervical vertebrae backwards but, keeping the head in alignment with the chest, elongate them upwards. After reaching maximum elongation and rotation take the trunk down to the right leg. However, as usual, go in stages, using the Mula Bandha breathing. On each inhalation elongate forward, and on each exhalation take the trunk further down. With the right foot still vertical turn the palm of the right hand forward and with the thumb and the four fingers form a ring. Place the dorsal side of the wrist in the outer arch of the right foot, turn the palm of the left hand also forward and insert the fingers of the left hand in the ring formed by the right hand. In this way there is the possibility of future elongation. Many people just clasp the fingers beyond the sole of the foot like in Head Balance, which means that there is no room for future elongation. In the way described the left hand can keep on sliding forward within the ring formed by the right hand, till the fingers of the right hand hold the left wrist or even further.

It is important to note that, with the right leg elongated forward, it is the right hand which forms the ring for the left hand to slide through. This is because, by placing the back side of the right wrist in the small arch, that pressure stabilizes the right foot in its vertical position. When going down onto the right leg, the lower abdomen has to arrive first on the right thigh, then the navel. The navel has to come to rest exactly on the midline of the right thigh. If this is not the case, but the navel stays on the inner side of the thigh, it means that you have not pursued the first part of this pose sufficiently.

After the navel, the sternum has to come to rest on the thigh, close to the knee. Here too, the sternum should be on the midline of the thigh, not on the inner side. The head is the last one to come and rest on the shin. You can either place the forehead on the shin, or, if you are more supple, the chin, so that the eyes look at the right foot. In both cases the neck, shoulders, shoulder blades and arms should remain relaxed and the head (and of course the whole trunk) should, with each Mula Bandha inhalation, move closer to the right foot.

Let us now look at *Ekapada Rajakapotasana I.* Sit on a blanket and extend the right leg straight back of you, with the foot and knee in line with the right groin. The right foot should be straight and the big and small toes should rest equally on the earth. The center of the right knee should rest on the earth so that the inner and outer knee at the back face straight up to the sky. Bend the left leg and place the left foot in front of the right groin. The left thigh comes out of the left groin at an angle of forty-five to the left, and the left foot should not be underneath the right groin, but in front of it.

In this position we have already a distortion of the pelvis, as the right hip is further back than the left. This is even aggravated if you do not keep the right leg back in a straight line, and if you do not rest it exactly on the center of the knee, but on the inside of the knee, shin and thigh (which many people tend to do). Proceeding with Ekapada Rajakapotasana I without correcting this situation puts great pressure on the right sacro-iliac joint and gives a wrong twist to the lumbar vertebrae.

In this wrong, twisted position, many people keep the weight of the body on the left hip, while the right hip is lifted up and twisted backwards. Thus, to correct this, you have to bring the weight of the body also onto the right hip, by shifting it to the right and at the same time taking the left hip slightly backwards. In this way we get an opening or an elongation in the right groin and hip joint. As the weight of the body is shifted onto the right hip, the left frontal hip bone also moves over to the right, while the right frontal hip bone moves over to the right to come into alignment with the outer edge of the right groin. Thus both the frontal hip bones will point evenly forward and have the same height from the earth. Simultaneously with moving the left frontal hip bone over to the right, the left femur has to be elongated out of the left hip socket. This includes a forward rotation of the left thigh, which means that the left knee is not only extended sideways, but is also rolled forwards on the tuberositas of the left tibia. As the trunk, from the navel upwards, has to face straight forwards, the right frontal hip bone, waist and rib cage should be rotated forwards at the same time as the weight of the body is shifted onto the right hip. Only in this way does the right sacro-iliac joint come into a better alignment with the left one, and is thus less compressed.

In this respect it is interesting to note that, if there is a problem in performing this preliminary movement, that is, elongating and rotating in the right hip joint, experience has shown that this is sure indication that the Back Bending is done from the lumbar vertebrae, not from the hip joints, and thus those vertebrae are placed under great stress and will sooner or later be weakened and give problems.

Once the right sacro-iliac joint is eased, the whole spinal column has to elongate upwards. This movement has to start precisely from those sacro-iliac joints, thus the urgent necessity to first bring those into alignment. Not only should those joints be in alignment, but the pelvis itself has to be brought as close as possible to a vertical position. As said just now, if there is no sufficient elongation in the right hip joint, the tendency is to let the pelvis fall forward so that the two frontal hip bones collapse into the groins. You can compare this to Virabhadrasana I, where many people tend to do exactly that, that is, collapse the pelvis forward into the groins, thus having to pull the body back up to a more or less vertical position out of the lumbar vertebrae instead of out of those same hip joints.

To bring the pelvis up to as close a vertical position as possible, you have to pull the two frontal hip bones back and upwards in the direction of the ribs (of course without twisting the right side of the pelvis backwards). Not only does the whole spinal column have to elongate upwards out of the pelvis but, as mentioned previously, as the tendency is to twist it towards the right, you have to pay attention to keep it centered. Then, using the Mula Bandha breathing, start elongating the spinal column upwards. On the inhalation, which starts always in the lower abdomen, the pelvis is, as it were, lifted up from the femur heads, while at the same time the buttock bones and the two thighs are rooted into the earth. On the exhalation the whole spinal column (and consequently the whole trunk), from the sacro-iliac joints upwards, is slightly turned towards the left, until the right shoulder, the right side of the rib cage, and the right waist are in alignment with the outer edge of the right groin. Thus the right frontal hip bone is above the groin close to the right hip joint, one third distance from that joint and two thirds distance from the pubic bone.

At this point, seen from the back, the spinal column should form an even groove from the sacro-iliac joints to the cervical spine, and should run straight without any sign of deviation to the left. In order to create the groove also in the upper thoracic spine, the ears have to be elongated out of the cervical spine, leaving, of course, the shoulders and shoulder blades down and relaxed.

In this initial upward elongation the head has to stay in alignment with the chest, and the cervical spine has to stay natural. Do not push the cervical vertebrae forwards or backwards but, keeping the head in alignment with the chest, elongate them upwards. Then bend the right leg and take the left arm up over the head to hold the right foot, keeping the right hand loosely on the blanket next to the right thigh. To do this, you have to first elongate the left arm out of the left groin/sacro-iliac joint, up to the sky. Never make short movements in yoga, so do not just take the arm over the head to hold the right foot, but first create that length and lightness in the left shoulder joint by elongating the left arm out of this joint. Needless to say that the drive for this elongation comes entirely from the breathing, which creates the wave of the movement from the base (the left groin and sacro-iliac joint) upwards. Then, on an exhalation, hold the right foot with the fingers of the left hand. Even though the left hand holds the right foot, this is only meant to give you a frame within which to elongate and rotate. Do not use the hand, the arm and the shoulder muscles to pull the spine and trunk upwards and to rotate them (towards the left).

Then, on a Mula Bandha inhalation, take the right arm up over the head, elongating it upwards from the right groin/sacro-iliac joint, and hold the right foot also with the right hand, keeping the pelvis straight and vertical. After reaching maximum elongation of the spinal column, start to bend the head and chest backwards in order to take the head towards the arch of the right foot. As usual, go in stages, using the Mula Bandha breathing. On each inhalation elongate upwards, and on each exhalation take the head and chest further back and down. Thus the movement is circular: the lower abdomen up, the chest up and back, the head back and down, so that at the front of the trunk there is one round line from the groins towards the collar bones. The line of the Back Bendings should always be seen at the front, and should be round and even. This will only be the case if you use correctly the wave of the Mula Bandha breathing. Keep the neck, shoulders, shoulder blades and arms relaxed and the forehead in the arch of the right foot.

2b.   *Uttanasana and Urdhva Dhanurasana*

Uttanasana and *Urdhva Dhanurasana* are both positions which start from Tadasana, and thus, if we prepare ourselves really well in Tadasana, those two positions should come accurately.

Standing in Tadasana and, rooting the soles of

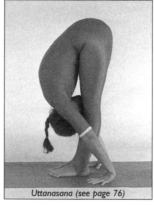
Uttanasana (see page 76)

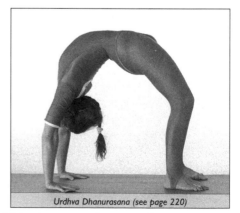
Urdhva Dhanurasana (see page 220)

the feet, rebouncing the body weight back upwards within the joints (lower and upper spring joints, knees and hip joints) against the pull of the gravity, we have to then rotate the pelvis forwards (Uttanasana) or backwards (Urdhva Dhanurasana).

One of the most important things to understand in yoga is that, to go *down*, one has to go *up*. Most people do not act with this understanding and thus, both in Uttanasana and in Urdhva Dhanurasana, one sees that the body just collapses under the pull of gravity, without creating any resistance or inner space, inner elongation. Before rotating the pelvis forwards (to go into Uttanasana) or backwards (to go into Urdhva Dhanurasana) one has to see if one can lift the pelvis up from the femur heads, creating that inner space or bounce within the femur-iliac joints before rotating those joints. Thus, when rotating, elongation is brought in the case of Uttanasana, in the upper part of the back of the thighs (the Biceps muscle), and in the case of Urdhva Dhanurasana, in the upper part of the front of the thighs (the Quadriceps and the Iliopsoas muscles). Thus, in Uttanasasa, the buttock creases in between the femur and the ischias bones are elongated, while in Urdhva Dhanurasana the groins are elongated.

At this point it is relatively easy to elongate the spinal column away from the pelvis against the gravitational pull (forward in Uttanasana, upward in Urdhva Dhanurasana) to go into the final pose. Thus, one has to maintain throughout this inner elongation, this space within the vertebral and pelvic joints, and not collapse them, thus losing the height and beauty of the pose.

An asana, or any other pose, is only beautiful if it is powerful, but this power is not in relation to somebody else or something else. Power, beauty, is where there is space in the body, in the mind. It is only there where the power of the muscle, the power of ambition, the power of thought, is absent. It is only there where mind and body do not look ahead to a future, to the fruit of its present actions, but when both mind and body are fused in the moment, in the pose, without ambition, without fear, with interest and joy. When that happens, even for a split second, there is an inner explosion of energy which transforms that pose into a thing of beauty, into a thing spiritual, in which the position 'does itself', in which there is no warfare between wanting to do it and resisting doing it.

Thus Asana and Pranayama have to mingle, and our attitude in Asana has to be the same as in Pranayama. In Pranayama one of the keys to a free and profound breathing is the release of the skin. If the skin on the chest and the rest of the body is hard, brittle, the body, the energy, is literally imprisoned within the skin.

Tension, under whichever form, is always from the periphery of the body towards the center. Clasping the arms as protection against cold (or as protection of the ego), frowning, the hunched-over position of a depressed mind, the so-called goose pimples on the skin itself, are all contractions of the body inward, an attempt, as it were, to make the body as small as possible within the surrounding space.

On the other hand, we 'heave a sigh of relieve', we feel as if a 'burden has been lifted from our shoulders', we yawn, stretch and smile in moments of relaxation, contentment, happiness, opening our body in all directions within the surrounding space, fusing, as it were, our inner energy with the surrounding energy. Thus, to elongate the body in the asanas, the first thing to do is to soften the skin, so that the underlying muscle and bone can expand. This is a mental process. We have to carefully and deliberately release the skin and the underlying tissues, moving the body from the bones and joints more than from the actual muscles, making, as it were, the muscles and the skin transparent, like an X-ray photograph.

In this process, the breathing is extremely important. If one can use the image of a surf board, the breathing is the wave which carries the surfboard a long distance. Without the underlying wave, the surf board and its rider would just be sitting in stagnant water.

Inhalation is an opening movement, a liberating movement, an expansion of the chest, of the body, in space. On the other hand, *exhalation* is an abandoning movement, a giving in to gravity, a controlled collapsing of the body. Thus, inhalation is that wave which carries the opening of the body, the elongation upwards (Urdhva Dhanurasana) or forwards (Uttanasana) before the act of going down, which, in its turn, is smoothed out by the exhalation.

For this, one should never be in a hurry. In each pose, take a couple of breaths to prepare for the elongation, opening the body on each inhalation and maintaining and consolidating that new position on each exhalation. Then, when the body has reached its maximum elongation, move with a smooth and controlled exhalation into the final pose. Doing things in this way, riding on the waves of the inhalation and exhalation, you will find that there is very little fatigue in performing the asanas and the body does not fight the pose. Then there is beauty, and power, and joy, and out of that flows the pose.

3. Beauty and freedom in yoga

In these two paragraphs, "Playing with Gravity" and "Front face - Back face", only a few asanas have been discussed. For fun's sake, find out for yourself all the different asanas that you can play these 'gravity games' with, or all the asanas that show a 'front face' and a 'back face'. Also, some asanas have a 'grounded' version as well as an 'elevated' version, like for instance Anantasana and Vasisthasana II, which are the same positions, the only difference being that in Anantasana the body rests on the earth, while in Vasisthasana II the body is elevated on one hand. Another such pose is Titthibhasana, which is the 'elevated' form of Kurmasana, or Urdhva Kukkutasana, which is the 'elevated' form of Yoga Mudrasana.

Looking at the asanas in such a way stimulates the creative vision and helps you to understand the poses better. As mentioned before, even though asanas are countless, the basic principles are few and simple. The important thing in all this is to look at yoga holistically, and not fragment either the asanas or yoga itself too much in a frantic search for more and more information. Information, beyond a certain point, beyond the 'point of no return', becomes a ballast, killing the very thing that you try to create, which is beauty and freedom in the asanas, in yoga.

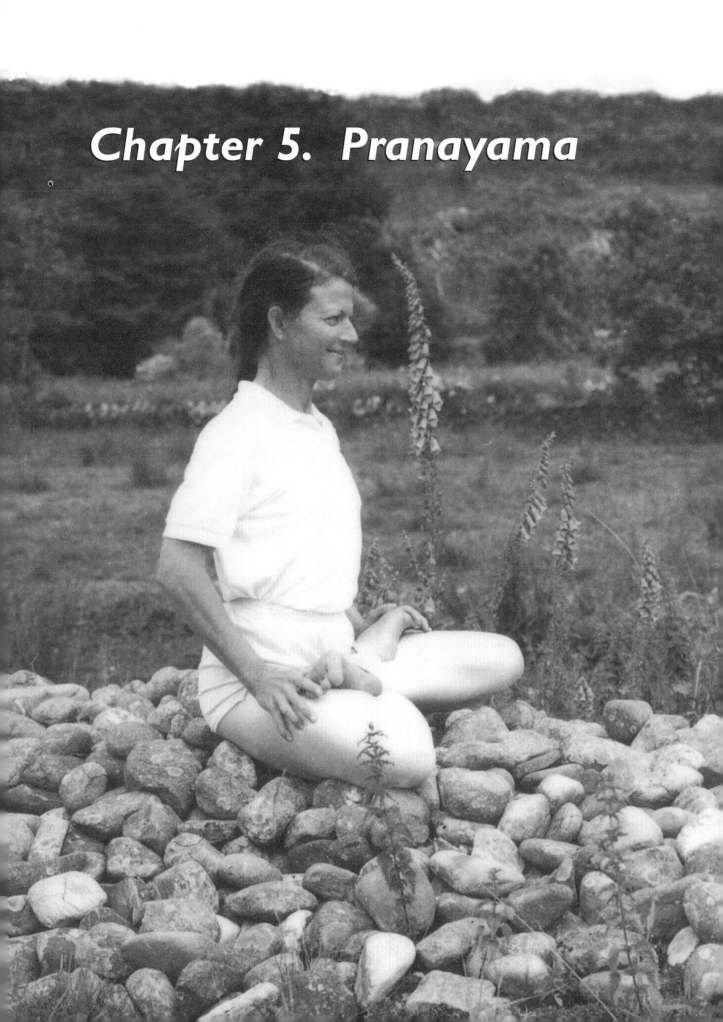

Chapter 5. Pranayama

5 Introduction: the Inner Logic behind the Technique

Before referring to the issue of *Pranayama* in itself we need to realize in general the connection between form and essence. Many times a tradition survives only partially because the outer, empty form of certain techniques and exercises are passed on, but their deeper meaning, their essence, is lost. These outer forms in yoga, Pranayama included, have no real future without understanding their inner logic and origins, for by going back to the roots of the technique we can often discover its essence, its raison d'être. Once we understand the roots, we can also see the route it is taking, and by the power of intent move forward in that same direction, thus enhancing the quality of the practice.

One cannot overemphasize the qualitative difference between a practice, which is but empty form, as opposed to a form that contains an inner direction, an intelligence, an intent. It is like making a comparison between Snow-white's beauty and that of her step-mother, the Queen. As often as the Queen asked: "Mirror, mirror on the wall, who is the prettiest of them all?", she never received a confirmation that she was the one. For, although she had achieved some form of outer perfection, she lacked the inner seed, the essence. Snow-white, on the other hand, though lacking in outer power and experience, always won that contest, because her outer form converged with her inner essence.

Let us return to Pranayama and try to discover its inner logic, and, through that, understand the direction it needs to take. To do that we need to, first of all, observe our natural breathing without any preconceptions or ideas, just as the first yogis did.

For the first yogis who observed the breathing there was no differentiation in the form of Ujjayi, Kapalabhati or Nadi Shodhana. These precise techniques developed at a much later stage. Rather, those yogis first became aware of their breathing the way it was, discovering through close observation its cycle and trying to pierce its significance. From understanding this natural breathing Pranayama was developed.

We too need to follow the same road and observe our natural breathing for a while. Lying on the back is ideal for this purpose, for in this position we need not make an effort to hold the body up, and so we can be completely the observer, without doing anything.

While lying down in Savasana (see page 286) and just observing the breathing, we first become aware of the movement of the abdomen. During inhalation the abdomen expands towards the sky; during exhalation it deflates towards the earth. This is the well-known abdominal breathing. It is our natural breathing and it is also the type of breathing that leads to relaxation. The area of the abdomen is, according to Oriental (Indian and Chinese) traditions, the stove of the body. According to these traditions, it is not only the main storage place of energy, but it is also the place from which this energy is distributed to all the other parts of the body. This oriental understanding of the abdomen coincides with the fact that it is here that food is digested. By the process of breaking down this food energy is released and distributed via the bloodstream to all the organs of the body.

It is precisely because the abdomen is such a center of energy that by watching and cultivating a soft quiet breathing in this area the body can relax and re-tune its energies. This was the first insight of the ancient yogis. In addition, if one wants to energize the body, to mobilize it, one can quicken the breathing in this area. This was probably the origin of *Kapalabhati*. Actually, Kapalabhati is abdominal breathing with a bit more emphasis on the exhalation and an acceleration of the rhythm.

We can experience this internal logic for ourselves by doing Kapalabhati very slowly: sit in a comfortable position and exhale fully from the abdomen, as is done in Kapalabhati. Let all the air out, and then do not inhale immediately by the will. Rather, wait until the inhalation occurs spontaneously. The abdominal muscles will release as if by themselves, as in natural breathing in Savasana. Repeat a few times to feel the connection between Kapalabhati breathing and Savasana breathing, and increase the rhythm. This process increases the heat in the abdominal area.

The realization that through Kapalabhati they could control and increase the heat energy in the area of the abdomen was the second insight of the ancient yogis. The question then arose was what to do with this energy that was accumulating. There were various answers to this dilemma which led to a radical new way of using the breath or *Prana*. (The word *Pranayama* means 'increasing the Prana or energy'. According to some traditions this mythical *Prana* is solar energy.)

In order to understand what was done with this increased energy we need to look again at the body. When sitting with the buttock bones rooting in the earth and the crown of the head reaching upwards towards the sky, and coming into contact with the energy in the area of the abdomen, this whole issue becomes less abstract.

It is the lower area of the abdomen, especially the long, snaky circles of the intestines that whorl around themselves, that promotes heat. It is from here that the spine arises as if out of a basket, to finally reach the skull which contains the brain. The brain too is full of winding passages which bear a striking similarity in shape to the intestines (the brain is actually much larger than it seems, and when you spread it out it takes the size of a pillow case).

All this is to say that one of the possibilities that the ancient yogis discovered was that this increased energy could be brought from the abdomen up to the brain via the spinal column. The question was how to do this.

Another observation showed how this could be done. The yogis noticed that there is a natural stop in the breathing after each exhalation and after each inhalation. Investigating further they noticed that after a long, full exhalation, if one lengthens this natural stop, the air (or Prana) rises up the spine almost by itself. This is how Kumbhaka (see page 271) after the exhalation, and inhaling upwards along the spine (the Mula Bandha breathing), became standard practice. Thus the yogis succeeded in their endeavor to bring energy in a most direct and powerful way from the abdomen to the brain.

They discovered also, however, that, on the way up to the brain, there are some blockages, black holes as it were, which swallow energy. These blockages or black holes had to be overcome so that the energy could rise up.

The ancient yogis called them *Chakras* - 'wheels' of tension, for when the energy reached these places it whirled around in them and could not move on. Only when these - unconscious - black holes were brought to the consciousness and unraveled could the energy be moved on upwards towards the brain. This was the aim, for this energy was capable of creating an alchemical change in the brain which the ancient yogis found increasingly valuable, as it produced a radical new way of seeing and being.

Observing the breathing and seeing the abdomen expand and deflate, is, in itself, not radical. Making, however, the exhalation very long and stopping afterwards, thereby creating a vacuum which pulls the air up along the spine to the brain, is radical. It is an idea which promotes transformation, change. It is a revolution, it is evolution.

Understanding this intent of the ancient yogis we can return again to that technique and use it in a more powerful way. In this context it is interesting to observe the different developments of the Chinese and Indian traditions. Although the original observation was the same, the difference in exercises reflect not just a technical diversity, but reflect the different goals that the Indian and Chinese yogis pursued. For while the Indian yogis became engrossed in exploring the frontiers of consciousness, the Chinese yogis were more practical-minded and thus found more practical uses for the energy they discovered.

The Indian yogis were consummated by the vertical line and its main channels. They were mainly interested in taking the energy up along the spinal column. While trying to improve this transference of energy these yogis noticed something which Western science has discovered only recently. That is the uneven breathing between the left and right nostrils.

Usually we are more dominant on one side or the other. These sides fluctuate every hour and a half, more or less. The most interesting observation concerning this was that, when the two sides were functioning evenly, the center channel along the spine was clear and the mind became quiet. Thus energy could flow up the spine without the least obstruction, and the brain was in the ideal mode to receive it.

From this observation it was only a matter of time before the yogis found a way to move the air from one side to the other to create this evenness between the two nostrils. Thus *Nadi Shodhana* - the Pranayama designed to clean out the channels on the left and right side of the spinal column (called the *Ida* and the *Pingala*), became one of the main techniques.

The Chinese yogis, on the other hand, were not so much interested in energizing the brain as well as in energizing all the internal organs and the limbs. This was because they were concerned with the quality of daily life itself, and thus they developed *Chi gong*, which implies energizing the organs and healing, and *Tai Chi* and *Kung Fu*, in which this energy is used for fighting. With these techniques the Chinese perfected the art of bringing *Chi* - Prana - energy to the necessary parts of the body.

Understanding the inner logic of Pranayama in this way will help us not to practice blindly the various techniques, but to extract from them the essence and thus enhance not only the practice itself, but the very quality of our daily lives.

As modern yogis we need not limit ourselves to one branch of this ancient knowledge, or to one culture only. Choosing from the various techniques available to us at this time we can search for and develop a new way which will help us not only to increase the energy in the brain but, by bringing this energy also to the rest of the body, revolutionize our practice of the asanas as well as our use of the body in general.

Pranayama

1. *Ujjayi*
2. *Kumbhaka*
3. *Kapalabhati and Bhastrika*
4. *Surya and Chandra Bhedana*

5. *Nadi Shodana*
6. *Subtle Pranayama*
7. *Savasana*
8. *Simply Sitting*

5.1 Ujjayi Pranayama

In the "Hatha Yoga Pradipika", Chapter II, sutras 51-53, *Ujjayi Pranayama* is described as follows:
- "Having closed the opening of the Nadi (larynx), the air should be drawn in such a way that it goes touching from the throat to the chest, and making noise while passing." (sutra 51)
- "It should be restrained as before, and then let out through the Ida (the left nostril). This removes phlegm on the throat and increases the appetite." (sutra 52)
- "It destroys the defects of the Nadis, dropsy and disorders of dhatu (humours). Ujjayi should be performed in all conditions of life, even while walking or sitting." (sutra 53)

In the "Gheranda Samhita", Fifth Lesson, sutras 69-72, *Ujjayi Pranayama* is described as follows:
- "Close the mouth, draw in the external air by both the nostrils, and pull up the internal air from the lungs and throat, retain them in the mouth." (sutra 69)
- "Then having washed the mouth perform Jalandhara Bandha. Let him perform Kumbhaka with all his might and retain the air unhindered." (sutra 70)
- "All works are accomplished by Ujjayi Kumbhaka. He is never attacked by phlegm diseases, or nervous diseases, or indigestion, or dysentery, or consumption, or cough, or fever, or enlarged spleen. Let a man perform Ujjayi to destroy decay and death." (sutras 71-72)

Technique

In Ujjayi Pranayama the sound of the breathing is heard in the upper throat. This is different from the Mula Bandha breathing, where the air passes directly through the bottom of the throat. Thus the upper throat has to be slightly constricted and the air, passing without making a sound through the nostrils, as it goes through the upper throat makes a slight 'wind' sound. This sound should not be rough, and should only be barely audible to the breather himself.

The difference between breathing with the sound (Ujjayi Pranayama) and breathing without the sound (Mula Bandha breathing) lies in the fact that, by constricting the upper throat, one creates also a slight constriction in the intercostal muscles. This means that the incoming air, as it touches the inner walls of the chest, has to, as it were, push against those walls in order to expand the chest.

On the other hand, in Mula Bandha breathing, where there is no sound because the breathing has been revolved inwards, the chest widens by itself before the air comes in, thus creating a vacuum into which the air is then drawn.

The trajectory for both is the same, however, with the inhalation starting in the lower abdomen, moving upwards along the inner line of the spinal column, and with the exhalation returning back into the lower abdomen. In this the three diaphragms are always active (Mula Bandha, Uddiyana Bandha and Jalandhara Bandha, supported by the power of the Pada Bandha).

Controlled breathing has been used in many disciplines, not only in yoga. For instance, if modern Catholic monks would have to sing the Gregorian chants in the way they were originally written, with a certain length for each sentence and exact stops for taking breath, they would not be able to do it. Those sentences were very long and demanded quite a control of the breathing and the muscles involved in it.

Controlled breathing has always been considered a means for arriving at the control of the mind. Thus, in Ujjayi Pranayama, it is important to regulate the rhythm in such a way that the exhalation and the inhalation have the same length, and that this length is gradually increased. This helps in calming the mind and bringing it to one-pointedness.

Most people breathe at an average of fifteen breaths per minute, that is, two seconds for each inhalation and two seconds for each exhalation. This rhythm should gradually be decreased to ten seconds for each inhalation and ten seconds for each exhalation, which makes for three breathing cycles per minute.

When one feels comfortable with this way of breathing and the rhythm, one can start adding Kumbhaka.

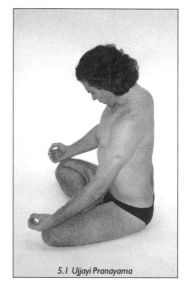

5.1 Ujjayi Pranayama

5.2 **Kumbhaka**

In the "Hatha Yoga Pradipika", Chapter II, sutras 45-46, *Kumbhaka* is described as follows:
- "At the end of Puraka (inhalation), Jalandhara Bandha should be performed, and at the end of Kumbhaka, and at the beginning of Rechaka (exhalation), Uddiyana Bandha should be performed." (sutra 45)
- "Kumbhaka is keeping the air confined inside. Rechaka is expelling the confined air. The instructions for Puraka (inhalation), Kumbhaka and Rechaka (exhalation) will be found at their proper place and should be carefully followed. By drawing up from below (Mula Bandha) and contracting the throat (Jalandhara Bandha) and by pulling back the middle of the front portion of the body (i.e. the belly), the Prana goes to the Brahma Nadi (Sushumna)." (sutra 46)

In the "Gheranda Samhita", Fifth Lesson, sutras 55-57, *Kumbhaka Pranayama* is described as follows:
- "The best is twenty Matras, i.e. Puraka (inhalation) twenty seconds, Kumbhaka (retention) eighty seconds, and Rechaka (exhalation) forty seconds. The sixteen Matras is middling, i.e. 16-64-32 sec. The twelve Matras is the lowest, i.e. 12-48-24 sec. Thus the Pranayama is of three sorts." (sutra 55)
- "By practicing the lowest Pranayama for sometime, the body begins to perspire copiously. By practicing the middling, the body begins to quiver. By the highest Pranayama one leaves the ground (levitation). These signs attend the success of these sorts of Pranayama." (sutra 56)
- "By Pranayama is attained the power of levitation. By Pranayama diseases are cured. By Pranayama the Shakti (spiritual energy) is awakened. By Pranayama is obtained the calmness of mind and exaltation of mental powers. By this, mind becomes full of bliss. Verily, the practitioner of Pranayama is happy." (sutra 57)

In the "Shiva Samhita", Chapter III, sutra 39*, Kumbhaka Pranayama* is described as follows:
- "When the yogi can, of his will, regulate the air and stop the breath (whenever and how long) he likes, then certainly he gets success in Kumbhaka, and from the success in Kumbhaka only, what things cannot the yogi command here?"

Technique
- The word *kumbha* means 'a pot', like the pot that the women in India use to carry water in. Thus the chest is like a pot, which has to be completely filled, and then the lid has to be put on it (Jalandhara Bandha).
- At the end of a deep Ujjayi inhalation hold the breath and perform Jalandhara Bandha. It is very important that the lungs are completely full, and that this pressure is maintained throughout Kumbhaka.
- In order to maintain that pressure, you have to continue, very gradually, lifting the thoracic diaphragm. During Kumbhaka you can feel that the pressure in the lungs diminishes, so you have to regulate the lifting of the diaphragm to that. This is important in order to protect the heart muscle. As the diaphragm keeps lifting, the chest keeps the same expansion and internal pressure as in the beginning of Kumbhaka.

- In the beginning keep the Kumbhaka only for a few seconds. Then gradually increase the time, always staying within the boundaries of comfort, though. Do not strain the lungs by overtiming.
- If Kumbhaka is performed within the Ujjayi Pranayama, you can obtain a good rhythm by keeping the Kumbhaka too for ten seconds. Thus one full cycle (inhalation - Kumbhaka - exhalation) takes half a minute, with each segment taking up ten seconds.
- Another possibility is to keep the ten second inhalation and ten second exhalation, but increase the time of Kumbhaka to forty seconds. In this case one full breathing cycle takes one minute.
- In Kumbhaka too the three diaphragms are always active in support of holding of the air.

Counter indications for Kumbhaka

For any major disease it is advisable to consult a doctor before starting to practice Kumbhaka. In general, it should not be practiced under the following conditions:
- During periods of menstruation or pregnancy.
- With high blood pressure.
- With heart problems in general.
- With ailments of the abdominal organs or lung disorders.

5.3 Kapalabhati and Bhastrika

One of the most well-known experiments in Pranayama breathing is called *Kapalabhati*. *Kapala* means 'skull' and *bhati* means 'to shine', so literally Kapalabhati means 'shining skull'. Another one is *Bhastrika*. *Bhastrika* means 'bellows' and, as it is very similar to Kapalabhati, it is often confused with it.

There is some confusion in the traditional texts regarding Kapalabhati and Bhastrika. The reason is that in various texts the same name was used to describe slightly different techniques. As explained before, this technique arose out of a wish to raise the level of energy in the abdominal area and is characterized by a series of intense exhalations in the area of the abdomen.

To this all traditions agree, yet there are differences in the amount of exhalations, their speed and the amount of time to be spent on each cycle. These differences are already evident in the old Hatha Yoga manuals. In order to make a connection between these and the way we practice today, it is interesting to have a look at these texts.

In the "Hatha Yoga Pradipika" (written about one thousand years ago) *Kapalabhati* is explained in the following way:
- "When inhalation and exhalation are performed very quickly, like a pair of bellows of a blacksmith, it dries up all the disorders of the excess of phlegm, and is known as Kapalabhati." (Chapter II,35)

Bhastrika is explained in the following way:
- "Padmasana (Lotus Pose) consists in crossing the feet and placing them on both thighs. It is the destroyer of all sins. Binding the Padmasana and keeping the body straight, close the mouth and exhale, carefully letting the air be expelled through the nose. Then inhale, filling the air up to the lotus of the heart by drawing it in with force, making a noise and touching the throat, the chest and the head. It should be expelled again and filled again and again as before as a pair of bellows of the blacksmith is worked. Then the air should be drawn in through the right nostril and when filled to the full it should be closed and confined. Having confined it properly it should be expelled through the left nostril. It quickly awakens the Kundalini, purifies the system, gives pleasure and is beneficial. It destroys phlegm and the impurities accumulated at the entrance of the Brahma Nadi. This Bhastrika should be performed plentifully, for it breaks the three knots, namely the Brahma Granthi in the lower abdomen, the Vishnu Granthi in the area of the chest, and the Shiva Granthi in between the eyebrows.' (Chapter II, 59-67)

In the "Gheranda Samhita" *Kapalabhati* is described thus:
- "The Kapalabhati is of three kinds: Vama-krama, Vyut-krama, and Sheet-krama. They destroy disorders of phlegm.
- Vama-krama: Draw the wind through the left nostril and expel it through the right, and draw it again through the right and expel it through the left. This inhalation and exhalation must be done without any force.
- Vyut-krama: Draw the water through the two nostrils and expel it through the mouth slowly.
- Sheet-krama: Suck water through the mouth and expel it through the nostrils. By this practice one becomes like the god Kama (the Indian god of love)."

In the "Gheranda Samhita" *Bhastrika* is described thus:
- "As the bellows of the iron smith constantly dilate and contract, similarly let the yogi slowly draw in air by both the nostrils, expanding the stomach, then throw it out quickly. Having thus inhaled and exhaled quickly twenty times let him perform Kumbhaka, then let him expel it by the previous method. Let the wise one perform this Bhastrika Kumbhaka three times. He will never suffer any disease, and will always be healthy." (Chapter V, 75-77)

From this written tradition various ways of practicing were developed in different schools. For our purpose we will mention four different ways of performing *Kapalabhati Bhastrika*:

3a. Classical Kapalabhati

1. Sit in Padmasana.
2. Watch the breathing until it has reached a calm rhythm.
3. Exhale deeply and wait for a second before inhaling. The inhalation should be passive and should happen as if by itself. Then exhale forcefully by contracting the Oblique abdominal muscles, without bending the back or spine. Repeat sixty times, or for one minute, and then exhale deeply again. Wait a second before inhaling again. The inhalation now should again happen by itself, flowing up along the spinal column until the lungs are full. Then perform Jalandhara Bandha and hold the air for as long as possible.
4. Exhale slowly and evenly, either through the two nostrils, or through the left nostril.
5. Repeat this cycle three times.

3b. Mild Kapalabhati

1. Sit in Padmasana.
2. Watch the breathing until it has reached a calm rhythm.
3. Exhale deeply and wait for a second before inhaling.
4. Inhale for five seconds and then exhale forcefully with the Oblique abdominal muscles without bending the back or spine. The subsequent inhalation should be passive and should happen by itself. Repeat twenty fast exhalations and inhalations, keeping the exhalations active and the inhalations passive. This should take approximately fifteen seconds.
5. Exhale deeply again. Wait a second before inhaling again. The inhalation now should again happen by itself, flowing up along the spinal column until the lungs are full. This should take approximately ten seconds. Then perform Jalandhara Bandha and hold the air for twenty seconds.
   During Kumbhaka it is very important to keep the pressure in the lungs, therefore one has to continue lifting the chest up from the diaphragm towards the throat, at the same time maintaining Jalandhara Bandha.
6. Exhale slowly and evenly through the two nostrils. This should take approximately ten seconds. The whole cycle should take one minute.
7. Repeat this cycle ten times.

3c. Gradual Kapalabhati

1. Sit in Padmasana.
2. Watch the breathing until it has reached a calm rhythm.
3. Exhale deeply and wait for a second before inhaling.
4. Inhale for five seconds and then exhale forcefully by contracting the Oblique abdominal muscles without bending the back or spine. The subsequent inhalation should be passive and should happen by itself. Repeat twenty fast exhalations and inhalations, keeping the exhalations active and the inhalations passive. This should take approximately fifteen seconds.

5. Exhale deeply again. Wait a second before inhaling again. The inhalation now should again happen by itself, flowing up along the spinal column until the lungs are full. This should take approximately ten seconds. Then perform Jalandhara Bandha. During Kumbhaka it is very important to keep the pressure in the lungs, therefore one has to continue lifting the chest up from the diaphragm towards the throat, at the same time maintaining Jalandhara Bandha.

6. This is a variation of the previous Kapalabhati Bhastrika. In this one you hold the air in the first two cycles for twenty seconds, then you do four cycles in which you hold the air for forty seconds, and then again you do the last two cycles holding the air for twenty seconds.

7. After each Kumbhaka exhale slowly and evenly through the two nostrils. This should take approximately ten seconds.

3d. Intense Kapalabhati

1. Sit in Padmasana.
2. Watch the breathing until it has reached a calm rhythm.
3. Exhale deeply and wait for a second before inhaling. The inhalation should be passive and should happen as if by itself. Then exhale forcefully by contracting the Oblique abdominal muscles, without bending the back or spine. The subsequent inhalation should be passive and should happen by itself. Repeat for ten minutes, and then exhale deeply again. Wait a second before inhaling again. The inhalation now should again happen by itself, flowing up along the spinal column until the lungs are full. Then perform Jalandhara Bandha and hold the air for as long as possible. During Kumbhaka it is very important to keep the pressure in the lungs, therefore one has to continuc lifting the chest up from the diaphragm towards the throat, at the same time maintaining Jalandhara Bandha.
4. After each Kumbhaka exhale slowly and evenly through the two nostrils. This should take approximately ten seconds.
5. This Kapalabhati breathing should be done softly and evenly, without exertion and without straining. If, after some time, fatigue or dizziness is felt, one should exhale and inhale a few times and discontinue this breathing.

In these four types of Kapalabhati Bhastrika one should pay attention to maintaining the right tone of the lower abdominal muscles. During the exhalation one should be careful not to overstrain these muscles. During the passive inhalation one should be careful not to inflate the lower abdomen, but to maintain the right tone. This is done by a slight holding throughout the entire cycle of the Mula Bandha as described in the Mula Bandha breathing.

> *Counter indications for Kapalabhati and Bhastrika Pranayama*
> For any major disease it is advisable to consult a doctor before starting to practice these *Pranayamas*. In general, they should not be practiced under the following conditions:
> • During periods of menstruation or pregnancy.
> • With high blood pressure.
> • With heart problems in general.
> • With ailments of the abdominal organs or lung disorders.

5.4   **Surya and Chandra Bhedana**

According to yoga tradition we have thousands of energy channels in the body. The most important of these is the *Sushumna*, the central channel that follows the line of the spinal column. Along this central channel there are two other important channels. The one on the right is called *Pingala*. It represents the sun (*surya*) or hot energy. The one on the left is called *Ida* and represents the moon (*chandra*) or cool energy. Based on this idea the ancient yogis developed two Pranayama techniques which specialized in raising either the hot or the cold energy in the body. These techniques were called *Surya Bhedana* (*surya* means 'sun' and *bhedana* means 'piercing') and *Chandra Bhedana* (*chandra* means 'moon').

Thus, in *Surya Bhedana*, all inhalations are done through the right nostril ('piercing' the right channel or *surya*, the sun), and all exhalations are done through the left nostril. In *Chandra Bhedana* all inhalations are done through the left nostril ('piercing' the left channel or *chandra*, the moon) and all exhalations are done through the right nostril. Which of these two techniques to apply at a certain moment may depend on the climate, the season, the time of day, the energy situation in the body or the task that lies before us.

Thus, if we live in a cold climate, or it is winter and we have a long day ahead of us, we may want to activate the hot energy in the body by practicing Surya Bhedana. Or, if we notice in the morning that our right nostril is blocked, we may also practice Surya Bhedana. If, on the other hand, we live in a hot climate, or it is summer, or if it is late in the evening and we are excited and need to relax, we may want to use Chandra Bhedana to activate the cooling energy in the body.

In this Pranayama too, like for Kapalabhati, there are slight variations in the descriptions in the classical texts.

In the "Hatha Yoga Pradipika" *Surya Bhedana* is described thus:
*   "Taking any comfortable posture and performing it, the yogi should inhale slowly, through the right nostril. Then the air should be confined within so that it fills the body from the nails to the tips of the hair. Then exhale slowly through the left nostril. This excellent Surya Bhedana cleanses the forehead (the sinuses), destroys the disorders of vata and removes worms. Therefore it should be repeated regularly." (Chapter II,48-50)
In the "Gheranda Samhita" *Surya Bhedana* is described thus:
*   "Now hear the Surya Bhedana. Inhale with all your strength the air through the Surya Nadi (the right nostril). Retain this air with great care, performing Jalandhara Mudra. Let the Kumbhaka continue so long as perspiration does not burst out from the tips of the nails and the roots of the hair. All the vayus ('winds' in the body), let him raise them up from the root of the navel, then let him exhale through the Ida Nadi (the left nostril), slowly and with unbroken, continuous force. Let him again inhale through the right nostril, retaining it as taught above, and exhale again. Let him do this again and again. In this process, the air is always inhaled through the Surya Nadi. The Surya Bhedana destroys decay and death, awakens the Kundalini Shakti and increases the bodily fire.' (Chapter V, 58,59,66,67,68)

In the above text Chandra Bhedana is not mentioned directly. Its technique is understood by reversing the process. Therefore in Chandra Bhedana the inhalation is through the left nostril and the exhalation is through the right one.

From this written tradition various ways of practicing were developed in different schools. For our purpose we will mention three different ways of performing Surya and Chandra Bhedana:

4a. Classical Surya Bhedana

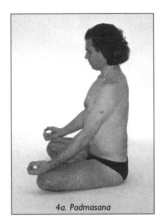

4a. Padmasana

1. Sit in Padmasana.
2. Watch the breathing until it has reached a calm rhythm.
3. Bring the right hand to the level of the nostrils with the index and middle fingers folded inside the palm and the thumb and the ring finger bent in such away that the tips of these fingers oppose each other, like a pair of pincers. The little finger adheres to the ring finger. Place the tips of the thumb and ring finger on the skin of the nostrils, about half way on the nose at

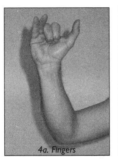

4a. Fingers

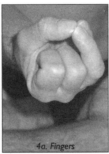

4a. Fingers

the precise division where the nasal bone ends and the nostrils begin. In order to place the tips of the fingers on the nostrils and at the same time have a free circulation of air between the face and the hand you have to keep the wrist slightly up, without raising the elbow. The right shoulder and shoulder blade stay down, level with the left shoulder and shoulder blade. Be attentive as not to turn the head towards the right,

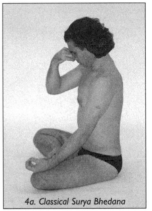

4a. Classical Surya Bhedana

but, keeping the face central, apply just enough pressure with the tips of the fingers in order to close one or the other nostril in such a way that the nostril is brought in contact with the septum without pushing the septum over to the other nostril. Thus the pressure of the fingers should be very delicate on the nostrils, and this can only be if the palm of the hand is kept relaxed with the wrist slightly raised. In Surya and Chandra Bhedana both finger tips stay always in contact with both nostrils, but only one finger tip is used to close the nostril. The thumb is used to close the right nostril, and the ring and little finger are used to close the left nostril.
4. Using the right hand close the left nostril with the ring finger, following the above technique, and inhale fully through the right nostril. Then place the right hand on the right knee and hold the breath, performing Jalandhara Bandha. At the end of Kumbhaka bring the right hand again on the nostrils and close the right nostril with the thumb, keeping the left nostril open and exhaling fully through it. This whole process forms one cycle.
5. Repeat this cycle five times, always inhaling through the right nostril, holding the breath and then exhaling through the left nostril. Each cycle should take approximately thirty seconds, with each segment of the cycle taking ten seconds.

4b. Classical Chandra Bhedana

In *Chandra Bhedana*, we close the nostrils with the right hand as in Surya Bhedana. Both finger tips stay always in contact with both nostrils, and only one finger tip is used to close the respective nostril. The thumb of the right hand is used to close the right nostril, and the ring and little finger are used to close the left nostril.

1. Sit in Padmasana.
2. Watch the breathing until it has reached a calm rhythm.
3. Bring the right hand to the level of the nostrils, close the right nostril with the thumb, following the above technique, and inhale fully through the left. Then place the right hand on the right knee and hold the breath, performing Jalandhara Bandha. At the end of Kumbhaka bring the right hand again on the nostrils and close the left nostril with the ring finger, keeping the right nostril open and exhaling fully through it. This whole process forms one cycle.
4. Repeat this cycle five times, always inhaling through the left nostril, holding the breath and then exhaling through the right nostril. Each cycle should take approximately thirty seconds, with each segment of the cycle taking ten seconds.

The disadvantage of doing Classical Surya and Chandra Bhedana is that by using only the right hand one creates an imbalance between the right and left shoulder and shoulder blade. In the case of right handed people, who tend to always use the right hand, and left handed people, who tend to always use the left hand, there is not only an imbalance between the right and left sides of the body as seen from a muscular point of view, but there is also an imbalance between the two hemispheres of the brain. Seen from this point of view it is advisable to practice these two Pranayama techniques not only alternating the nostrils to purify and balance the right and left nadis, but also to use the right and the left hand alternately in order to balance the two hemispheres of the brain.

4c. Two handed Surya Bhedana

1. Sit in Padmasana.
2. Watch the breathing until it has reached a calm rhythm.
3. After exhaling fully, bring the right hand to the level of the nostrils and with the tip of the ring finger close the left nostril.
4. Inhale slowly through the right nostril. Then place the right hand on the right knee and hold the breath. During Kumbhaka it is very important to keep the pressure in the lungs, therefore one has to continue lifting the chest up from the diaphragm towards the throat, at the same time maintaining Jalandhara Bandha.
5. At the end of Kumbhaka bring the left hand to the level of the nostrils. With the tip of the ring finger close the right nostril and exhale fully through the left nostril. This whole process forms one cycle.
6. Repeat this cycle five times, always inhaling through the right nostril, holding the breath and then exhaling through the left nostril. Each cycle should take approximately thirty seconds, with each segment of the cycle taking ten seconds.

4d. Two handed Chandra Bhedana

1. Sit in Padmasana.
2. Watch the breathing until it has reached a calm rhythm.
3. After exhaling fully, bring the left hand to the level of the nostrils and with the tip of the ring finger close the right nostril.
4. Inhale slowly through the left nostril. Then place the left hand on the left knee and hold the breath. During Kumbhaka it is very important to keep the pressure in the lungs, therefore one has to continue lifting the chest up from the diaphragm towards the throat, at the same time maintaining Jalandhara Bandha.
5. At the end of Kumbhaka bring the right hand to the level of the nostrils. With the tip of the ring finger close the left nostril and exhale fully through the right nostril. This whole process forms one cycle.
6. Repeat this cycle five times, always inhaling through the left nostril, holding the breath and then exhaling through the right nostril. Each cycle should take approximately thirty seconds, with each segment of the cycle taking ten seconds.

4e. Subtle Surya and Chandra Bhedana

This last form of *Surya* and *Chandra Bhedana* is the most subtle of all. The applying of the fingers to the nostrils in a correct manner in the practice of alternate nostril breathing often takes all our concentration. Thus we forget that the real emphasis is on inhaling along one side of the chest and spinal column and exhaling along the other side, and vice versa.

Limiting ourselves to merely alternating nostrils we greatly lessen the effect of these two types of Pranayama. To remedy this one can practice without the use of the hands, just visualizing the inhalation and exhalation through one nostril or the other as you breathe. In this way the two sides of the body are included fully in the process.

People who have problems controlling their fingers, or who have chronically blocked nostrils, can benefit from this way of practicing. After some minutes, when one feels clearly the flow from one side to the other, one can return to using the hands. In this way one increases the awareness and the efficiency of these techniques.

4f. Subtle Surya Bhedana

1. Sit in Padmasana.
2. Watch the breathing until it has reached a calm rhythm.
3. Keep the hands on the knees and concentrate on feeling the dividing line between the left and the right side of the body. Become aware of the left and right nostrils and their different ways of breathing. Then watch the backside of the body and become aware of the spinal column as a physical entity that divides the back into two.
4. Using only the mind, exhale through the right nostril. Air will also be exhaled through the left nostril, but more will be exhaled through the right if that is your intent.

Then inhale from the bottom of the lower right side of the back and from the right nostril. Keep your attention on the right side of the back and try to feel the air rising along this side. Then exhale on the left side of the body, from the top of the upper left side of the back and through the left nostril. Keep your attention on the left side of the back and try to feel the air descending along this side. This whole process forms one cycle. Each cycle should take approximately twenty seconds, with each segment of the cycle taking ten seconds.

5.   When you feel confident with this form you may add Kumbhaka between each inhalation and exhalation to make a full cycle. Repeat this full cycle of subtle Surya Bhedana five times, always inhaling through the right nostril, holding the breath and then exhaling through the left nostril. Each cycle should take approximately thirty seconds if each segment of the cycle takes ten seconds.

4g. Subtle Chandra Bhedana

1.   Sit in Padmasana.
2.   Watch the breathing until it has reached a calm rhythm.
3.   Keep the hands on the knees and concentrate on feeling the dividing line between the left and the right side of the body. Become aware of the left and right nostrils and their different ways of breathing. Then watch the backside of the body and become aware of the spinal column as a physical entity that divides the back into two.
4.   Using only the mind, exhale through the left nostril. Air will also be exhaled through the right nostril, but more will be exhaled through the left if that is your intent. Then inhale from the bottom of the lower left side of the back and from the left nostril. Keep your attention on the left side of the back and try to feel the air rising along this side. Then exhale on the right side of the body, from the top of the upper right side of the back and through the right nostril. Keep your attention on the right side of the back and try to feel the air descending along this side. This whole process forms one cycle. Each cycle should take approximately twenty seconds, with each segment of the cycle taking ten seconds.
5.   When you feel confident with this form you may add Kumbhaka between each inhalation and exhalation to make a full cycle. Repeat this full cycle of subtle Chandra Bhedana five times, always inhaling through the left nostril, holding the breath and then exhaling through the right nostril. Each cycle should take approximately thirty seconds if each segment of the cycle takes ten seconds.

5.5 Nadi Shodhana

Nadi Shodhana is another classical Pranayama. *Nadi* means 'channel', and refers to the energy channels in our body. According to yoga tradition we have thousands of energy channels in the body. The most important of these is the *Sushumna,* the central channel that follows the line of the spinal column. Along this central channel there are two other important channels. The one on the right is called *Pingala*. It represents the sun (*surya*) or hot energy. The one on the left is called *Ida* and represents the moon (*chandra*) or cool energy.

Based on this idea the ancient yogis developed a certain type of Pranayama which specialized in purifying and balancing these hot and cold energy channels in the body. This technique was called *Nadi Shodhana*. The term *shodhana* comes from the root verb *shuddh*, meaning 'to purify'. Thus *Nadi Shodhana* means 'the purification of the channels'. In the practice of Nadi Shodhana there are three main objectives.

The first objective is the one as explained by its name: to purify the channels, so that energy can freely flow in them without being obstructed. The most important is the free flow of energy through the central channel, the Sushumna. The second objective is the balancing of the hot and cold energies so that neither is dominant. The third one is the calming of the mind. This is the result of the previous two, namely the purification and the balancing.

Here too there are slight variations in the descriptions of this Pranayama in the classical texts.

In the "Hatha Yoga Pradipika" *Nadi Shodhana* is described thus:
*   "Sitting in Padmasana (the Lotus Pose) the yogi should fill in the air through the chandra (the left nostril), and keep it confined according to his ability (Kumbhaka). Then it should be exhaled slowly through the surya (the right nostril). Then, drawing the air slowly in through the surya (the right nostril), the belly should be filled, and after performing Kumbhaka again it should be exhaled slowly through the chandra (the left nostril).
*   By practicing in this way, through the right and left nostrils alternately, all the nadis become free of impurities after three months." (Chapter II, 7-10)

In the "Gheranda Samhita" *Nadi Shodhana* is described thus:
*   "The Sahita (Nadi Shodhana) is of two sorts: Sa-garbha and Nir-garbha. The Kumbhaka performed by the repetition of the Bija Mantra (seed mantra) is Sa-garbha, that done without repetition is Nir-garbha.
*   Let the wise practitioner inhale through the left nostril, repeating the 'A' sound sixteen times. Then, before he begins retention, let him perform Uddiyana Bandha. Then let him retain the breath by repeating the 'U' sound sixty-four times. Then let him exhale the breath from the right nostril while repeating the 'M' sound thirty-two times.
*   Then again inhale through Pingala (the right nostril), retain the breath and exhale through Ida (the left nostril) in the method taught above, changing the nostrils alternately.
*   Let him practice, thus alternating the nostrils again and again. When inhalation is completed, close both nostrils, the right one with the thumb and the left one with the ring finger and little finger, never using the index and middle fingers. The nostrils should remain closed for as long as one is performing Kumbhaka. The Nirgarbha Pranayama is performed in the same manner without the repetition of the Bija Mantra." (Chapter V,47-54)

In the "Shiva Samhita" *Nadi Shodhana* is described thus :
*   "The wise beginner should keep his body firm and inflexible, his hands joint in Namaste, and salute the gurus on his left and right side. Then let him close with his right thumb the Pingala (the right nostril), inhale air through the Ida (the left nostril) and keep the air confined for as long as he can (Kumbhaka). Afterwards let him breathe out slowly, not forcibly, through his right nostril. Again, let him draw breath through the right nostril, and stop breathing for as long as he can. Then let him expel the air through the left nostril, not forcibly but slowly and gently." (Chapter III,21-23)

From this written tradition various ways of practicing were developed in different schools. For our purpose we will mention four different ways of performing *Nadi Shodhana*:

5a. Classical Nadi Shodhana

1.   Sit in Padmasana.
2.   Watch the breathing until it has reached a calm rhythm.
3.   Bring the right hand to the level of the nostrils with the index and middle fingers folded inside the palm and the thumb and the ring finger bent in such away that the tips of these fingers oppose each other, like a pair of pincers. The little finger adheres to the ring finger. Place the tips of the thumb and ring finger on the skin of the nostrils about half way on the nose at the precise division where the nasal bone ends and the nostrils begin. In order to place the tips of the fingers on the nostrils and at the same time have a free circulation of air between the face and the hand you have to keep the wrist slightly up, without raising the elbow. The right shoulder and shoulder blade stay down, level with the left shoulder and shoulder blade. Be attentive as not to turn the head towards the right, but keeping the face central apply just enough pressure with the tips of the fingers in order to close one or the other nostril in such a way, that the nostril is brought in contact with the septum without pushing the septum over to the other nostril. Thus the pressure of the fingers should be very delicate on the nostrils and this can only be if the palm of the hand is kept relaxed with the wrist slightly raised. In the alternate nostril breathing both finger tips stay always in contact with both nostrils, and only one finger tip is used to close the nostril. The thumb is used to close the right nostril, and the ring and little finger are used to close the left nostril.
4.   Using the right hand close the right nostril following the above technique, and exhale fully through the left nostril. Then, keeping the right nostril closed, inhale fully through the left. Hold the breath (Kumbhaka) while keeping both nostrils closed with the thumb and ring finger. Then, keeping the left nostril closed, open the right one and exhale fully through it. Inhale again through the right nostril, and at the end of the full inhalation close the right nostril with the thumb and hold the breath (Kumbhaka). At the end of the Kumbhaka, keeping the right nostril closed, open the left one and exhale fully through it. This whole process forms one cycle (left, right, right, left).
5.   Repeat this cycle five times. Each cycle should take approximately one minute, with each segment of the cycle taking ten seconds.

The disadvantage of doing Classical Nadi Shodhana is that by using only the right hand one creates an imbalance between the right and left shoulder and shoulder blade. In the case of right handed people, who tend to always use the right hand, and left handed people, who tend to always use the left hand, there is not only an imbalance between the right and left sides of the body as seen from a muscular point of view, but there is also an imbalance between the two hemispheres of the brain. Therefore, with the modern understanding of the two halves of the brain and the body available to us it is important to use both sides of the body equally, first of all in the asanas and consequently also in the breathing and eventually in daily life. Seen from this point of view it is advisable to practice Nadi Shodhana not only alternating the nostrils to purify and balance the right and left nadis, but also to use the right and the left hand alternately in order to balance the two hemispheres of the brain.

5b. Two handed Nadi Shodhana

1. Sit in Padmasana.
2. Watch the breathing until it has reached a calm rhythm.
3. Bring the left hand to the level of the nostrils with the index and middle fingers folded inside the palm and the thumb and the ring finger bent in such away that the tips of these fingers oppose each other, like a pair of pincers. Close with the thumb the right nostril in such a way, that the nostril is brought towards the septum without pushing the septum over to the left, and exhale slowly through the left nostril. After exhaling fully, inhale again through the left, keeping the right nostril closed. Then place the left hand on the left knee and hold the breath. During Kumbhaka it is very important to keep the pressure in the lungs, therefore one has to continue lifting the chest up from the diaphragm towards the throat, at the same time maintaining Jalandhara Bandha.

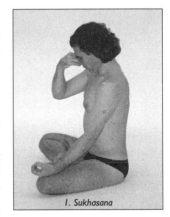

I. Sukhasana

4. At the end of Kumbhaka, place the right hand on the nostrils. Using the ring finger of the right hand, close the left nostril, following the above technique, and exhale fully through the right nostril. Then, keeping the left nostril closed, inhale again fully through the right. Place the right hand on the right knee and hold the breath. Then again place the left hand on the nostrils and, closing the right nostril with the ring finger of the left hand, exhale fully through the left nostril.

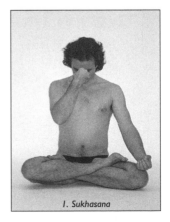

I. Sukhasana

This whole process forms one cycle (left-right-right-left.)
5. Repeat this cycle five times. Each cycle should take approximately one minute, with each segment of the cycle taking ten seconds.

5c. Kapalabhati Nadi Shodhana

1. Sit in Padmasana.
2. Watch the breathing until it has reached a calm rhythm.
3. Exhale deeply and wait for a second before inhaling.
4. Inhale for five seconds and then exhale forcefully with the Oblique abdominal muscles without bending the back or spine. The inhalation should be passive and happen by itself. Repeat twenty fast exhalations and inhalations, keeping the exhalations active and the inhalation passive. This should take approximately fifteen seconds and is described in Mild Kapalabhati.
5. The last fast exhalation should be a little deeper. Wait for a second before inhaling again. Then bring the left hand to the level of the nostrils and with the ring finger close the right nostril. Inhale slowly through the left nostril. Place the left hand on the left knee and hold the breath. At the end of Kumbhaka, place the right hand on the nostrils. Using the ring finger of the right hand, close the left nostril, following the above technique, and exhale fully through the right nostril. This should take approximately ten seconds. Then place the right hand on the right knee, inhale for five seconds normally and start the next round of Kapalabhati: twenty fast exhalations and inhalations. Keep the exhalations active and the inhalations passive. This should take approximately fifteen seconds.
6. The last fast exhalation should be a little deeper. Wait for a second before inhaling again. Then bring the right hand to the level of the nostrils and with the ring finger close the left nostril. Inhale slowly through the right nostril. Place the right hand on the right knee and hold the breath. At the end of Kumbhaka, place the left hand on the nostrils. Using the ring finger of the left hand, close the right nostril, following the above technique, and exhale fully through the left nostril. This should take approximately ten seconds.
    This whole cycle should take one minute. After each Kumbhaka you have to change hands and nostrils.
7. Repeat this cycle five times.

5d. Subtle Nadi Shodhana

This last form of *Nadi Shodhana* is the most subtle of all. The applying of the fingers to the nostrils in a correct manner in the practice of alternate nostril breathing often takes all our concentration. Thus we forget that the real emphasis is on inhaling along one side of the chest and spinal column and exhaling along the other side, and vice versa.

Limiting ourselves to merely alternating nostrils we greatly lessen the effect of this type of Pranayama. To remedy this one can practice without the use of the hands, just visualizing the inhalation and exhalation through one nostril or the other as you breathe. In this way the two sides of the body are included fully in the process.

People who have problems controlling their fingers, or who have chronically blocked nostrils, can benefit from this way of practicing. After some minutes, when one feels clearly the flow from one side to the other, one can return to using the hands. In this way one increases the awareness and the efficiency of Nadi Shodhana.

1.   Sit in Padmasana.
2.   Watch the breathing until it has reached a calm rhythm.
3.   Keep the hands on the knees and concentrate on feeling the dividing line between the left and the right side of the body. Become aware of the left and right nostrils and their different ways of breathing. Then watch the backside of the body and become aware of the spinal column as a physical entity that divides the back into two.
4.   Using only the mind, exhale through the left nostril. Air will also be exhaled through the right nostril, but more will be exhaled through the left if that is your intent. Then inhale from the bottom of the lower left side of the back and from the left nostril. Keep your attention on the left side of the back and try to feel the air rising along this side. Then exhale on the right side of the body, from the top of the upper right side of the back and through the right nostril. Keep your attention on the right side of the back and try to feel the air descending along this side. Following the above technique, repeat from right to left. This whole process forms one cycle (left, right, right, left).
     Each cycle should take approximately forty seconds, with each segment of the cycle taking ten seconds. Repeat this cycle five times.
5.   When you feel confident with this form you may add Kumbhaka between each inhalation and exhalation to make a full cycle. Repeat this full cycle of subtle Nadi Shodhana five times. Each cycle should take approximately one minute, if each segment of the cycle takes ten seconds.

5.6   Subtle (sukshma) Pranayama

In this *Pranayama* one does not work merely with the physical lungs, but emphasizes the movement of energy in the body. One can practice this Pranayama in any position, whether sitting, standing or lying down, and can eventually use it in the asana practice itself. But in the beginning it is easier to practice it in Savasana, as one does not need to hold the body up.

1.   Lie down in Savasana for a few minutes before starting to relax the body and to calm the mind.
2.   Watch the breathing in the area of the abdomen and tune yourself to it. Then focus your attention on the fingers of the right or the left hand, according to your preference. Become aware of the touch of the air on the hand, and feel the connection between the breathing in the abdomen and the air touching the fingers.
3.   Now imagine the fingers inhaling and exhaling in rhythm with the natural breath. It is as though each finger had a nostril attached to it, and the actual breathing is done through them. After some time you may notice different sensations such as tingling, prickling, heat, expansion and lightness in the area of the fingers and the hand.
     This is the right moment to go further and repeat this process on the other hand. The sensations should appear much faster as there is already a certain fluidity of the first hand, so that the second one follows the first one almost spontaneously. After some breaths one can usually feel the two hands breathing simultaneously.
3.   At this point one lengthens the inhalation as though bringing the air into the forearms and arms. With the inhalation the air rises up from the hands, with the exhalation it leaves the body through the finger tips. These first three steps need to be mastered before continuing.

4. Once subtle breathing is experienced in the hands, it is possible to continue one more step and let the sensations mentioned above, such as tingling, heat, lightness and expansion, slowly spread throughout the whole body. Do not make the inhalations and exhalations longer, but maintain the natural breathing. Rather, it is the mind which moves faster through the various parts of the body, thus allowing the energy to flow into and through them.

5. With time, the ability to bring energy to the whole body from the tip of the toes and fingers up to the top of the head becomes more natural and faster, and one can move the air along different routes. One can inhale through the toes and finger tips and in one inhalation cover the whole body. Then exhale the air again through the tips of the fingers and toes. Thus the exhalation too covers the whole body. Another possibility is to inhale through the feet (toes and heels) up to the crown of the head and then exhale through the hands and fingertips.

6. This whole process takes from five to twenty minutes, depending on the amount of time available and on your ability.

Although this technique seems mild, it can be a powerful tool and aid in cleansing and rejuvenating the body. For instance, if there is a pain or disease in a certain area, one can start as described above. Then, when one feels the free flow of energy and the relaxation of the body, one can direct this energy to the effected area to soothe and heal it. As the mind becomes more attuned to this process, one to three breaths are enough in order to direct energy to the required area.

In the same manner one can use this subtle Pranayama in the practice of the asanas, thus greatly enhancing the effect of these asanas on the body and the mind.

5.7 Savasana

sava=corpse

In the "Hatha Yoga Pradipika", Chapter I, sutra 34, *Savasana* is described thus:
*   "Lying flat on the ground, like a corpse, is called Sava-asana. It removes fatigue and gives rest to the mind."

In the "Gheranda Samhita", Second Lesson, sutra 19, *Savasana* is described thus:
*   "Lying flat on the ground like a corpse is called Mritasana (Corpse Pose). This posture destroys fatigue, and quiets the agitation of the mind."

7a. Classical Savasana

Physical Technique
*   Sit on a blanket with the legs bent in front of you, place the hands on the blanket behind you and lower the body onto the elbows, keeping the head up and the knees together. Supporting the body on the elbows, lift the pelvis up and rotate it backwards around the femur heads, so that the coccyx rolls towards the pubic bone and the two frontal hip bones are drawn up towards the ribs. Thus the lumbar spine is elongated. Then lower

the pelvis again on the blanket. Extend the legs, rest the heels on the blanket, and lower the rest of the body too. The inner ankles, pubis, navel, sternum, throat and the bridge of the nose are in line. The line on the back, starting in the center of the back of the head and ending in between the heels, passing through the spinal column, is straight, and the right and left side of the body rest evenly on the blanket.

- Extend the legs straight out of the hip joints, elongating the back of the legs and keeping the back of the knees in contact with the blanket. To bring the knees down, elongate the heels away from you and pull the toes towards you. Then relax the legs, letting the feet fall sideways, but keeping the heels together. Due to pelvic imbalance, one foot often turns out more than the other: be sure to rotate both legs out evenly.
- The pelvis rests evenly on the blanket. The line between the two frontal hip bones, across the lower abdomen, is horizontal; the pelvis should not be tilted up on one side. The lumbar area is broad and in contact with the blanket.
- Do not push the lower part of the chest (the lower ribs and the bottom part of the sternum) up to the sky. The chest is horizontal, and in line with the pelvis. The shoulder blades rest flat on the blanket, and the four corners of the chest (the shoulders joints and the lower ribs on the right and on the left) drop evenly down, so that the upper part of the sternum is lifted up towards the sky. Do not draw the shoulder blades towards the spine, but widen them sideways and move them down towards the waist.
- On an exhalation, elongate the heels away from the buttocks, and the back of the head away from the neck, so that the whole spine elongates from the coccyx to the back of the head. Elongate the back of the neck, so that the chin comes down; the back of the head rests on the blanket close to the first cervical vertebra, not close to the crown of the head. Thus the chin drops down automatically and easily: do not pull the chin in forcefully. Keep the face horizontal, with the forehead and the chin parallel to the earth. The neck is soft and natural and there is no strain on either the neck or the throat muscles. The face looks straight upwards, and the ears are at equal distance from the shoulders.
- Rotate the arms outwards, so that the biceps muscles rotate up towards the sky and the triceps muscles rest on the blanket. Elongate the arms out of the shoulder joints before placing them on the blanket, the inner elbows and the open palms facing the sky.
- Close the eyes, looking slightly downwards under the closed eyelids.

After having placed the body straight on the blanket as described above, proceed to the mental aspect of Savasana.

Mental Watching
Concentrate your attention on sinking the complete weight of your body into the earth, without withholding any of it. When we stand, sit or walk, there is always the risk of falling, so the muscles are in a state of alertness in order to prevent this. In Savasana, this risk is absent. As the body has already completely 'fallen,' there is no way it can fall further. Thus the muscles have no reason to grip or hold on to the bones. Gently 'convince' the muscles to let go of their grip on the bones, and to relinquish the entire weight of the body to gravity.

To do this, the brain has to be very alert; it should not go to sleep. The brain is the protector of the body, helping the body to release its weight. For some of us, though, the brain is not the protector of the body, but the attacker, and this attacking manifests itself in physical tensions produced by the agitation of the brain. Others go to sleep in Savasana, confusing this with a relaxed state of body and mind. Going to sleep is not the same as relaxing. It means the brain is not interested in watching, it is only interested in indulging in its own dull state of being. The brain should not be dull, and should not indulge itself, but it should be crystal clear, piercing the body with clarity and attention, helping it to release the parts where it has stored its anxieties. The brain should help the body to release those tensions, those anxieties, to *undo* them. In Savasana, the brain should become the protector of the body, it should neither attack nor indulge the body, but it should help the body to regain its own inner level of peace.

Watch inside, watch the upper chest between the shoulders, from one end to the other: tension is always from the periphery of the body towards the center. Watch how tension pulls the shoulders closer to the sternum, reducing the width across the upper chest: this is the psychological defense mechanism of the body. Gently, internally, you have to 'convince' the muscles of the upper chest to let go of the shoulders, to undo that tension that pulls them in towards the sternum. When the muscles release their grip, you can feel how the shoulders, by themselves, move away from the sternum, away from the thoracic spine, sideways, thus widening the upper chest across the front and the back.

You can do the same thing in the solar plexus. Most people have a certain tension underneath the lower ribs, a tightness in the solar plexus, a squeezing inwards from the periphery towards the center. Here also, watch that unnecessary tension, and gently, internally, see if you can release that grip, which is from the periphery of the waist to the center, so that the solar plexus widens as it releases.

In the same way, watch the skin, everywhere on the body. See how the skin is hard, how it forms a hard barrier between you and the space around the body, between the inner body and the external space. Relaxation of the body takes place when you separate the muscles, the bones and the skin from each other. Releasing the skin from the underlying muscle, mentally 'taking the skin away' between you and the external space, gives you a feeling as if the body swells up. That swelling is the relaxation of the muscles, which let go of their grip on the bones, so that the energy, which is locked inside them, can flow out through the skin into the space surrounding the body. You can compare this to a sponge: when you squeeze the sponge, it becomes smaller, harder, but when you let go of it, it swells up to its natural size. The same thing happens with the body: if you 'take the skin away', the muscles swell up like a sponge that is released.

Tension is always from the periphery of the body to the center, from the skin towards the bones. Relaxation is always from the center of the body to the periphery, from the bones towards the skin. By separating the bones, the flesh and the skin, from each other, tension is released and thus you have the sensation that the body 'swells up.' In Savasana, everything falls apart: the bones, the muscles, the skin, but not the brain. The brain remains very clear, not sleeping; if the brain sleeps, there is no intelligence in the body to help it undo its tensions. The brain is firm, clear, not oscillating: it penetrates all the parts of the body.

At the end of Savasana, turn over onto the right side, stay for a while quietly on the side, and then open the eyes and sit up.

7b. The Grounding Savasana

This type of *Savasana* is used to purify the body, and is very helpful in cases of physical fatigue and mental depression. It 'grounds' the energy and leaves the body rested and refreshed.

Technique
Follow the physical instructions as described above. Watch the breathing for a few moments, till it has become calm and rhythmical, and then start to focus your attention on the exhalations; the inhalations should be normal, not too deep and long, but easy and soft.

Gradually slow down the exhalations, without forcing; the exhalations, even though they are slower than the inhalations, should still be natural. As you exhale, visualize that you are not exhaling through the nose, but through the back of the chest: feel the air moving into the back of the chest, and then through the skin of the back into the earth underneath you. Feel how the earth absorbs that air, how the air seeps deeper and deeper into the earth. As the air drains out of the chest through the back, feel how is takes all the fatigue, the tensions, the 'old' energy with it as it sinks into the earth. Keep on repeating this until you feel that the whole chest is 'empty', that all the fatigue, the tension, the 'old' energy has been drained out and absorbed by the earth.

Then move your attention to the abdominal region and the pelvis, and repeat the same process, exhaling through the back of the pelvis, until the whole abdominal region and the pelvis are empty and free from fatigue and tension. The deeper you visualize the air sinking into the earth, the more the body is emptied.

Repeat the same procedure in the legs, the feet, the arms, the shoulders, the neck and the head. Keep the inhalations casual and the exhalations natural, even though you will find that in the course of this Savasana the exhalations will become spontaneously longer and deeper. With each exhalation, you will not only feel that the whole body becomes emptier, but it will also come closer to the earth, as if the whole body is sinking into the earth.

When you feel sufficiently refreshed and 'cleaned out' of 'old' energy, turn over on your right side, stay for a few moments on the side, and then open your eyes and sit up.

5.8 **Simply Sitting**

There is an old Hassidic story of a certain Jacob who lived in a small village in Poland. He was a poor Jew and owned very little. One night he dreamed that at a certain border pass between Poland and Russia there was a bridge, and under that bridge there was a treasure. He woke up amused and did not think much of it, only to have the same dream recur again and again the following nights. Finally, in spite of himself, he made the long journey to the border and located the bridge. Unfortunately there were sentries there, guarding day and night, and he could not think of a possible way to dig up the treasure. As he stood there, wondering what to do, the captain of the guard approached him and accused him of spying. Frightened he confessed to his dream, sure that the captain would search for the treasure himself. But the captain laughed and said mockingly: "You came here for a dream? I also dreamed that a poor Jew named Jacob from a small village had a treasure hidden in his backyard, but I did not go looking for it." Laughing, he sent Jacob away. Jacob returned home quickly, dug in his backyard and discovered the treasure.

This story is of course symbolic, but its end marks the beginning of this chapter: *Sitting*. For just sitting implies that we understand or know or believe that in our body and mind there lies a treasure, and it is up to each one of us to dig inside himself and to find it.

Simply sitting is not mystical or superior. It begins with sitting, with posture. When we sit, the first thing to keep in mind is the position - the buttock bones rooting into the ground, the crown of the head elongating upwards to the sky, the spine a bridge in between them.

Once the posture is established, we focus on the breathing, for the pattern of breathing is intimately connected to the patterns of the mind, and forms the link between body and mind. We bring the mind down into the body and stabilize it by watching the breathing at the area of the abdomen and the diaphragm. These are the initial instructions for simply sitting.

After the breathing and the mind have quieted down, we sharpen our listening: we listen as if we are sitting next to the key hole of a room where an interesting conversation is going on; we put all our intensity in listening, so that we can catch the words. We do not react to outer disturbances, other voices and sounds, for that would disturb the quality of listening. We simply intensifies our listening even more to hear what is being said on the other side of the door.

These two steps, quieting the mind (*nirodah*) and alert, intense listening (*ekagrata* or one-pointedness), are the basis of simply sitting. They are related more to observation and less to *doing*. This in itself is very important. For in simply sitting, we need to create an atmosphere in which nothing needs to be *done*. This is because doing is our usual pattern of mind, doing is what we know, doing is the waves of the mind in action. So the less we do, the better. Even saying: "Just sit and watch the posture and the breathing, just sit and listen attentively," is already saying too much, for these qualities are natural to the mind and would happen by themselves if we sat long enough without any instructions. The reason they are mentioned is that the nature of the Western mind is impatient and longs for instant gratification.

In fact, simply sitting is simply sitting - there are no rules, no right and wrong, nothing we have to do or not do, nothing to feel guilty about, nothing to wish for or reject. This is because, whatever happens in sitting - moody mind, sleepy mind, disturbed or dispersed mind, dull mind, collapsed or tense body - is OK. By *not* creating rules or objectives, we need not break them or adhere to them, and so we need not feel guilty or self satisfied. By *not* creating rules, we allow the nature of mind to present itself. From within, mind will show the way, and will help us discover new avenues, unknown to us.

Even so, when calmness and alertness are present and are intensified, certain processes may happen by themselves. They create the climate and atmosphere which precede the processes known as the 'inner limbs' of *Ashtanga Yoga*: *dharana, dhyana* and *samadhi*. These, according to yoga tradition, cannot be *done* voluntarily, but can develop spontaneously under the right conditions.

We all know that big fish swallow little fish, that big waves swallow little waves. In our daily life, the opposite occurs: the small fish swallow the big one, the small waves overtake the big wave. Usually we function out of the level of ego, which manifests itself as thoughts and emotions, memories of likes and dislikes, fears etc. All of these are *vrittis*, the 'waves' of the mind. These 'waves' are usually many, and because of them, something subtle inside us, the big wave underlying the vrittis, is unable to manifest itself, is being swallowed by all the small, daily affairs. The question is: how to make space for this big wave to express itself, to emerge and swallow the small waves. This happens when the mind, or consciousness, becomes empty and sinks into itself. One cannot force this process, yet one can create the circumstances where it may spontaneously occur.

Patanjali describes this phenomenon in his definition of *Samadhi* in Chapter III,3 of the "Yoga Sutras", where he says: "When the mind is as if empty of its own form (sva rupa-sunya-iva) and only the object shines, that is Samadhi." When the small waves of the mind start to calm down and the inner space within us can work like a vacuum, swallowing or sucking in or allowing the superficial mind to sink into it, then the mind is emptied of itself. Thus the big, profound wave swallows the small, superficial ones; the deep and subtle inner space, the vast, inner emptiness, shines forth.

After this kind of occurrence, where the superficial mind sinks or collapses into its deeper substratum, even only for a brief moment, we return to our normal functions of body and mind with great vigor; we see everything enhanced and are energized, because we have undergone an alchemical change. These experiences are often described as mystical, as if they belong only to the mind, but in fact they are physical and occur within the body as well. Through this experience, which flows out of a mental process, the brain itself and the body are also affected, and undergo a alchemical process, in which impurities of the body and brain are released for elimination, and we feel an effect as if we have slept profoundly and peacefully for eight hours.

Once we learn to sink the mind - even momentarily - into its substratum in this simple act of *sitting*, we can transfer that into our practice of the asanas and pranayama, and from there into our daily life. This is living our life in balance, when we know how to toggle back and forth between taking care of the superficial, small waves of daily life, and dipping into the deep, quiet wave underlying these small waves, so that body and mind are refreshed and rested.

Chapter 6. Becoming a Yogi

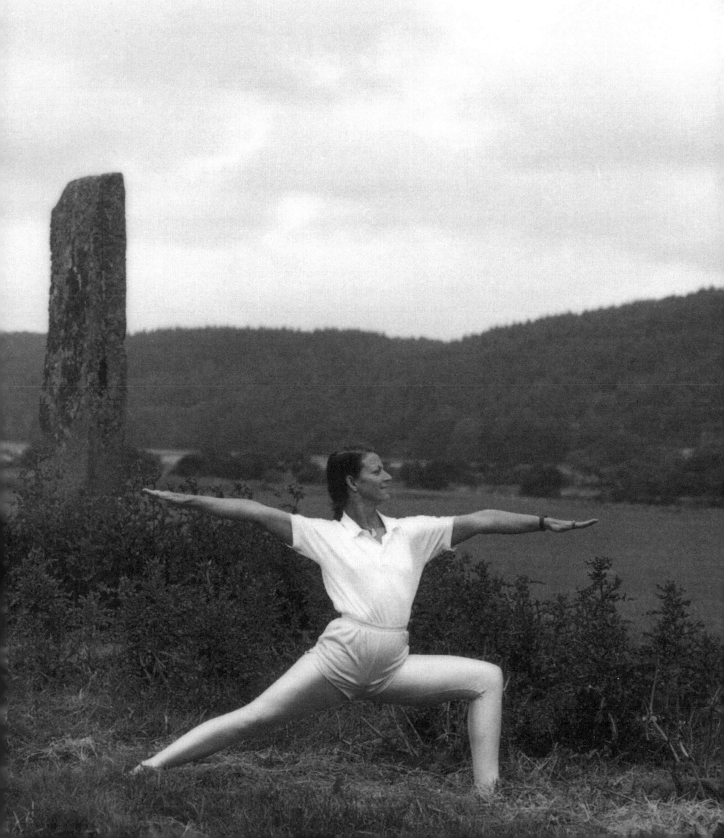

6.1   Wide Heart

In Chapters one and two of **Part One**, we described a path that integrates body and mind, thereby opening up the possibility of consciously experiencing and working with another level of being. This level, called the *Body of Light*, gives life to our physical body, and connects us to the Earth and the Sky and to the source of all life.

Working with the body and mind is only the first, if crucial, step. Yoga is about connections. A truly integral and holistic yoga will point towards ever widening and deepening vectors of connection. Intensification of practice does not have to lead to withdrawal from the world, from society; neither do we have to reduce yoga to mere physical exercise or mere meditation. As modern-day yogis, living in the global village, we must integrate the insights and discipline acquired through our practice, so that they transform our daily life, our ethics, our attitudes towards others near and far. Nothing less will be sufficient if we are to envision a truly vital future for the art of yoga.

Connecting our inner life - our emotional and ethical life - to the practice of *Empty Mind* and *Perfect Pose,* is the third component of a holistic yoga. We have called this component: *Wide Heart.*

This Chapter will begin close to home, with the relationship between teacher and student, and the attitude and lifestyle which contribute to successful practice. It will continue with an examination of the emotional and ethical life according to tradition. Finally, we will return to the individual self: the yogi artist.

6.2   Being a Student, Being a Teacher: Mind to Mind, Body to Body

There is an old Eastern saying: "No one except a fish knows a fish's heart; no one except a bird follows a bird's trace." If no one except a yogi knows a yogi's heart, how can one who aspires to be a yogi follow a yogi's trace? How does a student become a yogi, and how is yoga transmitted from teacher to student? Before dealing with this transmission, we need to discuss the characteristics of the teacher and the student in order to understand how it takes place.

About the teacher there is only one thing to say: he must be the example of what he teaches, of what he wants to transmit. The teacher cannot just be someone who has mastered the techniques of a few asanas and passes that on. Yoga does not deal only with the body and physical techniques. It deals with a profound integration of body, mind and heart. The teacher must be a living example of this integration.

Some teachers convey a general truth, but have not integrated this truth into all the facets of their lives. Other teachers are inspired. These are the teachers who, in their own practice, remain students, and share with others what they learn. The fire is alive in them; regardless of their age, they are totally engrossed in what they teach, and this, in turn, is intimately connected to their own practice. Such a teacher is not only an example of what he has mastered; he also serves as a model of someone who is still learning, who is still in the process of developing. This teacher uses words, explanations, theories, but they are fluid, and ultimately not of the greatest importance; his passion and the depth of his continued searching are more significant.

Setting the example of practice in himself, the teacher, in his dealings with the student, should interfere as little as possible. It is only when the student has done his utmost to overcome certain difficulties, but seems to make no progress, that the teacher should point out another way of seeing, a way which is creative and radical, and which helps the student to go beyond the present obstacle. Other than at those vital junctions, the less the teacher interferes the better, for by *not* helping he gives the student the opportunity to do as much as he can for himself, thus developing strength of character, determination and independence, necessary traits for a serious yogi. The teacher who takes over the path of the student by overly interfering, is unfortunately not teaching the student responsibility and independence, but non-thinking and dependence (upon the teacher).

The main focus should be on the learning process of the student, not on the knowledge of the teacher, for it is the student who is seeking knowledge, who is looking for another way of being. For the path to continue, for the teaching to be carried on, the teacher will have to rely on the student: not only does the student need the teacher, the teacher needs the student as well. If the teacher is like the tree whose fruits have ripened, he needs, at this crucial moment, somebody to pick these fruits. When this happens, there is a real meeting between teacher and student, in which both benefit and rise to their best.

Who is the keen student, and what are his characteristics?

The first characteristic of a dedicated student or any creative person is that, when confronted with something that needs to be understood and manifested, *he does not stop until he 'gets it'.* The keen student is often not the one who 'gets it' immediately, but the one who doesn't. This student does not care to just please the teacher, but has a real need for knowledge. He is not satisfied until he really 'gets it'. This may take much longer than trying to understand something merely intellectually. For a long time he may feel unsatisfied and insecure, and for this reason keeps on practicing. In this he is not mechanical, blindly following the instructions of the teacher, but is constantly searching for the wholeness of the asana or the breathing movement. Because he is never satisfied, he finally reaches a high level of practice and understanding.

The second characteristic of a keen student is his *ability to empty himself.* In the beginning, the student tries to imitate the teacher, to understand what is being taught. To receive true knowledge, though, the student needs to be empty. He has to learn to let go of his under-standing, his knowledge and his fear; to stand empty in space and listen from there, allowing his body to echo the knowledge that is being transmitted to him. His keenness is a powerful tool, an enormous, infinite eye or ear, observing and listening with the whole body and mind.

The third characteristic is *persistence.* The faith that there is a way, and the determination to walk it, are vital in order not to lose heart. There will, of course, always be difficult moments, but experience shows is that it is impossible to move away from yoga if one has real love for it. Someone once asked Sir Edmund Hillary why he climbed Mount Everest. His answer was: "Because it is there." In the same way, the keen student acts, in final analysis, not for the sake of power or success, but simply because yoga is there, and he is for some inexplicable reason drawn to it.

We have described the teacher and the power of his or her personal example, as well as the characteristics of the keen student. Now we need to look at the way yoga passes from the one to the other: the transmission. This transmission takes place on two levels: *mind-to-mind transmission*, and *body-to-body transmission*.

To understand *mind-to-mind transmission,* let us use an example from the tradition of Zen. Dogen, a Japanese Zen master who lived in the 12th century, felt that in his time Zen had degenerated, because people had become willing to accept words and intellectual understanding as transmission of real knowledge. He criticized many of his contemporary teachers for falling into the trap of using empty techniques and words, thus deadening the 'way'. After going to China, where he received true mind-to-mind transmission, he returned to Japan to revive the tradition of Zen.

Mind-to-mind transmission does not go through the channels of words and intellectual understanding. Only when a teacher is so immersed in his teachings that they have become part of his being, internalized, can the student 'catch' something of vital importance that emanates from this teacher. This kind of interaction was traditionally considered the true link between teachers and students.

Indian tradition mentions five ways in which knowledge can be passed on: through ritual, through verbal explanation, through touch, through eye contact, or through merely being in the presence of the teacher. Whereas in the first two ways the teacher relies on words or techniques to convey his teaching, in the last three he transmits his knowledge by rather being in a particular state of mind and body. Knowledge passes over, as it were, by a process of osmosis, not through a specific technique, after which it is up to the student to integrate that knowledge into his own life. This way of teaching, through direct transmission, has kept yoga alive throughout the centuries, and is the true link in the teacher-student relationship.

Not only mind-to-mind transmission needs to be revived, but *body-to-body transmission* as well. Traditionally, the techniques of yoga and martial arts were conveyed, in the beginning stages, through the eyes, with the student imitating the teacher, or through touch, with the teacher correcting the student physically. Only in a later stage of the teaching, when the student had acquired a certain degree of understanding in his body through repeatedly performing the postures, did the ears become important, with the teacher giving verbal instructions. In the same way as knowledge of the mind was passed over, in the beginning stages, without words, so the knowledge of the body was passed over from body to body, directly, with the explanations as the last stage.

For true knowledge to be transmitted, we do not need so many words and explanations. Rather, what is needed is a teacher who embodies his teaching and cares to transmit it, and a student who is keen to receive it. In this, the main emphasis is on the student, giving him a great deal of responsibility, with the teacher figuring mainly as an example, a transmitter. There is a reason for this. We are all students on the path of yoga. This path is an endless one, and, no matter where we are on it, we are but small links in an evolutionary chain which will carry yoga into the future as an ever developing discipline. The student needs to take responsibility because, for the path to continue, he needs, in his turn, to become a teacher.

As such, he needs to develop his skill of learning, and integrate this - only then can he become an inspiring teacher himself. Otherwise he will but repeat the situation which Dogen deplored so strongly in the world of Zen in the 12th century, and true knowledge will be lost:

- *"When a bird flies in the sky, beasts do not even dream of finding or following its trace. As they do not know that there is such a thing, they cannot even imagine it. However, a bird can see traces of hundreds and thousands of small birds having passed in flocks, or traces of so many lines of large birds having flown south or north. Those traces may be more evident than the carriage tracks left on a road, or the hoof print of a horse seen on the grass. In this way a bird sees birds' traces."* (Dogen)

6.3 Yoga in Daily Life

In the beginning of the book we discussed the passage from East to West, and the tree of yoga replanting itself and flourishing in the West, stipulating that for this to be successful all the components of yoga should be developed simultaneously - the physical, the mental, the emotional and even the ethical. In choosing not to choose between body, mind, and heart, we choose to walk the path of a complete yoga, which develops and refines all parts of our being.

We have also talked about the role of the teacher, and the responsibility of the student to integrate the teaching transmitted to him in his practice. To integrate the practice in daily life is the final challenge of the modern yogi living far away from the cave and the monastery, but it needs to be aligned with a certain inner attitude so that we don't acquire clarity and energy in the practice only to lose it when we come in contact with disagreeable people or situations in daily life. Rather, the practice, coupled with the inner attitude, create the courage, strength, vigor and energy we need for the rest of the day.

To attain a certain inner attitude we begin our practice by sitting quietly for a moment and becoming aware of our present mood. We then need to choose the specific attitude which deals with this specific mood. In this way we can, in a more conscious fashion, use our practice as a technique for emotional and spiritual transformation.

There are three major moods that yoga recognizes and deals with.

- The first one is called: *Negative mood.* There are times when we are dealing with an emotional crisis or with an unpleasant interaction with other people. These moments are often accompanied by feelings of defiance, guilt or anger, which make the body and mind feel dull or nervous. When we are in this mood, there is no need to feel helpless. These feelings occur often in relationships and in daily life, and we need to accept them, but we need not indulge in them. In these moments we can use our practice as a way to purify ourselves; thus our objective in the practice here is *purification.* Each breath, each movement, is done with purification in mind, so that by the time we have finished our practice we feel cleansed and optimistic.

- The second mood is called: *Positive mood*. There are other times when we feel lighthearted and happy; everything seems perfect just as it is, nothing needs to be done or changed. In this case, the objective in our practice will be to enhance this optimistic feeling of '*just being*', to revel in it, feeling the harmony with each moment. We thus intensify this way of being and come out of our practice shining and energized.
- The third mood is called: *Creative mood*. Finally there are times when we are in a creative mood, ready for change, for transformation, for a leap into something new, unknown; we are excited and full of energy. In this case, the objective in our practice is *creativity and transformation*. We may discover and see the same practice from different angles, from new dimensions. We may take a quantum leap forward.

These *objectives - purification*, *just being*, and *transformation*, have a double effect. They connect us to our moods and pay heed to them; rather than suppressing, ignoring or indulging them, they interact with them in a creative way, and linking them to our practice is the best preparation for our day as we cleanse, tune and energize ourselves. Each of these objectives is equally important, as we need each one of them at different moments in our lives.

At the same time they imply a deep spiritual purpose: as we move from our practice into daily life, we need to remember that it is in daily life that our challenges lie. The sign of slow, but sure, progress is when we close the gap between the practice room and our daily life.

6.4 Reversing Negative Emotions

In spite of the momentary relief that working with the *objectives* brings, there can linger deep emotional patterns that need to be dealt with in a more specific and lasting way. Otherwise there is the danger that we use the practice of the asanas and the breathing and sitting techniques, as temporary sedatives, instead of as a lasting cure.

How do we deal with such powerful thoughts and emotions as love, hatred, anger, jealousy and fear? Two thousand years ago, when the classical yoga texts were written, emotions were no different from today. What was the ancient yogis' view on the emotions and how did they deal with them? What place did the heart have in their practice?

Bhakti means 'devotion' in Sanskrit. One of the classical types of yoga, called *Bhakti Yoga*, deals specifically with the emotion of love and devotion, and became, as we saw, one of the three components of Aurobindo's *Integral Yoga*. This yoga became one of the most powerful types of yoga and at the height of its popularity swept through the whole of India. Some of its leading adherents were famous poets, who sang of love and surrender, giving thanks to their chosen god or goddess. These yogis did not aim at uniting with their chosen god or goddess, neither did they aim at reaching a transcendental state. All they wanted was to be close to their god or goddess. Ramakrishna, a famous modern Bhakti yogi, expressed it thus: "I do not want to be sugar, I want to eat sugar." This devotion often brought a transformation in the emotional foundation of its practitioners, in which the love for their chosen god or goddess was transformed in the end into an attitude of love towards all of God's beings.

In the West, *Hatha* and *Raja Yoga* are often used as psycho-physical techniques, but there is no specific emphasis on how to deal with the emotions. The assumption is that these same techniques will work on the emotions as well. This is not necessarily true. Some meditation practitioners, who experience transcendental states of mind in the East, find, on their return to the West, that their emotional patterns are still intact, and rise up at the first occasion. To deal with these, they often have to integrate modern psychology in their practices. Certain classical texts do give an outline of how to deal with emotions, though. These techniques can and should be integrated with the *Hatha* and *Raja Yoga* techniques in order to provide the third component of Perfect Pose and Empty Mind: *Wide Heart.*

More than two thousand years ago Patanjali, who is still one of the most quoted authors of yoga today, gave precise outlines in his "Yoga Sutras" on the emotions, and on ways to transform them. The first group of sutras that deal specifically with the emotions, shows how turning the mind inwards through meditation and awareness brings us, on the one hand, inner stability, and on the other hand, makes us aware of our psychological patterns. The second group of sutras deals with changing our behavioral patterns in order to adjust to our new view of life.

One can categorize these sutras into four *Practices* that focus on the emotions; their aim is to develop the quality we have called *Wide Heart*, the third component of the triangle Perfect Pose, Empty Mind and Wide Heart.

The first *Practice* is called: *Awareness.* We become aware of our patterns, watching our emotions rise and fall during sitting, pranayama and asana, as well as in daily life. Watching without judgment, without trying to change anything, simply accepting these emotions as they are, is the first step.

The second *Practice* is called: *Returning to the Source (pratiprasava).* In order to explain this Practice we need to understand the origin of our thoughts and emotions. According to Patanjali, patterns of thought and emotion arise from two different sources. One source is our innate tendencies, the personal traits we are born with; these are called *vasanas.* The other is the imprint of the time and culture we live in, the experiences we collect during our life; these are called the *samskaras.* The vasanas and the samskaras form together our personality, our way of seeing the world, and our way of acting in it.

In order to clarify this, we can use a simple example. When looking at a wasp, we do not just see an objective wasp. Simultaneously with seeing the wasp as an outer object, an 'inner wasp' comes to the surface of the mind. This 'inner wasp' is composed of all our memories of past wasps, how they affected us and other people: this is the samskara. In addition to this, our innate tendencies or vasanas also rise to the surface: we may be by nature more courageous or more fearful, and this too will effect the way we see the wasp, and the way we react to it. Therefore, the vasanas and the samskaras contribute as much to the picture of the wasp in front of us as does the wasp itself, but they are lodged so deep inside the mind that they cannot easily be dealt with in a direct way.

To weaken the samskaras, we need to bypass them and return to a deeper place within the mind; this is done through deep meditation. In deep meditation we are released from the power of the samskaras or imprints, as we reconnect to that part of ourselves which existed before they came into being. Patanjali calls this practice of deep meditation the 'inner limb' of yoga, and we have dealt with it in the description of *Empty Mind*. The practice of the asanas, the breathing practices, the ethical conduct, and the turning of the senses inward (called *pratyahara*), which Patanjali collectively calls the 'outer limb' of yoga, are activities we can and must do with conscious effort. The 'inner limb' cannot be 'done' with conscious effort. Instead, they are the outcome of all the other practices. While practicing the 'outer limb' our feeling of stillness and focusing inward begin to intensify. Then consciousness sinks back into itself. This is deep meditation, which we cannot 'do'. We can only prepare the ground for it.

The third *Practice* is called: *The Cultivation of the Opposite (pratipaksa bhavana)*. According to Patanjali, negative behavioral patterns can also be dealt with in a more active way. When we are troubled by certain strong emotions, which have a negative effect on ourselves or on others, the solution is neither suppressing them, nor indulging in them. Rather, we can deliberately choose to cultivate the opposite emotion. For instance, if we are inclined to losing our temper, instead of acting that out or trying to suppress it, we can choose to practice patience. Usually one chooses to deal with one behavioral pattern at a time. As soon as we target the behavioral pattern that we wish to transform, we have to imagine how we would like to behave instead. Then we begin to practice this alternate behavior. Being creatures of habit, we believe that we cannot change. This is not true. Just as we can transform our physical habits through intelligent and persistent practice, we can transform our behavioral habits too if they disturb us or others. This is an integral part of yoga, for disturbing patterns of behavior consume energy and cause suffering to ourselves and others.

The fourth *Practice* is called: *The Four Attitudes*. Patanjali believed that our emotions will adjust themselves to a great extent to the attitudes we cultivate towards others under various circumstances. He recommended that students internalize the following character traits in their dealings with their fellow men: friendliness (maitri), kindness (karuna), happiness (mudita) and equanimity (upeksa). When coming across happy people (sukha), he recommended the attitude of friendliness (maitri). When coming across suffering (duhkha), he recommended kindness in thought, speech, and action (karuna). When coming across somebody or a situation of goodwill and virtue (punya), he recommended that we rejoice (mudita). And finally, when coming in contact with somebody or a situation whose actions cause pain and sorrow (apunya), he recommended that we choose to abstain from judging and condemning (upeksa).

With time and practice, these Four Attitudes can help us find a new way of seeing the world and reacting to it; merely understanding them intellectually is not enough. When we apply them in daily life we are rewarded with a wide, open heart. With this *Wide Heart*, yoga finds and re-integrates its initial wholeness and again becomes the path of *Perfect Pose*, *Empty Mind* and *Wide Heart*.

The last issue is the lifestyle of the aspirant yogi. The more we become aware, the more we see that everything is connected. A good practice does not exist in itself, but is the outcome of a good night's sleep, which, in turn, is the outcome of having eaten healthy food and being in a happy mood. The outcome of a balanced interaction with the world around us is thus a positive one, and therefore we will, naturally, begin to feel the need to adopt a lifestyle that does not deplete us of our energy and insights. This issue may be a rather difficult one for some people to solve, due to the habits, the commitments and the fast living that have become part and parcel of modern society. Even so, it is an essential one: the inability or unwillingness to introduce changes in lifestyle may eventually produce stagnation in our practice, as both the body and mind need certain rhythms to function optimally. Each person needs to find the particular rhythm of sleeping, eating, working and recreation that suits his body and mind best, so that *Perfect Pose, Empty Mind* and *Wide Heart* can flower undisturbed.

6.5   Creative Ahimsa

We have looked at psychological issues and recommendations for transforming our emotions. What about ethics; did the ancient practitioners have anything to say about ethical standards and practices? If yoga is primarily a technique for achieving a healthy body, a calm and still mind and a wide heart, where does the idea of good and evil fit in?

In Patanjali's "Yoga Sutras" we find the *yamas* and *niyamas,* which deal with the yogi's behavior towards society (the yamas) and towards himself (the niyamas):
*   "Non-harming, truthfulness, non-stealing, chastity and lack of greed are the yamas."
*   "Purity, contentment, austerity, self-study, and devotion to the lord are the niyamas." (Patanjali Yoga Sutras II,30-32)

Ethical codes, far from being removed from spirituality, were among the first considerations. These codes were meant to be road maps, but the ancient yogis realized that they were relevant only to the beginning stages of the path, and were meant to help the aspirant behave in certain ways which were conducive to his progress.

From their own experiences they knew that, as one progresses on the spiritual path, one eventually encounters another mode of 'seeing' the world, and therefore another mode of behaving. This other way of 'seeing' makes one realize that Reality is ultimately beyond the duality of right and wrong, and renders socially constructed ethical codes obsolete, as it leads the yogi to the natural humane kindness, which goes beyond the individual instinct for survival, and which is not coerced through a fixed set of rules. Thus, where in the beginning stages of the practice of yoga ethical behavior is a result of obeying outer rules, at a later stage it flows naturally as a result of 'seeing.'

Most of us, however, relate to the middle part of the path, where we begin to see beyond the white and black aspect of right and wrong, beyond duality, yet haven't fully realized its implications in our daily interactions. It is crucial at this point to practice within the framework of the yamas in the web of relationships that make up our life. In this, the first *yama, ahimsa* (nonharming, nonviolence) is our point of departure.

Classically, *ahimsa* has been interpreted as 'not hurting' others by thought, word or deed. We can go one step further, though, towards a more holistic view of ahimsa. To do this, we have to look at its opposite, *himsa*. *Himsa,* which means literally 'hurting' or 'harming', is an interaction between two or more participants. The hurter and the hurt, the slayer and the slain, they all are bound to the same thing: himsa, pain.

Instead of having one person 'hurting' another, we can create a situation where 'hurting' is avoided or brought to an end altogether, for the benefit of all concerned. This is because the act of 'hurting' is never an isolated phenomenon; rather, it is part of a chain reaction. The hurter was probably hurt before, and is acting out his pain. The one who is being hurt now will probably in his turn inflict pain on another, sooner or later. This never ending chain of pain and suffering has to be brought to an end, for everyone's sake.

Gandhi's first principle of action was ahimsa. This was usually understood as nonviolence towards others, specifically towards the British. But maybe Gandhi was saying something more profound. Was he not saying to the British: "I won't allow you to hurt me and my people, but I also will not allow hurting you. This vicious circle must come to an end."

Gandhi was a genius of what we will call here *Creative Ahimsa*. He understood that when we say no to 'hurting', we are not only protecting ourselves, but are also protecting the person who is about to inflict injury on us (and harm himself by that too), as well as those that would almost certainly be hurt by our reaction. *Every time we stop a hurt, we create ahimsa*, we create an island of peace in the world. Therefore, in a hurtful situation, whether thought or spoken or done by you towards another, or by another towards you, or by you towards yourself, be determined not to hurt, but to act creatively to stop this hurting. This is the cultivation of Creative Ahimsa.

To act creatively to stop himsa implies two things. In the first place we need to be convinced that we should not be hurt. This is for the good of everyone, therefore we should not allow anyone to harm us. This is part of the yogic path and is, in the words of Patanjali, the *Great Vow* that binds all of humankind. In the second place, as creativity implies vision, we realize that this hurt is not just against us. Perceiving the whole situation with wide caring eyes, we try to stop it with as little pain as possible for all involved.

This is a radical way of understanding ahimsa. It is vital, however, for without understanding it in this way we are drowned by ideals of love, kindness and forgiveness. These are perhaps high ideals, but often cause us merely to suppress our real emotions, without really transforming them. Eventually this creates more suffering.

By applying Creative Ahimsa in our daily life we will eventually find ourselves closer to the emotional and ethical refinement described by Patanjali in his "Yoga Sutras":
* *"When the yogi is grounded in ahimsa or non-harming, hostility is abandoned in his presence.*
* *When grounded in satya or truth, action and its fruit depend on him.*
* *When grounded in asteya or non-stealing, all jewels come to him.*
* *When grounded in brahmacarya or moving-towards-Brahma, he obtains vitality.*
* *When standing in greedlessness, he receives knowledge of the 'whyness' of his birth."*
  (Patanjali Yoga Sutras Chapter II,35-39)

6.6 The Yogi Artist

After having broadened our view from the aspirant yoga practitioner, to his teacher, to the people around him, and finally, to the whole globe, we return full circle again, to the single yogi artist, to you:

- *"Every man is the builder of a temple, called his body, to the god he worships, after a style purely his own, nor can he get off by hammering marble instead. We are all sculptors and painters, and our material is our own flesh and blood and bones. Any nobleness begins at once to refine a man's features, any meanness or sensuality to imbrute them."* Henry David Thoreau

It seems that human beings have spent a lot of time and energy perfecting the 'habitat' of the body, cushioning it from all sides with material well-being and comforts. Yet the body itself has been overlooked to such a degree that in spite of increased external comfort, the body seems to be nowadays less comfortable than ever before in the history of man.

If it is true for all things that what is added on one side is chipped off from the other, then it must be that the more the body is cushioned, the more it is robbed of its own native power and resources. Thus, in spite of added security in the outward world, the body itself has become less secure.

Together with this diminished bodily security, having been robbed of its power and resources, it seems to have lost that beauty and grace that is natural in tribal people. This does not mean to say that we have to go back to primitive living conditions. Rather, it may be the right time, now that we have acquired a certain amount of material and habitational security, to turn our eyes back to the primal habitat of the human being, that is, his own body, in which he lives and acts from the moment of birth to the moment of death.

What is the source of our anxiety over bodily security? Looking at ourselves in daily life we can easily see how we have become totally dependent on the 'experts', in whichever form or field. For everything that goes 'wrong' in our life, we seek the aid of somebody, or something, else to solve the problem. Thus, gradually, we let ourselves be robbed of that most precious of human resources, creativity, which permeates the totality of us, from the simplest cells of our body to the deepest core of our being.

We all know that, when there is a cut in the flesh, the cells of the body immediately 'know' what to do. Given the right conditions, which are to keep the cut clean and the body rested, the cells will busily start to repair the damage and in no time the body will be again as good as new. The key to this bodily restoration work is to surround the body with the right conditions - rest and cleanliness. The body is a self-healing organism: this is the creativity of the cells, the innate intelligence of the body which can deal with most problems that occur on a daily basis.

This creativity is not confined to the body alone. In final analysis, the body itself is the result of creative activity on another level. Day in day out, we build the body to conform to our thoughts and emotions, from the most superficial to the most profound. Each thought, each emotion, is etched on our face, in our body, till these become the book from which others can read us, if they wish.

Not only have we become heavily dependent for our bodily security on the 'experts.' In our mental and emotional life as well, we no longer trust our own innate intelligence and creative powers. In other words, we seem to have lost the strength to fully assume our place in this world, standing joyfully alone, face to face with the world. Religions, philosophies and gurus have proliferated to an astounding degree. They teach us how to live in the world, they give us a rule, a measure, by which we are to measure ourselves in relation to the world, and if we fall short of the rule, short of the measure, we are called to account.

We are no longer encouraged to live creatively, using as a measure the world itself and our own relation to it. Our link to the world is bent and looped through a church, a sect, a philosophical concept, to then be re-attached to the world itself, and we look at the world through this loop, and are therefore no longer capable of seeing directly what there is all around us.

Where does yoga and art fit into this? Both yoga and art aim at the same thing, that is, to re-establish our personal connection with the world around us according to our own inner creativity. To render body and mind a conduit through which the creative energy can flow freely, unimpeded by outer restrictions, in the trust that this energy, being part of the universal energy, is ultimately 'pure' and joyful.

'Purity' does not meant prudishness, but implies a sense of innocence. The word 'innocence' comes from Latin and means 'not-harmful.' This is also the first concept in the ancient yoga texts: *ahimsa*, or nonviolence, non-harmfulness.

True artists, as well as true yogis, have their being in this innocence and joyfulness, which come from standing alone in the world, looking at it with eyes which are empty of rules and measures, and reflecting this innocence and joy in body, mind and emotions. This is the stamp of really great artists. And, in ultimate analysis, each one of us is an artist. The work of art that we create is our own life, our body, our mind, to render it beautiful, graceful, and above all, free. Or, out of fear or timidity, yield to the overwhelming need for security and thus sell our aloneness for the safety of company, whether this is physical or mental.

As such, the path of yoga, if followed in all earnestness, is the same as the path that the artist has to follow. In yoga, each asana is a small work of art, and, like music and dance, it is ephemeral, a small ripple in the vastness of the world, like leaves dancing in the wind, before they fall. Nothing is left but the memory of joy, of a body moving in freedom, alone, with only the Earth and the Sky as witnesses. And yet, something has changed, some perfume lingers in the air, and maybe, some day, that will affect another human being. Someone else may recognize the call, and risking all, may follow it toward freedom.

This freedom is, however, not what most people think. For most people freedom means to throw all restrictions to the wind, to pursue the path of pleasure. This is not what freedom in art or yoga means. Freedom means to pursue perfection for its own sake, without expecting any recompense for it. Perfection, beauty and grace have their own rules, which have to be obeyed, but this obeying should be done for its own sake, only then will it turn into freedom. Thus the artist and the yogi, scorning recognition from society, will pursue the only worthwhile recompense: the knowledge of having laid their highest creativity on the altar of perfection, with the only aim of serving that same perfection.

To reach this perfection, however, the artist, the yogi, the human being, has to go, like in all good fairy tales, through fire, water, earth and air, before the Universe will open its gates. He has to be purified by the elements, but, like in the fairy tales, these elements are real, not imaginary, not mental. It is not enough to go through some process mentally - the body has to be transformed too. The mundane, ordinary human being has to become a prince in order to be able to claim the princess at the end of the tale. For this, there needs to be a total transformation, involving body, mind and heart.

Fire and *Water* represent the passions and the unconscious thoughts and emotions, which stand in the way of this transformation. Each of these elements has a positive and a negative side, and the real art is to convert them from negative to positive. Where human passions are often violent and at the service of the ego, passion in itself is a necessary ingredient for the yogi artist, because without passion there is no power.

Fire is the driving force that underlies action, but where, in mundane life, fire underlies ambition to achieve something in the world, in art it is the driving force to search for perfection. Without passion there would be no search.

Similarly, *Water* symbolizes that part of us with which we do not deal on a daily level, but which nevertheless conditions all our life, from the simplest physical actions to our deepest thoughts and feelings. This part has to be brought to the surface, so that we can look at it, and deal with it directly. This can be an extremely painful process - which human being does not have a closet full of skeletons? Yet, without dealing with this part of himself, the yogi artist cannot proceed on his path, and will be caught forever in the maze of his own making.

Luckily, instead of dealing with each unconscious thought or feeling separately - something that would take years - one can go directly to the root. This root feeling, that underlies all human thoughts, feelings and acts, is a real sense of alienation, an unbearable longing for 'home'. As we do not recognize this, or do not want to deal with it directly, we express this longing in many different ways, from broken marriages and friendships, to a desperate grasping after money, position, power, and violence, even to madness and suicide. Not until we consciously recognize this sense of alienation and longing can we embark on the path of yoga, or art.

Like in the fairy tales, at the end of the road there is the princess, but she has to be won, not conquered. And she can only be won after a journey of transformation. This is the ultimate message of the element of Water.

Once the yogi artist has kindled that passion and recognized that he needs to go 'home', he encounters the next element, *Earth*. Part of the alienation that human beings feel lies in the fact that we have placed ourselves outside nature, so to speak. We have split the world into nature and us, the Earth and us, thus placing ourselves outside and above all other creatures and things that the Earth has produced, even placing ourselves above the Earth itself. This, in final analysis, cannot be. Like all other creatures that crawl, walk, swim, and fly on the Earth, we are a product of the Earth. We are all children of the same mother. All that we are and have belongs to the Earth, to nature.

The yogi artist has to, first and foremost, seek to regain his place in nature. Foregoing all philosophies and theories that tempt him to consider himself removed from the Earth, he has to place his body here again, reconnecting his energy to that of the Earth. Whether it is in dance, music, or yoga, our energy, once it is reconnected to the energy of the Earth, draws its power from the Earth. Where the hands reach out on a horizontal level to grasp the things of the world, the feet are rooted in the Earth and draw power vertically up through the soles. Once that connecting link is established, that power is stored in the center of gravity, in the lower abdomen, at the height of the sacred bone, the sacrum. This center of gravity is the true center of humility, the midpoint between Earth and Sky, where the energies of the Earth and Sky meet.

Humility and being humble are not the same thing. All religions, all philosophies, all gurus advocate that one has to 'be humble', without realizing that the very fact that one 'is humble' is a grotesque form of arrogance. It is another form of being 'something,' a more cunning way of wanting to be recognized as separate, unique, special. True humility is that moment in time and space when the yogi artist, having re-established his connecting link to the Earth and recognizing himself as an integral part of nature, joyfully re-aligns the spinal column on the vertical line of energy. The sagging or bragging posture is abandoned, and the body lifts up with the energy flowing in through its roots, the soles of the feet. At the same time that the body lifts up, the eyes are also lifted from an inward gaze to an outward one. For the first time the yogi artist begins to see the world, not as something alien, different, separate, but as part of himself. Or rather, he sees himself as a child of the world, with all the rights and all the duties that any child has towards its mother.

It is only when the yogi artist has thus taken his rightful place in nature, and has aligned the spinal column on the energy flowing upwards from the earth, that he can proceed to the fourth purification, that of the element of *Air*. This is the moment when, instead of abandoning the body like many religions advocate, the yogi artist has to start transforming the gross physical body into a body of air, a *Body of Light*. As the feet have again made contact with the energy of the Earth, the rest of the body should again make contact with the surrounding energies.

The skin, which over the years has become a formidable barrier, has to lose its hard edge. Instead of keeping the internal energy locked up inside and the external energy locked out, the skin has to again become a membrane which allows free exchange between those inner and outer energies. The more the skin becomes, as it were, transparent, the more there can be an intermingling between the inner and outer energies as the inner energy, locked within the tightness of the skin, can expand and flow out freely into the space surrounding the physical body. As this energy is allowed to expand, it will loosen the very atoms of the physical body, until the whole body feels as if it is expanding. Thus, gradually, the body will lose its sense of separation from the surrounding space, as the dividing edge between body and space is dissolved, and the body is transformed into a body of air, of energy, of Light.

At this point the yogi artist is ready to open the last gate, the one at the top of the head, at the very end of the spinal column. This opening is called the fontanel, or little fountain. It is the gate that, in upright human beings, points straight up to the sky; a lens through which the human being looks up at the rest of the Universe. It is through this lens that the yogi artist finally realizes that he is not only a child of the Earth, but, in final analysis, a child of the Universe itself, and thus takes his rightful place in this vaster 'home'.

Having taken his rightful place in nature, and having kindled the internal energy and reconnected it to the Earth, the Sky, and the four cardinal directions, he now arrives at the most important point. That is, he now has to find out what his role is in this vast Universe.

Each human being has, as it were, pre-programmed on some kind of psychic DNA, a particular task, a particular talent, a particular destiny. Kindling the energy itself has no great significance, unless it is connected to the fulfillment of this destiny.

What is this destiny? It is a particular talent, a particular bent for something. For one person it may be painting, for another it may be music, for another yoga. If this particular talent is not recognized, or worse, not taken into consideration, the person will spend all his life in activities that have nothing to do with his deepest core. His whole life will remain out of alignment.

To bring one's life in alignment with the Universe means that we have to recognize and respect that particular bent or talent, and employ all the energy that we have previously kindled towards the fulfillment of this talent. The ultimate task of fulfilling one's potential, and traveling one's own unique path, is something that is each person's individual responsibility.

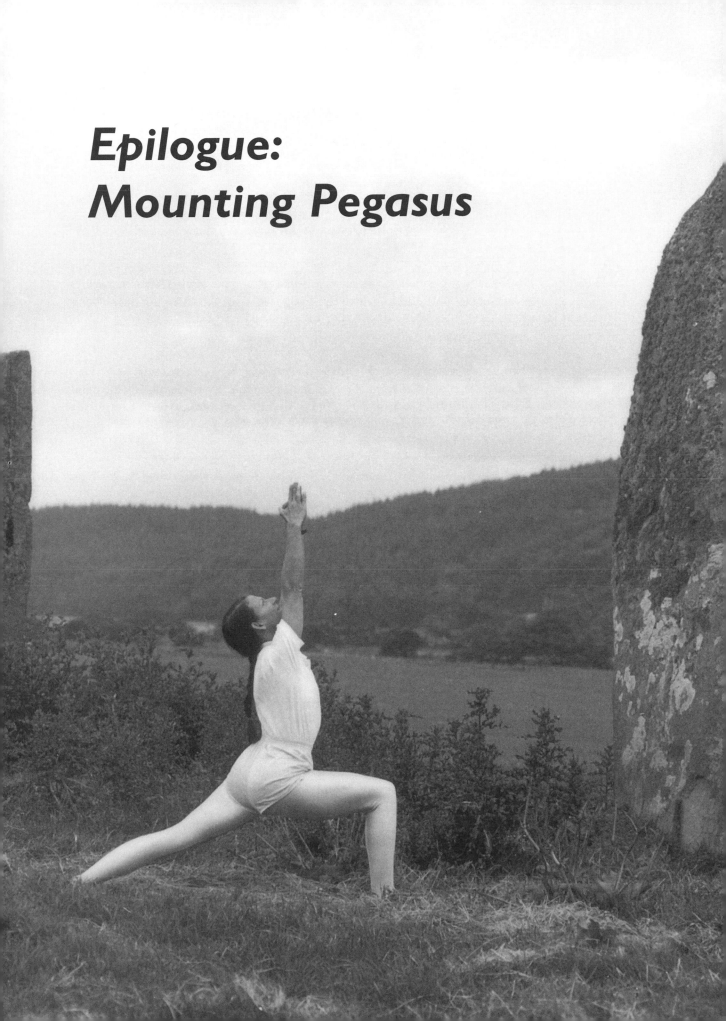

Epilogue:
Mounting Pegasus

Mounting Pegasus

In this book we have discussed the two different levels of the body: the purely physical part and the energy body which makes this physical part move, which gives it life, and which, at the moment of death, is severed from the physical part, so that the person is declared 'dead'. This we have called the *Body of Light*.

The physical body needs to be taken care of, as it is that part of the totality of us that serves as the vehicle for the rest to live and move in this material world. This does not mean that it should be indulged, though. The real needs of the physical body are few and very simple: food, shelter, exercise, and rest, in that order.

On the other hand, the needs of the mind, for the most part imaginary, are endless. It is the mind that needs all the extra things that go beyond these simple physical necessities. It is also the mind which can eventually overload the body to the point that the body can no longer repair the damage done to it by over-feeding, over-luxurious living, over-resting and even over-exercising.

The twin body of the physical one, the Body of Light, also needs to be cared for well. The Body of Light, as the name says, needs, in the first place, light. Sunlight. Starlight, the light which is locked in the air we breathe. Breathing is as vital to the Body of Light as eating is to the physical body; breathing the outdoor air, sun-bathing, walking underneath the moon and the stars on a clear night, this is food and exercise for the Body of Light. But it is not enough.

Both of these bodies, the physical body and the Body of Light, are in the middle of a giant tug-of-war between opposing forces. On the one side is the social part of us, that part which was born in a particular culture, in a particular time. This culture, this moment in history, made its imprint on us the moment we were born, and conditions us for the rest of our lives. This imprint forces us to live, think, and feel in a particular way, and unless we become aware of it, our whole life will be programmed according to its rules. Our beliefs, our feelings, our thoughts, even our choices, are conditioned by the society in which we live.

Something in us, however, remembers vaguely that there is another side to us, that there is another part in us, which is not born in a particular time or culture, and is not conditioned by these. This part in us is not bound by any rules other than the rule of *Being*. This is the real Light within each one of us that blazes in no-time and no-space, but which, for some reason, has chosen to immerse itself in the experience of time and space, thus becoming split. Part of it turns into the social person, caught and trapped in the rules of the particular time and space it finds itself in, and part of it remains in the background, untouched, unchanged. These two parts, for the duration of one's life, pull at the physical body and the Body of Light. This is the tug-of-war that goes on all the time.

The social person, being vaguely aware of having traded something precious - its awareness of no-time, no-space, for the illusion of time and space - turns to the only defense it knows: self-pity, the feeling of alienation, of being separated from this Light within, and not knowing how to get back to it. The manifestations of these feelings are countless: anger, fear, frustration, hate, obsessive love, addictions, all emerge out of this sense of alienation.

The first step in going beyond these feelings is to become aware of them in daily life, to become aware of how much of our emotional life and our thoughts are like birds flying out of the nest of self-pity and alienation. Only after we have gained this awareness, can we turn our eyes back to the other part of us, the part of us that did not split itself off to become the social person. This part of us remained as it always was, a Light which is not caught in the web of time and space, with its rules and regulations.

This is the riddle that we all have to face: how to walk the tight-rope between finding this Light and cultivating it, making it shine stronger and stronger through the physical body and through the Body of Light, and at the same time maintaining, with our social being, our life in this world.

Falling off the tightrope to either side means death, either the death of the social person, or the death of the Light. Our real art as human beings is to find and maintain that balance; there is no path, no road, which we can easily follow, nobody can do it for us, nobody can guide us. To find the Light inside, and to establish a balance between this Light and our social persona is a task that each one has to accomplish alone.

As human beings we are taught, from childhood on, to survive in a world which is at once complex and simple. Complex in the sense that all our relationships, whether these are with people, things, or nature, take place on a horizontal level. We reach out horizontally to the world around us on an exchange basis, a basis of give and take. For every action we expect a result, for everything we give we expect something in return. This is the simplicity of our world, that however complex our relationships are, their basis is simple: reciprocity.

Cultivating the Body of Light, without changing the blueprint of our horizontal life connections, often gives fuel to this lifestyle, turning us into overpowering tyrants. This is not a desirable state.

The awareness of the Body of Light, and the capacity to enhance and use it, has to be guided by something else. This something else is the capacity to suspend our horizontal life style and to reach out vertically into something that is beyond our daily activities, even for a moment. Sometimes this vertical reaching out happens accidentally, or is caused by something not man-made, like a beautiful sunset, or a bird singing, or any natural manifestation. At that moment, the world of exchange, of give and take, is shut off temporarily, and something within us is touched at an inconceivable level. This is always felt within the body, and it is only afterwards that the mind 'computes' the experience and says it had a vertical or mystical experience. We realize that in this moment there is no sense of a separate self, just a mass of being, on a par with and part of everything else. This is a burst of energy, a burst of Light, which is outside the scope of the rational mind and the emotions. In this moment we are touched by something that can be called joy, or love. It is an experience which is impersonal, and yet intensely personal.

Where the various physical and mental yoga practices enhance the energy level of the physical body and the Body of Light, it is the capacity to reach out vertically and let oneself be touched by joy which enhances the Light within.

A certain form of radiance can also come about through horizontal interaction; for instance, people in love can be 'radiant'. Yet this radiance is dependent on an outside agent within the daily world: the other person. When the outside agent fails, the radiance too fails and falls away. True joy or love, though, which is experienced in a moment of vertically reaching out, is not part of the horizontal, daily world of exchange, and is not dependent on an outside agent. It just is, and by its very being, and even by its very 'uselessness', it is capable of transforming the person who has the experience.

Finding the Light and cultivating it, so that it shines ever stronger through the physical body and the Body of Light, is that vertical reaching out which links us back to our home in no-time no-space. Living our social life out of this awareness, letting this Light shine through in our daily life, is that horizontal reaching out to the world of time and space around us. It is only by establishing this fine balance that we trade our feeling of alienation back for joy.

Joy is the natural expression of a life in which the Light blazes within the human being, within the social person. This joy does not have any aim, is not missionary. It does not want to impose itself; yet by its very being it lights up all that it comes in contact with. This joy is the passionate love for both the world of time and space and the world of no-time no-space; it is the realization that both are equally important, that neither of these two can exist without the other. It is this love which finally cuts the tightrope between the two worlds and welds them back together again into one unbroken whole.

Having resolved the illusion of duality, instead of leaving the body behind in our search for spirituality we have to give it wings. In Greek mythology, the great winged horse *Pegasus* rescues the princess Andromeda from the fate of being devoured, and for this act of courage is placed by Zeus as a starry constellation in the sky. When we mount our physical body, mind and emotions, onto our own Pegasus, the Body of Light, we can escape our fate of being devoured by the world and can fly up towards the heavens on the wings of joy, to become one with the luminous dance of the Universe.

Book agent
- Johanna van der Schaft   : jschaft@xs4all.nl, information on wholesale and retail

How to order this book
- Europe   : Johanna van der Schaft, jschaft@xs4all.nl
- Israel   : Orit Sen-Gupta, omyoga@netvision.net.il
- USA, Canada and Mexico   : Sylvia Strike, yogspks@pacbell.net

Websites
- www.donaholleman.com   : homepage of Dona Holleman, information on workshops
- www.klik.nl   : homepage of Buro Klik, Intermediation
- www.spiritual-art.nl   : homepage of S. Bob Tomanovic, who painted the cover art
- www.liqua.nl   : homepage of Liqua, bureau for text and graphic design